Praise for *Ian Gawler: The*

'Ian Gawler: The Dragon's Bless⸱   and
determination to go beyon⸱   . This
frank and inspiring acc⸱   physical
and spiritual healing   ⸱ffering can
be transformed to br⸱   ⸱ility to benefit
others.'—Sogyal Rinpo⸱   ⸱etan Book of Living
and Dying

'The broad outlines of his story   well known. Young man's leg is amputated as a result of cancer, severe secondaries occur but gradually disappear. After his "miraculous" recovery, he writes about how meditation can cure cancer and sets up a foundation to teach these principles. It's an inspirational story. What makes this biography interesting, though, are not simply the inspirational facts of Ian Gawler's life, but his struggles, set-backs and flaws. He is not a guru. He has got things wrong along the way, often driven by his impulse to live on "the edge" … It is Gawler's hope that his story will function as a "teaching story" and that it will serve as "another nail in the coffin of my ego". Well-told and thought provoking, *Ian Gawler: The Dragon's Blessing* has achieved its aim.'—*The Age*

'In my encounters with Ian and his work, I have found them both inspirational and deeply pragmatic. This book is both those things. Its value extends, I believe, well beyond people dealing with the profound challenges of cancer, to many of us who may face personal medical challenges or professional or policy responsibilities around medicine, health care, prevention, healing, recovery, and caring—or simply have an interest in being well and healthy and getting the most out of life.'—Sue Pieters-Hawke, author of *Hazel's Journey*

'A tranquil tale of mortal combat.' —*Herald Sun*

'Ian Gawler is a man who has lived the message. He is an inspiration to all those who are confronting their mortality due to serious illness. His story shows us how we can make a difference and participate in our lives, our health and our ability to survive. Exceeding expectations and being a survivor are related to personal factors and Ian's story and life are an example of self-induced healing.'—Bernie Siegel, MD, author of *Love, Medicine & Miracles* and *Help Me To Heal*

'Guy Allenby has written a beautiful biography of one of the greatest pioneers of integrative cancer therapies. Ian Gawler has made an historic contribution to the great quest to understand deep healing. This book should be required reading for all who care about healing and cancer.'—Michael Lerner, President, Commonweal, co-founder, Commonweal Cancer Help Program, California.

'Like many, I suppose, I had relegated Ian Gawler to the lunatic fringes of alternative medicine without knowing much about him, except that he was a skeletal, kaftan-wearing, one-legged man who favoured organic produce ... I took the opportunity to challenge my prejudice and I'm glad I did. The Gawler portrayed by Allenby is no effete, mung-bean-eating hippie. Rather he's a competitive, fast-driving, meat-eating decathlete, a pragmatic, married, hard-working veterinarian who gets bone cancer in 1974 when he is just 24.' —*Canberra Times*

IAN GAWLER
The Dragon's Blessing

GUY ALLENBY

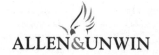

ALLEN&UNWIN

This edition published in 2010
First published in 2008

Allen & Unwin
83 Alexander Street
Crows Nest NSW 2065
Australia
Phone: (61 2) 8425 0100
Fax: (61 2) 9906 2218
Email: info@allenandunwin.com
Web: www.allenandunwin.com

National Library of Australia
Cataloguing-in-Publication entry:

Allenby, Guy.

 Ian Gawler : the dragon's blessing / Guy Allenby.

 978 1 74237 265 5 (pbk.)

 Gawler, Ian, 1950- Gawler Foundation. Cancer—Patients—Attitudes.
 Cancer—Patients—Australia—Biography.

362.1969940092

Printed in Australia by McPherson's Printing Group

10 9 8 7 6 5 4 3 2 1

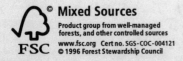

Mixed Sources

Product group from well-managed
forests, and other controlled sources
www.fsc.org   Cert no. SGS-COC-004121
© 1996 Forest Stewardship Council

FSC

The paper in this book is FSC certified.
FSC promotes environmentally responsible,
socially beneficial and economically viable
management of the world's forests.

Trained as a journalist, Guy Allenby was a feature writer and editor at the *Sydney Morning Herald* for a number of years. His work has also appeared in *The Age* and *The Australian*. *Ian Gawler: The Dragon's Blessing* is his first biography. He lives in Sydney.

Foreword

To be the subject of a biography is to challenge the ego. A biography presents the opportunity for the ego to run wild. What will be said? Who will read it? What will they think? What will it lead to?

There are two witnesses to our life: our self and others. In Richard Bach's wonderful book *Illusions*, there is a statement . . . *Live never to be ashamed if anything you do or say is published around the world—even if what is published is not true.*

What is that all about? Perhaps it is speaking of being content with what you have done in your life, and being unaffected by what others say of you. That what is most important is how you see yourself—which would be helped if you were not too ego-driven, too neurotic, too emotional!

Of course, emotions and thoughts can be quite valuable and they can seem quite real at times. However, His Holiness the Dalai Lama tells us that even an emotion as simple and common as anger can distort our perception of reality by 90 per cent. That is, anger distorts what we see, believe we have heard, or witnessed; what we believe to have happened.

When we examine our thoughts, we soon realise they come and go very quickly. There is nothing permanent about a thought.

So when it comes to telling a story, that story will be based upon what really happened, and then it will be filtered, modified, overlayed and adapted, according to the participants' and witnesses' perceptions, states of mind and emotions. And as time goes on, memories fade, merge, metamorphose, and become something new.

Stories encompass fact and creatively work a version of truth into something that aims to be entertaining and instructive. So the fact is that all that is written here may not be true in the strictest sense of the word.

Guy may not be too happy about me pointing this out as I know he has earnestly and conscientiously aimed to recount a version of the truth concerning a story that in a way actually did take place. But even my personal diaries—some involving very detailed accounts of events recorded on the day they happened—only present my experience, my recollection, my perspective of what occurred. There is a famous story of a group of blind men coming across an elephant each one bumping into a part of the elephant and then being asked what it was. Some described a trunk, another a tail, another a leg and yet another a huge tummy. All true. All parts of the truth. All a version of the truth.

So my own wish, in agreeing to this story being told by Guy, was twofold. The first, as already explained, was to confront my ego yet again. My approach to the story has been to respond to Guy's prompting as openly and fully as possible and to trust in his ability to do something useful with what was said. The people with whom I did speak directly about the possibility of being interviewed for the book were all encouraged by me to take the same approach.

My second and more important motivation was in fact to explore the truth. Looking back over the events of this life described, I have found it extraordinary to be the one living the story. Many of the events depicted in these pages go beyond what can be characterised as 'ordinary'. Some seem even a little incredible to me—and I was the one experiencing them at the time!

So why bother to record it? Well, for many years it has been felt that there was almost a duty to tell it. This story, particularly the early part to do with my healing journey through cancer, was so remarkable, so extraordinary, that it did feel at the time that it was guided by a higher purpose. As fortuitous coincidence followed on more and more fortuitous coincidences, it felt natural to believe there was a need to share with others what I was learning and what was helping my particular recovery.

Yet when I did begin to run groups in the early 1980s, mind–body medicine was in its infancy. For the average person, meditation was more likely to be associated with a risky cult than a valuable therapy. And psychic phenomena, Filipino faith healing, subtle energy healing: all that was tainted as mumbo-jumbo.

And there was more than this. As well as wanting to be taken seriously as a participant in those pioneering days of mind–body medicine, I felt an urge to empower people to use their own healing resources. To draw on inner healing, in a way that complemented the medicine of the day. In a way that added to what was possible.

So why would you bother to read this book? Well, hopefully it is at least entertaining. And a little mind-blowing in parts! If it does serve to shake up some concepts about how life is, what is real and what healing really is made of, it may be useful.

But I have greater hope: that the real purpose of the book will be fulfilled to some degree. It is intended as a teaching story.

If it is a teaching story, what are the lessons, you may well ask? Well that clearly is the point of the book! Read it and find out if there are any, and if so, how they might be helpful.

Perhaps a hint: the stories of the life that is herein described— how real do they seem? How do they resonate with your own sensibilities? What do they spark in you? Contemplation? Feelings? Emotions? And what do they point to? Is there anything relevant that you might take usefully into your own life?

Finally, for me—two wishes. Firstly, that the book serves as another nail in the coffin of my ego; then perhaps I can be of more use to others.

Secondly, the wish that something here inspires and serves you to focus upon finding the Truth in your own life. The story concerns a relative truth—something that happened and people's versions of how it can be recounted. But perhaps there is a deeper, more fundamental Truth. Not the truth of our daily lives—what we did, where we went and what happened; but the Truth of who we really are.

So the fundamental wish is that you do come to experience directly the Truth of your innermost nature, and find a way of living in the light of that experience.

Many thanks to Guy Allenby for initiating this project and pursuing the story with enthusiasm, professionalism and such a good heart. Thanks to all who gave their time and contributed in many ways. And of course a special thanks to the love of my life Ruth, and the light of my life, Sogyal Rinpoche, and all the members of family, friends and spiritual teachers who have helped and supported me in so many ways.

Ian Gawler
Yarra Junction, Victoria
February 2008

Contents

To everyone who devotes their lives to the service of others

1

The Edge

It was a familiar dance on country roads. Tight corners. Braking. Accelerating. Dodging potholes. No time, no bounds, only the thin ribbon of bitumen ahead.

'It was one of those perfect Australian days when the sky is not content to be blue and cloudless; but vibrates with its purity,' wrote Ian Gawler in his journal. 'The air was still and warm and did little to slow our progress, as Gail and I sped to the Rock on the MV.'

Ian was savouring the big sky, the rushing wind and a potent trust in his fortunes as he pushed his beloved new MV Agusta 750 motorcycle—and his girlfriend—to the limit.

The speedo edged 160km/h in the straight.

Gail Kerr, on her first ever ride on a motorbike, attached to Ian's back as tight as a rock climber's rucksack, felt little more than the thump of her heart in her throat. Her hair whipped out in long auburn strands from beneath her helmet.

The country was flat—a collage of yellows and ochres. The dry paddocks were scattered with fresh hay bales. At the end of the road was the Rock—Hanging Rock—the plug of an ancient volcano, poking impressively out of Victoria's Hesket plains as Ian, young veterinarian, athlete and lapsed Anglican with an unrepentant passion for going fast, swept towards it with the then terrified, but usually unflappable, Gail.

It was New Year's Day, 1975.

The couple motored up to the racecourse on the Italian superbike to find a mile-long queue of cars outside. Police were turning cars away at the entrance gates as they eased to the top of the line—Gail, eyes wide and face flushed from the full-throttled turns along the narrow roads. Fortunately there was room at the races for just two more on a motorbike. It had become a yearly habit for Ian to attend the event ever since Frank, the Clerk of the Course, a lean, greying and dignified man and member of the older generation of Australian stockmen, had taught him to ride.

Ian patently preferred the power and speed of two and four wheels to four hoofs but seeing Frank and attending the races every year 'was a delight, and it rapidly became a matter of honour to front each year, regardless of the hour New Year's Eve celebrations ended'.

More than that though, Ian had come to love the magic of nearby Hanging Rock, rising 100 metres above the surrounding plain. While working as a stockman at a farm at nearby Woodend during university holidays he would often run the steep path that winds its way to the top, seeking the stillness and majesty he found there. 'Up there is a central, relatively clear area ringed by huge rock sentinels,' he wrote. Set in clusters, these sentinels rise up 6 or more metres each from an oval base.

> Once, I had crouched under the shelter that the megaliths offered as a rainstorm vented its fury on the rock. Nature in all its awe. More frequently, however, I delighted in running through those dark corridors, blocked off from light and sound with the feeling of space and time suspended and not knowing what the next turn might bring. Often I would round a corner and pull up sharply, breath cut short. In front would be the panorama of the outstretched Australian bush. At my feet would be the precipice and the drop to the plain below.

And it was the profound stillness and magic of the rocks and the mind-arresting sweep of this panorama—more than the races— that would draw Ian once again this particular morning. The following day, 2 January, he was booked in to St Vincents Hospital in Melbourne for tests on his sore and swollen right leg. He had said little to Gail about the soreness until the previous week when, after Christmas lunch, he had taken aside his elder sister Susan, a physiotherapist, to take a look at the leg.

She had not liked what she had seen.

Ian had first met Gail, a veterinary nurse, the previous year while he was filling in at a fellow veterinarian's practice in Geelong. At that time he was only a few months out of university and was busy running his own practice in the small neighbouring community of Bacchus Marsh—an attractive rural town nestled in a fertile valley midway between Melbourne and the gold-rush town of Ballarat.

Ian's first impression of Gail was that she was pretty, intent on her work and a little aloof. Her long reddish-brown hair was drawn back in a ponytail and she had an angular face with high cheekbones, silver-rimmed glasses and 'a penetrating gaze that added to her efficient air and gave a hint of severity'. In those first few days, Ian discovered that this look was, in fact, determination. Perhaps there was also a hint of something else, as Ian noted in his journal at the time: 'The glasses couldn't hide the spark that the eyes contained and I sometimes found myself wondering what would happen if they were to come off and the hair was let down.'

Ian ran his Bacchus Marsh practice with a friend and fellow recent graduate, Kathy Humphrey; they had taken over the lease for the small practice together in January, 1973. The owners, committed Christians, had headed to Korea for two years to work on a mission development farm. The plan was that upon their return, the four would go into partnership together.

As part of the deal Ian would do occasional locum work at the Geelong practice where, it turned out, Gail worked. This practice was owned and run by Daryl Sefton and his wife Nini, who were also re-establishing vineyards in the area. At harvest time, Ian was asked to step in for a couple of weeks to keep the veterinary practice running.

Back at Bacchus Marsh, Ian's real passions in veterinary science were surgery and horses. One of the main reasons he had been drawn to the town was because he knew there was not a vet in the immediate area working specifically with horses. The only problem was that he was fresh out of vet school. He had a lot to learn about the subject. Not that that was anything to put off the then eager young vet.

At first, business was slow. And then on 25 February—Ian's twenty-third birthday—he had his father and stepmother over for lunch. Kathy and Ian had decided to take turns to be on call during the weekends and this particular weekend, despite the birthday, it was Ian's turn to be on duty. The surgery itself was attached to the little house shared by the two young vets. It was not long after Ian and his parents had sat down to the birthday lunch that the doorbell rang.

Ian opened the door to two concerned-looking men and instantly recognised one of them. It was Alex Katranski, proprietor of a large Australia-wide rental car company and owner of Underbank, the biggest horse stud in Bacchus Marsh. Ian masked his excitement, secretly thrilled that Katranski was maybe, just maybe, about to ask for help with one of his horses.

'Do you know anything about horses?' challenged Katranski, more than a tad unsure of the likely experience of the tall, long-haired and youthful vet standing before him.

Ian looked him straight in the eye, smiled, and said: 'That's my main interest'.

Apparently satisfied, Katranski explained that he had two horses that he was concerned about and asked Ian to look at them.

'I didn't want to appear too eager. So I told him I would finish lunch with my parents first. My sense was that he would respect this too. In fact, I was keen to get out there as fast as I could go.'

One horse had an injury and the other had an illness. After Ian examined them he was not entirely sure what was wrong with either of them. He told Katranski that he did not have the things he needed with him to treat the horses and that he would need to go back to the surgery and return the following day with what was required.

Ian went straight home and rang Dr Geoff Hazard, a friend, fellow veterinarian and mentor from his school and university days. He described the symptoms of the two horses to Hazard, who told him exactly what he thought was wrong with them and, if so, what to do.

Ian went back to Underbank the next day to treat them. The treatments worked.

Katranski was delighted. Unbeknown to Ian, he had already had his usual vet out to treat the horses—but to no avail. Katranski transferred all his work to Ian.

Horse people have their own network and soon, through word of mouth, other studs and horse owners in the area began calling him in rapid succession. If things got really tricky, Ian continued to seek out Geoff Hazard's advice as he needed it.

'I also worked out that it was best if I didn't say too much [when treating animals] because the farmers loved talking,' says Ian. 'As a young graduate, a lot of those old horse guys knew heaps more than I did. They'd tell me what was wrong most times. What they wanted was reassurance—someone to say that what they were doing was okay.'

Ian soon found himself learning invaluable folk medicine— techniques and remedies—from the old-timers; sound knowledge that had been tried and tested and passed down through the generations. He began to develop a deep respect for these elders who knew things that veterinary school simply had not taught.

'What they helped me to realise was that animals had an innate ability to heal themselves,' he says, 'and that, as a vet, half the time your job was not to do too much to interfere with this process and to let nature take its course and help it along its way.'

Ian relished getting out and working with horses, but he loved working in the surgery just as much. 'With both the horses and the dogs and cats I was able to do a wide range of challenging and interesting things,' he says. 'The technical side was wonderful.'

Soon he recognised that although the vet school had taught a particular methodology, there were in fact other ways of treating illness that were often 'cheaper, easier and had less side effects'.

THE DRAGON'S BLESSING

Clearly in many situations the modern techniques worked really well, but it was exciting to learn of other possibilities.

Ian was soon a sought-after and effective vet working long hours every week. He was loving it, particularly the horse work. And then, in the middle of 1973, the emerging practice suffered its first real setback. Ian and Kathy's veterinary nurse suddenly gave two weeks' notice one Friday.

'It was really bad news because we were working flat out,' says Ian. 'A veterinary practice can't practise without a good vet nurse and they are hard to train. You can't conjure one up overnight.'

The following Sunday morning, Ian was catching up on a little much-needed rest when he was awoken by a knock on the front door. It was Gail.

Ian, rubbing his leaden eyes as he opened the door, was taken aback. Gail's hair was down and she was wearing an old fur coat and faded denim jeans. 'She looked really attractive,' he wrote in his journal. 'Gone were the hard lines of uniform and clinical manner. The glasses were still there but they only added to the feminine appeal.'

According to Gail, the young vet had lent her money when he was last in Geelong and she had dropped in to return it. Also, for reasons she put down to Ian's quietness and complacency, Gail had assumed that he was married.

At the time Ian was sharing the house with Kathy, but the pair were merely business partners and friends—nothing more—and it was convenient for them to live at the place where they worked.

Straight away it was clear that there was chemistry between Gail and Ian. He thanked her for returning the loan, hesitated for an awkward moment, and then invited her in for a lunch he had cooked of steak and boiled vegetables.

What the twenty-year-old Gail did not bother to tell him was that she had been a vegetarian since she was five years old. Ian, on the other hand, a lean and muscular athlete, with a 6-foot 2, 12-stone frame and an appetite to match, 'ate anything that moved'. Gail, it turns out, had sworn off eating living things ever since she had come home from school one day to discover that the pet sheep that she kept in the backyard had inexplicably vanished. That night the Kerr family had lamb chops for dinner. Gail was heartbroken and resisted all attempts to eat meat from that day forth—at least until this Sunday fifteen years later, when she chose not to reveal her strongly-held dietary preferences. What she did mention casually though, between mouthfuls of steak, was that she had quit her job at the veterinary practice in Geelong.

Gail had strained her back while drumming in the Geelong Scottish pipe band. Her boss, Daryl Sefton, took a dim view of this injury as it meant that Gail now found it too difficult to lift heavy animals onto the table. Daryl could not lift either because of arthritic knees, so they had taken to bickering over which of them would do it. She told Ian they could not sort it out and had reached an impasse. Gail had subsequently resigned and was looking for a new job.

Giving up her job was particularly devastating for Gail as her schoolgirl ambition had been to go to university and study to become a veterinarian. There was no doubt she had the requisite intelligence and application, having topped her class year after year. When Daryl Sefton had offered her the job as a vet nurse in her final year of school, she had wanted to refuse the work and continue her studies. But Gail's parents, Bob and Olive Kerr, who were old-fashioned working people, saw little value in a higher education and pressed her into taking the job.

Once in the position, Gail actually enjoyed the work tremendously. In her own words, the Seftons 'were really good people and they were like parents to me'. So while she had been sad to leave them, fate had now seemed to smile on her with a new appointment. She started at Ian and Kathy's practice two weeks later.

In her new job it was soon very apparent that Gail was well trained, enthusiastic and efficient. 'She set about organising the practice procedures, freeing us to concentrate on our cases,' says Ian. 'Also she had an almost photographic memory and clients loved the fact that she remembered them, their animals' names and most of their details as well.'

The relationship between Ian and Gail was simply professional at first. However, Ian had no steady girlfriend and, at the end of

1973, he asked her out to join Kathy and her boyfriend to celebrate the first anniversary of the new practice.

Gail remembers how they returned to Ian's home afterwards and he asked her, very tentatively, if she wanted to spend the night. 'I said no,' she says, 'and I stayed in Kathy's room, because she was away with her fellow for the night.'

At that time the young nurse was sharing a house with a group of teachers in Bacchus Marsh. This had made it a lot easier than living with her parents in Geelong and commuting to work, 45 minutes away by road. It had also given her the opportunity to gain more personal freedom.

During the course of 1973, Kathy, who was really interested in working with cattle, became increasingly frustrated with the region's extremely patriarchal old farmers who were reluctant to have a woman veterinarian tend their animals. She moved to northern New South Wales, leaving Ian on his own. The workload at the practice, now run by a solitary vet rather than the original two, was even more hectic.

As 1974 began it was another hot and dry summer. By now Ian and Gail's work day would typically start with Ian leaving at 6 am with horse stud work, followed by a small animal clinic back at the Bacchus Marsh surgery from 9 am, until mid-morning. Then there would be surgery to complete on the dogs and cats who needed it, before he would jump in the car with Gail for a quick dash to the other small animal surgery he conducted at Melton, 16 kilometres away.

'My record for getting there was five minutes,' he says, 'which is an average of about 120 miles [190 km/h] an hour. I had a rotary [engine] Mazda then and I could get it up to 130 miles an hour [210 km/h]. It barely touched the ground. It probably was fairly dangerous but I always felt quite bullet-proof.'

In the afternoon Ian would do more horse work, returning to the surgery later to check on the animals he had operated on that day. Then there was an evening clinic. Meals were usually on the run and there were often emergencies late at night. The Saturday morning clinic completed, Ian would then be on call all weekend because now there was no-one else to share the workload.

Eighty-hour working weeks were typical.

'That was the pace I was tearing around at and I loved it,' he says, adding that he found time to fit in a couple of hours of training most afternoons.

'He used to get tired. Really tired,' says Gail.

Ian, it turns out, had made time to play centre half-back in the local Australian Rules Football team during the winter of 1973 and did so again in 1974. Still, his real passion since early schooldays had been for athletics and he represented Victoria in the decathlon in three national championships. He was hoping to be in the state team again in 1975.

It was a busy life, to say the least, and one with little room for a developing romance. And in matters of the heart, he had been burnt before. In his university days there had been a love affair with a girl named Liz. After three years she left him suddenly for another man. Ian admits to have taken away from this first serious romantic involvement the pain 'that attachment can bring' and a determination to become less involved and give less of himself in the future. When he met Gail he recognised her inherent strength and accordingly presumed she might be able to handle a no-commitment type of relationship.

And so in December 1973, very early in their new relationship, Ian invited Gail to visit his land overlooking Bacchus Marsh. The vet had bought the 40 acres early in his working life. The entire amount, including the deposit, was financed by a bank loan arranged by friend and financial adviser, Tony Bongiorno.

Lying back on the grass, gazing out over the plains below, in a rare moment of stillness and tranquillity in their hectic lives, Ian decided it was a good time to set out his intentions directly.

Ian told Gail that he was interested in the possibility of a relationship with her but that he did not want to have 'any sense of permanence or attachment or anything like that. I did one of those things that probably never works: I said if you are interested in a relationship with no conditions, no sort of commitment—then I am happy. If not, let's stop now.

'One of the reasons I was attached to her was that she was a really, really strong woman. I felt quite screwed up emotionally, so I thought she could handle me. I thought she was emotionally tough.'

'He was a very cautious and a very quiet guy,' says Gail. 'He didn't say a lot in those days.'

One of the things that Ian kept to himself was the fact that he had never been able to imagine himself beyond the age of 27. He also had a vague awareness that life was going to serve up a major change; that life was going to take a totally different direction to the one he was currently headed in. 'I even had vague notions that this involved heading off to some type of spiritual retreat, or becoming a hermit or something,' he explains. 'It was a peculiar feeling which was strong without being defined.'

For all these reasons Ian felt he could not commit and he felt it best to lay it all out to Gail. 'I did not want to offer any sense of permanence or security.'

'It was fine,' says Gail, 'because neither did I.'

It was, nevertheless, a naïve view of the nature of serious relationships, particularly as they were soon living together. Very quickly it became clear, at least to Ian, that Gail had fallen deeply in love, while he tried to keep his 'side of the bargain by remaining somewhat detached' he says. 'It was lopsided at the start.'

Gail agrees that she thought she had fallen in love with Ian, but adds that she had a 'funny thing' with love in those early days. 'I had what they call agape. It's a sort of unconditional love which is given freely to people. It has a high rate of conscience and heart in it and I think I mistook that, in my tender years, for love,' she says. 'There's love and *being in love* and I don't think we were ever *in love*.'

Besides, from Gail's point of view her new boyfriend 'just seemed a very silent person about emotional things. I don't think he ever actually held my hand in our relationship.' To complicate matters, Ian was also still quite attached to the memory of Liz. 'He was having a lot of trouble letting go,' Gail maintains. 'I think he found that very difficult.'

This created real problems for Gail and she reacted to it quite strongly. Liz dropped in to say hello at their Bacchus Marsh home a couple of times in the early days and the two of them kept in touch by phone, much to Gail's displeasure. Ian remembers her pulling the connection out at the wall one day when Liz rang.

Throughout 1974 work became busier and ever more hectic. Living together and working side by side, the bond between Ian and Gail steadily strengthened. Yet, as Ian remembers it, the uneven nature of their relationship in that first year together was an occasional source of background conflict and, along with other issues, difficulties were starting to emerge.

'It was a very unusual relationship at the beginning,' says Gail. 'You can look back with a great deal of introspection but it seems like we were thrown together.' It was almost as if it had more to do with fate than real romance.

By the end of 1974 the couple who owned the veterinary practice, Kevin and Jo Bell, were due to return from Korea. The plan was that Kevin and Jo would move back into their house, Ian would go into partnership in the business as agreed, and Gail and he would have to find somewhere else to live.

They settled on an old—if somewhat neglected—pioneer settler's home. 'Kippen Ross' was halfway between Bacchus Marsh and the neighbouring town of Melton.

Set on a flat plain, it was huge and of solid brick, thick with creepers and surrounded by verandas. It was at the end of a 400-metre driveway flanked by gum trees. It had many large rooms, each with its own fireplace, leading off a wide central corridor. The timber floors sagged a little. 'The lounge room was immense,' says Ian, 'with a fireplace you could almost stand up in.' Outside was a rose garden, overgrown lawns and paddock where Gail could keep her horse, Tabooka. In the chook shed meanwhile they installed ducks and bantams, two rabbits and a guinea pig. The couple also kept a cat and two dogs—Ian's Saluki and Gail's Afghan.

And then Christmas rolled around.

The Gawler family always celebrated the festive season with all the trimmings. There were presents under a tree dripping with tinsel and a roast turkey lunch was served on a large table outdoors.

However, Christmas 1974, unlike previous years, was held at Ian's sister Susan's and her husband Ross Macaw's house in Melbourne instead of the Gawler family home. This was because Alan, Ian's father, had just flown to Canada with second wife Glenyss and Ian's younger sister Helen, to take up a two-year posting.

While it was a happy day, Ian was carrying a niggling concern. His right thigh had been getting bigger and increasingly sore for most of the previous month; something he had not really considered to be a serious problem up until then. He had assumed it was a pulled muscle. Now he was not entirely sure.

He quietly took Susan aside for her opinion. Ian and Susan, as the only offspring from their father's first marriage, had grown close by Ian's early adulthood. Susan, an experienced physiotherapist, remembers her brother dropping his trousers to reveal a right thigh that was quite noticeably bigger than the other. She was deeply shocked, although she kept the full extent of her concern to herself.

'I took him into my little treatment room so that I could examine it more clearly.' She palpated it, pushing the skin down over the swelling on Ian's thigh with her finger to see how it responded. 'Normally if you palpate the skin like this, you make a dent and then, as you take your finger off, the skin changes colour and it bounces back,' she says. 'But this was solid. I could hardly push my finger into it at all!' Susan remembers that she did not actually know what it was but she knew there was something seriously wrong and that Ian needed to do something about it as soon as possible. 'I told him you had better go and see a doctor.'

The two rejoined the family at the table and the festivities continued late into the evening. When Ian and Gail finally arrived back home at Bacchus Marsh, a 40-minute drive away, they were tired and ready for sleep. However Ian was called out immediately to assist a dog that was having trouble giving birth. He performed a successful caesarean section and finally fell into bed at 4 am.

The next morning, Boxing Day, was another clear blue summer's day. Ian decided to try and shake off the previous long day's weariness and overindulgence, with a training run around the Bacchus Marsh oval with his dog, Sara.

Sara nearly always trained with Ian; training that usually consisted of a three-mile warm-up run followed by countless laps of interval work—jogging, sprinting, jogging, sprinting, jogging, sprinting.

Ian's chosen event was decathlon—ten events competed over two days. Athletics was his summer sport and during the winters at Bacchus Marsh Australian Rules Football kept him fit. Running long distances was a daily habit.

When Kathy Humphrey had left the practice earlier that year the demands of work had left him less time to train as he had liked. So when the 1974 football season had finished in September Ian had decided to take a two-month rest from training. It was the first time he had taken a real break from training in about eight years.

During the break, Gail remembers he confided in her that he had felt something about the 'size of a walnut' in his right thigh. He had assumed it was scar tissue from a previous pulled muscle and thought little of it.

Curiously though, earlier that year another warning note had sounded. Ian and Gail had called in to browse around a shop that sold antiques and old wares while visiting friends in Adelaide. 'It was a very unusual shop,' says Gail. After the pair had been looking around for a little while, the proprietor approached them and, out of the blue, enquired of Ian if he was 'well'. Then she said that she felt sure there was something 'going on', explaining that she was an iridologist and could see from his eyes that he had problems. In those days neither of them even knew what an iridologist was. 'Ian thought she was a crackpot,' says Gail. And then the shopkeeper mentioned that her husband was a therapist who performed his 'diagnoses and treatment using a little black box and a piece of hair'. Apparently, he was next door and Ian was asked if he minded if he had a look at him too? Rather bemused, and a little curious, Ian agreed.

The woman went off and returned a short time later with her spouse. He examined him (without the aid of his little black box) and agreed there were possible problems. 'The poor bloke was a bit embarrassed by my obvious scepticism,' says Ian. And then, just before they left, the woman turned to Gail and said: 'Promise me one thing, young woman ... go and get him a total all-over checkup; something is going on.'

When they got home, Gail suggested he book himself in with a doctor, but Ian was adamant there was nothing wrong with him. Gail kept nagging and eventually he agreed. Ian spoke with some of his medical friends and discovered that an organisation called the Shepherd Foundation was just what he needed. It had been established recently with the express purpose of carrying out exhaustive health checks intended to diagnose and prevent illnesses before they arose. Ian booked in and completed a full medical late in October of 1974. The results found nothing wrong and he was told he was a 'fit and healthy young man'.

Gail was not so sure. 'He was sallow, he was jaundiced-looking, he was tired, he did not look good,' she says. 'All those sorts of things were going on for the last months of '74.' Gail kept at him for further tests, but now he would not discuss it, citing his recent clean bill of health. And then when Ian had returned to training in November he had noticed that a soreness had developed in his right thigh during the down time. 'Perhaps it was related to the walnut lump, but really I thought it was a strained muscle and that it would clear up as I ran more,' he says. But instead the pain grew steadily worse and the leg began to swell up. By mid-December he could hardly get over the hurdles and running became increasingly difficult.

And so on Boxing Day, with the weariness of the previous day and night adding to things, Ian struggled to complete even a single lap of the Bacchus Marsh oval.

'Now I was sure it had to be something more than a mere pulled muscle,' he wrote at the time. 'Dejected, I stopped and walked back to the car. Sara followed reluctantly.'

The very next day Ian sought help from his local doctor and friend, David Stewart. The GP scrutinised his leg closely and very quickly recommended he see a specialist in Melbourne at the earliest possible opportunity. Ian remembers asking him what he thought it was. Stewart avoided his gaze and then mumbled—without looking up—'There's definitely some new growth there. Perhaps it is lipoma [a benign fatty growth and the most innocuous of tumours].' The comment filled Ian with dismay. 'I didn't know what the lump was, but one thing I did know for sure was that it was not a lipoma. Also I knew that David would have to know that it was not a lipoma. Therefore, it seemed obvious that he was trying to reassure me in a way that was quite ineffective. It hit me that this had to be something serious. It had to be some sort of cancer.'

Until this moment Ian had somehow managed to avoid facing the possibility that the growth on his leg might be a benign tumour, let alone a full-blown cancer. After all, he was young, he was super-fit, he felt invincible. The notion of serious illness seemed an utter impossibility to him. Coming out of Dr Stewart's surgery a completely new feeling enveloped him. It was a deep sense of dread. No panic. No real sense of fear, but a powerful sense of apprehension. And a numbness.

The following day Ian had an appointment to see Mr John Doyle, a surgeon in Melbourne and he motored off there on the MV. He parked it on the kerb outside the surgeon's Collins Street rooms.

Ian describes Doyle as a gentle soul and a strong Catholic. Doyle, for his part, remembers Ian as extraordinarily calm.

That day Doyle reviewed his history and gave him a physical examination. According to his notes, Doyle asked Ian how long the swelling in his right thigh had been present and he replied 'eight to ten weeks' and that he could not remember any recent trauma to that region.

'I thought it was a very nasty swelling,' says Doyle, 'and was suspicious of it from the beginning.' No malignancy could be formally confirmed that day—and Doyle, like Stewart before him, did not reveal the true depth of his suspicions.

He sent Ian around the corner to be x-rayed immediately and said that he would not be drawn on what he thought might be wrong with the leg until the x-rays were assessed. Even then he suggested further tests would have to be undertaken to diagnose anything conclusively.

However, once the x-rays were taken, Ian pressured the radiologist into allowing him to have a look at them. What he saw, as he explained it at the time, was that in the middle of his thigh there was a mass of new bone growth spreading out from the main bone like fragments of a grenade caught at an early stage of explosion. 'If the leg can be saved, I would say it will make interesting reading.'

With the sense of dread deepening and still feeling numb, Ian climbed on the MV and roared off down Collins Street. Instead of returning to Gail, he swept off in the other direction; down the coast to visit his old friend Tom Barrett, who was staying at his grandmother's beach house at Sorrento.

It was a beautiful day, with a surreal edge to it. The sky was clear, the air warm and it was a good road with gentle curves—near perfect conditions for a big new bike. And there was this throbbing in the right leg. As the trip flowed on it became increasingly difficult to even use the leg.

'He rode down on his bike to have his Will signed,' Barrett remembers, adding that his friend appeared to be maintaining his natural calmness, despite the extraordinary gravity of the situation. Barrett did not share his best friend's serenity. 'It was a shocking day. It was just so unexpected that it could happen to someone so fit.'

The next day, Mr Doyle phoned Ian with the results of the x-rays.

'I said I was very worried about it,' says Doyle. 'I thought that it was a malignant tumour and I wanted him to come into hospital as soon as possible.'

Not at all surprised by the news or the instructions, Ian booked into hospital straight away. Further tests, with a biopsy on the swollen thigh and lymph nodes in the groin, were planned for Saturday 4 January 1975.

The subsequent days passed in quiet apprehension, although Ian and Gail did not dwell on the impending investigations or likely outcomes—in fact they did not talk of the leg at all.

They spent New Year's Eve at the Maddingley Football Club's

fancy dress ball. The couple turned up in their ordinary clothes and left early.

New Year's Day dawned. It was a sharp, still and cloudless summer's day. One to fully embrace the annual tradition of attending the Hanging Rock Picnic Races—not to mention the opportunity to really open the bike up, to push it to its limits and to challenge fate at a time that seemed more relevant now than ever before. Gail was coerced into being the reluctant passenger, under the guise of 'a nice day at the races'.

Ian says he had come to feel over the years that the race day was partly his own. Nonetheless, 1975 boasted a bigger crowd than he had ever remembered attending before.

Once inside the gates, the couple parked the heavy bike, pushed through the massive crowd and found Frank. Ian made his annual reacquaintance with the old horseman—and then proceeded to back three losing horses, before deciding he and Gail would be better served taking off up The Rock.

Ian trudged up the narrow path to the top with a pronounced limp—such a contrast to the times only a few short months before, when he would bound up to the peak in a matter of minutes.

The view from the top was familiar, with the added colour and movement of the horse races below. It was familiar but breathtaking nonetheless. Also it offered a comforting sense of the wider, open scale of things, as Ian himself teetered on the edge of a very immediate, personal unknown. As Ian wrote in a later journal,

Looking over the precipice onto the spectacle below is one of those floating images that comes before me now and then. Muted memories of the hazy forms of horses, careering before the colourful crowd. A tableau that lacked both clarity and sound. The silence, particularly I remember the silence . . .

2

Checking in

On the way to hospital in Melbourne from their home in rural Melton, Ian Gawler stopped his car on the side of the road, dropped his trousers and insisted that his girlfriend take a photograph of his legs.

Passing cars honked their horns as they went past, Ian standing by the side of the road in his y-fronts, trousers around his ankles. It was a surreal scene in what must have been one of the most anxious days of his life, but it bore the mark of Ian's particular brand of humour and determination. He was also keen to have what already he was sensing might be a last record of his two legs.

As the young couple laughed and the photo was taken, nobody passing by would have guessed what menacing shadows must have been sweeping through his mind that day.

Ian was an intelligent, intense and driven young man, full of confidence and ambition. Then again, like many people who have taken some serious knocks in early life, he was more comfortable playing up to a sense of the ridiculous than peeling open the darker corners of his mind.

Walking into St Vincents Private Hospital, a crisp and shiny new building with granite steps, a carpeted foyer and large reception desk, only underlined an air of absurdity for Ian. He remembers feeling more like he was checking into a five-star hotel than a facility for tending the wounded and infirm.

But this was no ordinary hotel. Soon he was handing over his wallet, his keys, all the personal belongings he had with him. He struggled with an overwhelming sense of disempowerment, as the numbness crept ever deeper.

He was taken to room 725. It had a heavy door and more of the clinical air he was expecting. The bed was stainless steel, the blanket white and the walls finished in patterned and shiny off-white wallpaper. There were cupboards, benches, telephone, an air-conditioner, radio and an oval TV—all in white. Opposite the end of his bed was a simple chrome crucifix. Christ appeared as a stylised moulded form; again in white.

After he was settled in, Gail headed home and left him alone with his journal.

Since he was fifteen, Ian had kept a journal off and on because it provided him a way of airing feelings and observations he could not, or did not want to, express to others. Now it gave him a chance to cope with the yawning depth and brutal suddenness of what was happening to him. In those days there was no offer of professional support and counselling to cope with the emotional or psychological trauma that so commonly attends major surgery and life-threatening illness.

Ian's first journal was burnt in a 'fit of embarrassment' at the age of sixteen and he did not keep another until he was nineteen. From then his thoughts were self-consciously locked away in an old army munitions box he had bought and carefully restored.

And then someone fiddled with the lock while the young vet was on an extended trip away working in country New South Wales.

'What a betrayal of trust. Perhaps I make too much of nothing,' he would write in a later journal. 'At the time I felt like a knife had been passed midline below my chest and twisted around my diaphragm.'

Hurt and 'disenchanted', he did not log his private feelings for another couple of years and it 'was only when I became sick that I started writing again,' he says, declining to suggest who might have taken an uninvited stroll through his psyche.

His musings in hospital flow between thoughts on meditation, karma, reincarnation, the levels of consciousness, parapsychology and the work of pioneering quantum physicist Niels Bohr. Ian had also taken two books with him into hospital. Both had been sitting on his shelves for many months, waiting to be read. The first was *Meditation in Action* by the Tibetan lama, Chogyam Trungpa. It was the first specific book on meditation Ian would read and now he started dipping into it, hoping to gain some ease and comfort through improving his very basic experiences of meditation.

The second book was the *Bhagavad Gita*, a key volume in the Hindu epic the *Mahabharata* and it had an immediate and powerful effect on the young man. It crystallised for him a deep unease, a growing sense that he had, until now, been lost in the outer world of experience and utterly ignored his inner one.

As he wrote about his early discoveries in the *Bhagavad Gita*,

It says it so clearly: 'Thinking of sense objects, man becomes attached thereto. From attachment arises longing and from longing anger is born. From anger arises delusion; from delusion, loss of memory is caused. From loss of memory, the discrimination faculty is ruined and from the ruin of discrimination, he perishes . . .'

Ian had always been a contemplative person by nature, but it seems his unlimited energy and taste for hard work had also left the young vet with little time for reading or introspection. The enforced hospital rest soon left him feeling, in a way that seems quite extraordinary, 'truly relaxed' and deeply contemplative.

'How long and pleasant these two days have been,' he writes of those first days in hospital while tests were run on his swollen thigh. 'When the future is so uncertain, one can concentrate fully on the present.'

Now his mood was buoyant and curious—the tone tinged with a little of the pomposity of youth. It seems that his earlier dread and melancholy was rapidly transformed. After just a few days in hospital resting, reading and reflecting, he seemed less given to wallowing in anxiety and apprehension, rather observing with detached and clinical interest what might happen next to his body. Despite his predicament, the time and circumstances to ponder spiritual things were clearly both comforting and nourishing. That said, his darker thoughts were now of an existential, rather than physical, flavour.

> The thought that really scares me ... is that I believe malignancies to be an imbalance in cell mechanisms. They are to me an outward sign of an inward disorder. Certainly a cause–effect type relationship between the inner man and the physical body. This being so, and presuming my problem is neoplastic, I have obviously more problems than I imagined.

This inward disorder is one Ian touches on a lot in those early days in hospital. He interpreted his predicament to be the result of a fundamental schism between the sort of life he had been living and the one he felt he *should* be living. He had the clear sense that he had become swept up in the material world, when he already knew deep down that his true drives were towards a more spiritual life. After leaving university and starting his veterinary practice, Ian had enrolled in a part-time Arts degree at the University of Melbourne—to honour his interest in this aspect of his nature. However, his practice flourished and within months he made what he now regards as a major decision. He dropped the Arts degree and, along with it, the spiritual focus. He justified this new, intense working life in his own mind by figuring he could establish financial security by working hard for a few years, and *then* in the comfort that would bring, he could swap to spiritual rather than secular advancement. The *Bhagavad Gita* only confirmed his suspicions that his choice had been misguided.

> Perhaps in so doing, I have committed greater folly than someone who sets out from the beginning to pursue materialism. Having an inkling of the purpose of life and then to turn away from it, even temporarily, sounds utter foolishness; more so in retrospect.
>
> Perhaps I am being melodramatic. I am scared because I know I have bastardised myself for material gain. It would have been fine

to work and develop at the same time. But to give all to work, to chase the material world so openly, this is a bad thing. I enjoy my work, like to think I help the animals and their owners and feel I am reasonably competent at it, but I should have left room for my self as well.

On the surface Ian apparently remained his usual cheery self. Ian chose not to confide his vunerability and his deepest fears, even with the people he was closest to—including Gail.

'Gail and I didn't talk about death at all,' he remembers today. By then the couple had been living together only twelve months and the relationship was still, as Gail characterises it, 'very casual'.

The couple might have been companions, but they were not each other's confidants.

'I didn't talk much at all. It was part of the nature of myself at the time and this is fairly typical of people with cancer in general. There was an aspect of not wanting to trust people with that heartfelt information. And I think for me it was also about the intensity of what I was going through, and how I coped. There was this feeling that I had confidence in my own resources. I think if I had wanted to talk to somebody about it I probably would have. But Gail and I only talked about the things that we had to. We talked about the practical side of things but we didn't talk about our concerns, our fears. We didn't talk about death. It was unexpressed. The journals were important. They were where I expressed myself.'

Mr Doyle visited on the afternoon of Friday 3 January, talking hopefully of possible alternative treatments to surgery, including radiation and chemotherapy, but Ian could not help but notice the concern in his voice. Mr Doyle asked Ian if he knew what a sarcoma was.

I guess he is not to know that animals have the same problems and that I have amputated the legs of quite a few dogs with bone cancer.

The biopsy was to be performed at 9 am the following morning and Ian was resigned to bad news.

He slept well, refusing the night nurse's strong demands to take sleeping pills, and woke at around 7.30 am. At 9 am he was wheeled, groggy with a tranquilliser, to theatre. At 3 pm that afternoon he woke, unsure if the biopsy had been performed, but a huge bandage on his leg and a jab of pain assured him that it had.

Later on, Dr Donald Cordner, Ian's sister's godfather, a general practitioner and ex-champion Aussie Rules footballer (he won the code's top honour—the Brownlow medal—in 1946), called in with his wife.

Dr Cordner told him it was 'almost certainly' a sarcoma, a particularly virulent form of cancer.

> Gail was in too, probably before Donald and maybe the love that she shows towards me is far in excess of my deserve. It makes me feel awkward sometimes. I cannot remember much of her visit however.

Later in the afternoon Gail returned and Ian shared with her what Donald Cordner thought was the likely prognosis.

> She prefers to wait for the biopsy result and we joke over the film Sunshine. It concerned a young woman with the same problem who refused amputation and had a drawn-out death over two years. Each to his own. I want to get the whole thing over with and get back to coping with life as soon as possible.

The couple had been to see *Sunshine* late in the previous year. They had retired to a Mexican restaurant in central Melbourne and analysed the movie together in depth. Ian thought that the woman had given up too easily and was pretty weak. Gail believed that the husband, whose way of coping was to have an affair with a neighbour, 'should have done a lot more than he did'.

The results of the biopsy and a scan on his groin were unequivocal. 'The groin was clear,' according to Doyle, 'but the tumour itself came back consistent with osteosarcoma.'

Osteogenic sarcoma (or osteosarcoma for short) is a bone cancer that most commonly occurs in adolescent boys and is often found in the legs or arms. Until the late 1970s the standard treatment was amputation and the prognosis was poor. At the time of Ian's diagnosis, the usual course was for the cancer to recur quite quickly, most of the time in the lungs. And once it did recur, it was almost invariably rapidly fatal.

In more recent times surgeons have developed a technique whereby they first give chemotherapy to shrink the cancer, then they remove the affected area and graft in a new piece of bone (usually taken from a deceased donor). This surgery is then commonly followed up with a further course of chemotherapy. Recent studies suggest that ten-year survival rates can be as high as 70 per cent among those diagnosed with osteosarcoma. It is one area of cancer treatment where the advent of chemotherapy has brought substantial benefits. But at the time Ian was diagnosed, the statistics were substantially grimmer.

'In 1974,' says Doyle, 'there was probably a 10 to 12 per cent cure rate of osteosarcoma—following surgery—and it might have been even less than that.'

John Doyle consulted with Mr Kevin King, an orthopaedic surgeon (who later became head of orthopaedics at the Royal Melbourne Hospital), and Mr Rowan Webb, a senior surgeon at the Royal Melbourne, about the next course of action.

Dr Cordner was also present at the discussion. It was Cordner who had been keeping Ian's parents, Alan and Glenyss, only recently arrived in Canada, in touch with what was going on with their son from a medical standpoint.

Ian had rung his father when he first realised the seriousness of the illness.

'I can see us sitting in that hotel room,' says Glenyss. 'Alan was talking on the phone and I could only hear his end of the conversation, but I could see his expressions. It makes me shake just thinking about it. It was terribly shocking.'

Alan and Glenyss and daughter Helen had left for Canada those few days before Christmas. For the time being they were staying in a hotel until more permanent accommodation became available.

'To be so far away and to have to rely on other people's impressions or passing on information—it was a terrible time,' says Glenyss.

Alan's instinct had been to return immediately. He asked Ian if he wanted him to, but Ian had said not to bother and Alan agreed. Meanwhile Sue rang her father and told him that she thought he should come. 'I didn't ever tell Ian I'd rung,' she admits.

On 4 January the surgeons, with Cordner present, examined Ian on a ward round and retired to agree that amputation was Ian's only chance.

'There was no sign of it spreading,' says Doyle, 'but we all thought privately that it would spread. They always do.'

It was Doyle who was charged with having to tell Ian the terrible news.

> It is an osteogenic sarcoma. The leg is to come off. Poor Mr D seemed quite distressed in having to tell me.

The operation was scheduled for 8 January, four days later.

Outwardly, Ian appeared 'extraordinarily calm', says Doyle. Inwardly, his thoughts were of the road back to wellness and the work he would have to do to get there.

> I think it is important to set times to meditate and to learn and that these times must become an essential part of the day, as when I trained for athletics so seriously and the one or two hours became a routine to be accommodated with each passing day. It is not going to be easy as so many people are pressing me to do this and that.
>
> I am still unsure how Gail will see my thoughts. I am sure she is not aware of them and if I can convey them to her and make her understand, it will be a good start. I owe her too much to offend her, but it is going to be difficult. I do not feel she is of the same ilk. I fear my relationship with her because I know I am not conducting

myself properly. I feel it is too one-sided, she is so good to me. I begin to feel awkward in asking her to help me.

One of Ian's surprising thoughts in the journal is that he felt that others' compassion for him, although welcome, was undeserved. This apparently stemmed from his deeply-held belief that by following a material path in the previous few years, instead of the spiritual one he had long felt as his true calling, he had somehow brought the cancer upon himself.

I am like a man under death sentence who has been given a chance to make a sacrifice and to work his way out of prison.

It was a terrible judgement to lay at one's own feet, but he bore it with a clear-eyed certainty of what had to be done to re-balance his life. It seems to have given him a meaning and a sense of purpose that transcended the very real trauma he was going through. More importantly, though, it was an early sign of Ian's iron-willed resolve, as well as his sense of personal responsibility, for treading the long path back to health and equanimity—whatever the difficulties.

I hope I can weather the sacrifice in the days to come and go on to begin the work.

On the morning of the amputation Sue and Gail both came in to see him. They left just after 11 am. Ian was grateful for their visit but felt that he could better keep his calm and equanimity on his own. He opened his journal and composed a letter.

Wednesday, January 8, 1975—To my leg
How well you have served me for nearly twenty-five years. I remember long treks through the mountains of Gippsland and how you led the way to jump over six-feet-four. That soaring feeling you gave rise to as you swept up into the air, leading the rest of my body into flight. Just the joy of running was so dear. I was fortunate you were so strong and coordinated. I guess I shall never again feel my mobility to be normal.

You carry scars of days gone by. Below the knee is a small raised up thickening of skin that reminds me of a tip in Longueville, Sydney. How when a friend had his leg caught in the rubbish, you carried me running half a mile for help and only then let on that you were bleeding so badly. On the knee itself is a jagged, ill-defined, purplish scar. A reminder of that foul football match at Sebastopol [near Ballarat] the year before last. It took weeks to get all the gravel out. There are two other scars on the lower leg which are reminders of hockey days, flying sticks and pain that was not so easily subdued. More recently there is the bandaged biopsy site and its resultant swelling.

My mind wanders over the many happy times. There are no complaints as the only time you fell short of my expectations was when my pride and ambitions were too great.

That you are to be lost to me in a few hours leaves me feeling empty. I feel drained of feeling. I hope I still go forward with expectation. I am apprehensive and fear I may shrink before the challenge. So melancholy. I must lift my spirits.

Ian spent most of the rest of the day in quiet, melancholic but calm contemplation and redoubled his efforts to meditate in an effort to buoy himself up. Raised as an Anglican he remembered earlier times when repeating the Lord's Prayer over and over as a twelve-year-old, he had entered the early stages of a meditative state—and it was this technique he returned to once more that day. He also remembered the advice of Dr Raynor Johnson about meditation from a series of lectures he had given at veterinary school that had made a deep impression on Ian.

Johnson had talked of using a mantra, notably the Lord's Prayer, in repetition as a skilful way to focus the mind and keep it from wandering.

I am repeating the Lord's Prayer, and with eyes closed, trying to fix my concentration between my eyes and to keep my mind clear. The only thing that has any certainty is the repetition of the Prayer. Most of the time thoughts come bursting in over the top of it, cascading ideas through my head. I am still full of resolve, but the more imperfections I see, the more awesome the task.

The prayer and his journal were his only anchors at a time when many might have dropped into bottomless depths of utter despair, or worse, succumbed to a blind and terrible panic.

Ian remained calm as he was wheeled to his appointment with the surgeons.

I went down to an anaesthetic room where I had to wait about 20 minutes. The delay was good as it gave me time to set my mind at rest and pray for strength. After being transferred from my bed onto a narrower table, a blanket was draped over my surgery gown and I was left to wait.

The room itself was quite narrow and cluttered. My head was at its entrance, my feet pointed towards the operating theatre. At my left stood the anaesthetic machine in all its pseudo complexity. On the walls beside this were benches stacked with intravenous fluids, same as the ones we use. Against the opposite wall was a stark bench and cupboard with who knows what in it. From the ceiling hung suspended a huge operating light on articulated beams. There were hinged swinging doors into the operating theatre and, periodically, as people came and went, I caught a glimpse of more lights all focused on the operating table.

Finally my anaesthetist arrived, appearing somewhat apprehensive. I still cannot decide if she was just unsure how to conduct herself with someone who was about to lose a leg or if she was concerned with the technical aspects of the coming procedure . . .

I was soon wheeled into the surgery and manhandled onto the operating table. Then there was much slapping of my left hand by the anaesthetist, presumably to get a vein up. This annoyed me, being quite unpleasant. Anyway, finally we were under way.

I tried to keep meditating and praying as I went under . . .

Mr John Doyle, assisted by Mr Kevin King, amputated Ian's right leg at the hip. It was barely two weeks after Ian had first realised, on the Bacchus Marsh oval, that something might be seriously awry.

'It was a very difficult and long operation,' says Mr Doyle, now retired, reading from his notes from the operation. The surgery took almost three hours. 'Most amputations are just below the knee or just above the knee,' he says. 'This was through the hip joint. I don't think I'd ever done a disarticulation through the hip at that stage. These things are pretty uncommon. Kevin had done two, which is why we joined forces.'

The incision went from the outer side of his hip to a point between his scrotum and his anus. The gluteal muscles ('arse to anyone else,' wrote Ian at the time) were folded up and around and sutured to the front of the leg. Nothing at all remained of his right leg. Although as Ian recorded: 'The end result therefore, is quite pleasing to the eye and I am sure will be practical in terms of sit-on-ability.'

The most extraordinary thing about Ian's writings at the time is that the young veterinarian seemed to balance a deep intuitive sense of how the loss of his leg might fit into the bigger picture, with lightness and humour. His predominant thinking at the time seems to have been that the amputation was a fateful reckoning for a wilful ignoring of his spiritual leanings and for letting himself be wholly swept up in a worldly existence—but there was no self-pity.

It could be an atonement, a cleansing or sacrifice for past errors like my misuse of the past year or so.

Whatever the truth, the surgery certainly changed the course of both his inner and outer life in a swift and radical way. Indeed, Ian's life could now be divided neatly into phases and he talks in terms of this feeling like 'separate lives'.

Before the operation Ian had led a consciously outer life, concerned with all the aspects of achievement, enjoyment and material acquisition. After the operation, and in no small part due to his readings in the *Bhagavad Gita,* 'an inner way dawned,' he says. After the operation, it was as if his old life had ended—died—and now a new one was about to begin. 'It was almost like a conscious reincarnation.'

So it was—waking up groggy, disoriented and in sharp pain on the evening of 8 January—that Ian was reborn into his second life (or at least, initially, into the state of purgatory that immediately preceded it) as a 24-year-old with one leg.

The surgery completed, first he drifted out of a 'deep narcosis' and wondered if it 'had all been done'. Three spasms of excruciating pain near the incision left him in no doubt that it had. He was drugged again and slipped back into oblivion.

Gail was the first person he saw and she told him that his sister Sue had already been in to visit. Ian had talked to her apparently, but he could not remember. That following night was a long one, clouded and defined by a four-hourly dose of strong painkillers.

The first two hours of each cycle of the painkillers' effect, Ian remembers he spent dozing. The next half-hour to an hour he experienced a 'half awareness of pain and a mounting apprehension' and then in the last hour, before the next dosage, the pain returned. 'Usually the pain was centred on the inside of the leg—I mean stump—and radiated from it.'

As he steadily regained consciousness, Ian realised that he was in Intensive Care, on an intravenous drip and surrounded by monitors. As clarity returned, clouded by pain, he noticed the man in the next bed to him. Ian remembers noticing how ill he looked and shuddered when he realised that he too was on the critical list. Then his companion's monitors went silent. Quite suddenly Ian was in the room by himself.

And then an immediate, most pressing, dilemma. With the trauma of the surgery, passing urine seemed nigh on impossible. As the hours wore on, the pressure became extreme. Until Mr Doyle came to the rescue. 'Pass urine in the next hour, or when I come back I am going to catheterise you!' This was all Ian needed to hear. Immediately overcoming his fear of moving from the apparent safety of his bed, and aided by two caring nurses, he gingerly swung his leg over the side of the bed and stood for the first time. Remembering how the sound of running water helped to make horses pee when he had wanted to collect a urine sample, Ian asked another nurse to turn on a nearby tap. As the water poured down the sink, Ian tentatively emptied his bladder into a waiting bottle and the first hurdle had been overcome.

Even as Ian's pain peaked and troughed and he returned to his private room, his thoughts were firmly focused. It seems that he was transforming, even transcending, his own very human drama by interpreting it within a spiritual context.

My God though, I am scared to die. At times the terror comes over me like a wave of hot, cloying air, stifling me and transfixing me in sweating fear. Usually I can control it; but the thought remains if secondaries do appear it means I have failed my second chance and what a low level of development I must be at. All through this I have this unshatterable belief in myself; that I am such a good person. I am so, so self satisfied, I do not know how to beat it. It must be done away with. I am so smug, notwithstanding my difficulties. I fear I secretly enjoy the martyred youth image and tremble at the consequences of such thoughts. This is the problem with so many visitors. They bolster my spirits to the point where I overlook the cause and become preoccupied with the effect. I must accept them only as people keen to see me back on the road to recovery, both physically and spiritually.

When Ian had first been diagnosed he had assumed deep down that Gail would leave him. His mother had died suddenly during his childhood and at the time this had felt like desertion. All his teenage girlfriends had eventually left him too. He had never been the one to end a relationship. And then long-term girlfriend Liz had left him for another man. Now Ian expected Gail to be the next woman to leave him.

As Ian puts it, 'It really was unconscious at the time, but in retrospect I am sure that I thought I would get in first.' So he was telling her to go—repeatedly.

'He would say: "Go. What are you doing around here? Just go,"' says Gail.

Gail's friends, meanwhile, gave her similar counsel.

Nevertheless, Gail felt that she could not leave. Ian's sister Susan (his closest family) was pregnant with her second child and was about to give birth; his parents were on the other side of the world in Canada. 'There was nobody else,' says Gail. 'What was going to happen to him?' Even if she had decided it were better that she left him, she says she 'couldn't have done it; my conscience wouldn't have allowed me.'

Before the diagnosis, Ian says, their relationship was 'definitely in trouble', or as Gail had put it, the romance had remained 'very casual' in those early days. The illness changed everything. Now she was loving, attentive and patently willing to devote herself utterly to his recovery. Ian was deeply grateful and found enormous comfort in Gail's love and unqualified support. But, he was also troubled by knowing that the amputation represented the end of his old life and the beginning of a completely new and different one.

3

First Life

Ian James Gawler was born in Melbourne on 25 February 1950.
In a lift.

Billie, Ian's mother, went into labour and was rushed to hospital
sure that she was about to give birth at any second. She made it
to the hospital safely, was placed on a trolley and wheeled into
the elevator (it is not clear who was with her in there, although
husband Alan was likely parking the car). By the time the doors
opened again at the labour ward a few floors up, one more little
soul had made his impatient entrance into the world.

Ian was Alan and Billie Gawler's second child. Their first, Susan
Lee, was born in June 1947, three years before Ian.

Alan Gawler, Ian's father, was first son to Oswald and Doris
Gawler, a solidly middle-class couple of British lineage and old-
fashioned, Victorian sensibilities. Oswald was an actuary and
Melbourne stockbroker who famously predicted the Great
Depression. He was the last person to sell his seat on the stock
exchange before the crash and subsequently sold all this stocks and
shares in the nick of time. Then he quite deliberately moved his
family to take up a safe job as State Statistician for South Australia.
Later he became the Victorian Government Statistician.

Alan studied civil engineering at university and then, in late
1940, enrolled in the Royal Australian Air Force, graduating as

a navigator, with the rank of pilot officer, in February 1942. In April he was posted to No. 32 Squadron on the northern tip of Queensland. He was the eldest of four children (three boys, one girl) and his younger brothers, Bob and Douglas, also enlisted for active service during the war. Bob was killed in 1944 during only his second bombing mission over Germany.

'Poppa Gawler—which was what we called him—used to dote on Alan and Bob,' says Pat King, who was married to Oswald's other son, Doug, who died of leukemia in 1959.

Pat, Ian Gawler's favourite aunt, was a radio actress in her younger days and remembers her in-laws as very conservative and not given to easily embracing change.

'All the daughters-in-law had washing machines and proper refrigerators while Nanny Gawler [Oswald's wife, Ian's grandmother, Doris] was still getting ice from the ice man and washing the clothes in a copper. I think Alan and Doug eventually shamed Poppa into getting a washing machine for her and some other more modern things.'

Alan went on to serve in Australia and New Guinea and clocked up over 1000 flying hours in a number of different types of bombers. While he was directly involved in engaging the enemy a number of times, it was learning how to fly the aircraft that had proven equally perilous. Once flying in close formation during training, Alan Gawler's plane touched wings with the one alongside. The neighbouring plane nosedived into the ground, killing all on board. Gawler's pilot somehow was able to nurse their plane back to earth for a heavy crash landing, with its crew only just managing to scramble to safety before the bomb-laden plane blew to smithereens. The commanding officer sent Gawler's crew straight back up the following morning to fly in close formation with him—this being the accepted, if somewhat brutal, way his generation got on with the job. Counselling was simply unheard of. There was a job to do. Emotional reactions were suppressed. Self-control was the order of the day.

Ian recalls, 'I talked with my dad a couple of times about what it was like to deal with people getting shot and blown up and he said "you just got on with it". Dad told me he had so many close encounters with death that he soon lost all fear of it.'

The other thing that confronting your own mortality daily did typically do was to underline the sweet taste of romance and the urgency of new love.

In August 1942, No. 32 Squadron was transferred to Camden near Sydney to provide convoy escort and surveillance. During one rare night of leave, Alan and his colleagues went to a nearby dance and it was here that he met Majorie (Billie) Gray. Billie and Alan were both twenty years old.

Like Alan, the vivacious Billie was descended from British stock that had immigrated to Australia in the 1820s. She was the daughter of Charles and Mima Gray and had one elder brother, Brian.

Alan Gawler and Billie Gray's courtship lasted a couple of years and during that time they saw each other as much as Alan's job in reconnaissance, and then as an instructor, would allow. Then in April 1944 he was posted to New Guinea. The pair decided to get married a few days before he left for the uncertainties of the north.

'There were probably some people who thought there would be a birth in less than nine months,' reflected Alan in a journal charting the family history he would compile in his later years. In reality though, first child Susan, 'had a gestation period of about three years'.

After Alan Gawler's discharge from the RAAF he finished his studies at the University of Melbourne (during which time Susan was born) and then began work as a research engineer with Rocla Concrete Pipes in the engineering department at Springfield, Victoria in 1949.

Ian was born in the February of the following year. When Ian was three, in 1953 the young family moved to Sydney where Alan took up the position of works manager at the concrete engineering firm's Belfield branch. Then in 1957 the Gawlers moved to Blackheath in the Blue Mountains, just west of Sydney, where Alan supervised the construction of a 50-kilometre underground pipeline stretching from Oberon to a power station at Wallerawang.

Ian Gawler remembers having a lovely few years living in the Blue Mountains and out of that experience he has retained a real love of the bush. He would often pedal his pushbike on the narrow walking tracks near his home, sometimes alone and sometimes with schoolfriends. Ian remembers being filled with awe at the rugged natural beauty of the distant mountains, the deep valleys, the rocky escarpments and the dense bush that characterises the countryside near Blackheath. On the weekends he would sometimes camp with his father near the pipeline the company was building through the bush.

It was also at this time that the family inherited a stray skinny black dog that had wandered into one of the company factories. Ian named him Bimbo.

'He was an absolutely magic dog,' says Ian. 'He was an extremely intelligent black kelpie-cross type cattledog mixture. He was a very dear friend for a long time.' One of Bimbo's distinctions was that he was directly responsible for Ian Gawler's first exposure to the prospective profession of veterinary science, thanks to something that was discovered hanging from the poor dog's backside one day. 'It was very impressive,' laughs Ian. 'So there was quite a panic call to the vet as to what this particular thing was. He assured us it must have been a tapeworm, and came personally with the appropriate treatment.'

Aunt Pat says Ian was pretty wild as a child. Once, on a visit, she remembers him tearing around on his bike and making 'a terrific noise. He was full of beans. Alan told him to stop and of course he didn't,' she says. 'I felt so sorry for him because Alan shut him in the car and he had to stay there for about half an hour.'

Ian Gawler was an energetic boy with a growing interest in animals. Later after the family moved to Adelaide (in 1960, as the very capable and efficient Alan Gawler was promoted ever higher in the Rocla hierachy) he would often take off for a day at the zoo on his bike with his best friend who shared his obsession with living things.

At around the age of twelve Ian developed a strong determination to become a veterinarian. Initially he was keen on making a career as a doctor, but he remembers wondering how he might deal with the emotional issues that he imagined would inevitably arise amongst his patients. He observed the doctors that he knew through the family and quickly realised that most of them seemed to cope by becoming clinically detached. 'I couldn't see how you could do that and, in fact, I didn't want to do that.' Ian reasoned that animals would not have the same issues. 'So with the naivety of a twelve-year-old I thought: right, I'll do that. I'll become a vet.'

It was also around this time that a sequence of terrible events would change his family's life forever.

One day in late 1961 Ian arrived home from school to find his mother missing. Normally she was in the garden or the kitchen, ready to greet him with afternoon tea. This day all he found was an ominous silence. Troubled, he called out but there was no answer. Moving into the house he discovered terrifying smears of blood all along the walls of the main corridor.

Entering his parents' bedroom he found his mother in bed barely conscious with her face bashed up. He ran immediately to the neighbours next door and they called an ambulance.

Meanwhile Susan remembers waiting to be picked up from school that day and her mother never appearing. She waited and waited and then finally walked home. She, too, was shocked by what she found. 'We were told then that she must have fallen over in the bathroom. Nobody knows what happened,' she says.

Ian remembers it being discussed at the time that somebody had broken into the house and beaten his mother up. But it was not talked about more than that. The police investigated and there were no charges laid. Susan later found a newspaper cutting about the incident in her father's wardrobe saying it was an accident. 'If any one knew [any different] we weren't enlightened,' she says.

A few months later far worse was to come.

In early 1962 Alan was sent away to Melbourne to spend five intensive live-in weeks doing administrative training. He only had one weekend off during the entire length of the course and then returned home for good again in late February. Once home his most pressing domestic duty was to tackle the oxalis weeds that had taken hold in the back garden while he was away. He set to it the next free weekend with garden tools but had not finished before he had to go back to work on the following Monday.

A few days later, one hot weekday in early March 1962—with Alan at work and the children at school—Billie decided to tackle the remaining weeds. As the story goes, she mixed up one jug of weed killer and filled another similar jug of water with which to slake her thirst and took them both outside. It appears she must have taken a swig from the wrong jug. Realising her terrible error, she rang her husband to tell him what had happened and was rushed to the Royal Adelaide Hospital critically ill.

That night Ian remembers praying fervently into the night for his mother to get well.

Ian was raised as an Anglican (the family regularly attended the local church on Sundays) with a strong sense of moral responsibility, underpinned by an unquestioning faith in a just and loving God.

Billie had lapsed into a coma at the hospital and she died early the following day. Her death certificate, dated 7 March 1962, lists the cause of death as 'acute arsenical poisoning', the arsenic being confirmed as coming from the weed killer.

After his wife's death, Alan went first to daughter Susan's school to tell her the shocking news. Then he drove with her to find Ian at his school. 'He left me in the car to get Ian,' she remembers, 'and while he was looking for him, Ian's class walked past from sport. So I called out to him and then I went over and told him what had happened.' By now Alan, unable to find Ian in the school building, had returned to the car. When the two returned, they found their father, sitting somewhat dumbfounded in the car.

Ian's impression of the day was very different. He remembers sitting on a stony bench in the school and his sister coming over to him. She broke the terrible news and then the two of them went back to where their father was waiting in the car. Not surprisingly, Ian grew up thinking that his father had sent Susan in to deliver the news because he could not face doing it himself.

It was only during the researching of this book that the truth came out that Susan had, by accident, been the one to break the distressing information to her brother. That this extraordinary and crucial piece of information did not emerge at the time, let alone in the years that went on, is symptomatic of another extraordinary fact.

After Ian and Susan had joined their father in the car and they drove off shocked and silent that terrible day in March 1962, Alan did not talk about Billie or mention her name with his children until years and years later—and even then, only at his offspring's insistence. The lessons learnt as the child of straightlaced Victorian parents, which were further ingrained, as an imperative in war, carried on into Alan Gawler's civilian and married life.

Meanwhile, the fact that his mother had not got better, despite Ian's impassioned prayers the night before, 'had as much effect on my view of morality and the way the world worked as did the loss of my mother itself,' says Ian. 'Before her death I had a very strong and quite simplistic belief that if you said your prayers and did the right thing, then things would happen the way you wanted them to.'

With his boyhood belief system in tatters, Ian also slipped into a state of denial, a state which was exacerbated by his father's silent grief for his wife. 'I can't remember Dad talking about anything to do with the death after that,' says Ian.

'It was all very hushed up,' says Aunt Pat. 'The Gawlers never really discussed these things.'

Alan Gawler was coping the way he knew best by just getting on with it. It was an approach that included not wanting his children to go to the funeral, held on 9 March at the Centennial Park Crematorium, Springbank. Ian insisted that he go—and did; Susan acquiesced. 'I was given a sleeping pill and stayed at home,' she says. Meanwhile both the Gawler children were left with the uneasy feeling that their mother had simply vanished off the face of the earth.

Billie's ashes were eventually placed under a native Australian shrub at Woronora General Cemetery, near the place of her birth and upbringing, at Sutherland in Sydney.

'It was like I'd look around and she'd come back,' says Susan. 'We didn't have the opportunity to see her before she died because it was all so quick.'

Ian remembers the impact as a brutally swift chain of events. He remembers going to school one day, coming home to be told his mother was ill in hospital, going to school the following day and being told by his sister that she had died, going to a funeral and then coping with the terrible reality that his mother was gone. And all of this without seeing her either sick or after she had passed away.

As a twelve-year-old he could not accept that his mother had died and thought that she must have disappeared to take care of something important. Perhaps she was a spy, he fantasised, and she had to 'make up some excuses not to be around. For six months I was really quite convinced that it was all a put-on and that it was not real.'

Ian was growing up in a family where, not uncommonly for the day, he was taught that boys did not cry. He never really expressed any overt grief for the loss of his mother at the time. He was numb. In fact he never really felt the effect of his mother's death and after that first six months, he came to accept it like a 'defensive anaesthetic wearing off. It just sort of gradually filtered through,' he says, until finally he was left with the sense that 'perhaps it was real'.

Perhaps it was an expression of his anger, grief and inner turmoil, perhaps it was just his nature to get into scraps, but at school after his mother's death, Ian was drawn into fist-fights almost daily. It was, he says, at a time when there was a lot of violence inside and outside the classroom of the school he was attending. The masters would regularly rap pupils over the palm of the hand or knuckles with the student's own wooden rulers. In an attempt to cope with this and make light of it, Ian and his friends would carve a notch into their rulers, as a matter of honour, every time they were hit in front of the class. 'I think I had 78 notches at the end of one year,' says Ian. 'It was bloody ridiculous. Quite extreme.'

Ian was also left with an uncomfortable feeling that there had to be a link between his mother's bashing and her sudden death a few months later. 'It never sat well with me because it was such a weird conjunction of events,' he says today.

Years later, in 1978, he asked his father for the 'real story'—

thinking it possible he might have bent the truth at the time to protect the then twelve-year-old Ian.

'But Dad was really adamant that the version of events I got as a twelve-year-old was in fact the right version. I challenged him as hard as I could but he stuck to the story.'

A year or two later he made another attempt to confront his father.

This time Ian told his father he found it very hard to believe that the events had transpired as they did. He asked him if he thought Billie had committed suicide, as well as asking him who had beaten her up and why the two events had happened around the same time. Again, Ian was not told anything by his father that he had not already heard.

Still not content, he visited the Coroner while living in Adelaide in the 1980s and had a look at a copy of the inquest into his mother's death. The timing of her poisoning and her admission to hospital on the report varied from what he recollected his father had told him.

It puzzled Ian deeply and it only added to the mystery. 'But people do forget,' he says in his father's defence, 'although they would be pretty strong details, you'd think.'

Mollie Stock was Billie's best friend and is Ian's godmother. She is now quite elderly and remembers nothing of the events of 46 years ago. Nonetheless, at the time of her mother's death Susan remembers Mollie, who lives in Sydney, questioning her repeatedly to try and make sense of the events around that time. Also Ian remembers Mollie telling him, a number of years ago, that his mum was never really happy in Adelaide.

'I asked her whether there was a possibility she was having an affair or something like that and they got sprung and that sort of precipitated all this,' he says. 'She said she had wondered about it herself, but she didn't know.'

Another intriguing and quite remarkable fact was that Billie's brother Brian, who had been at the Royal Adelaide Hospital at the time of her admission, called on Gail a couple of days after Ian had visited the Coroner (and while Ian was out), and was keen to know why he was interested in his mother's inquest. Somehow, Brian knew almost immediately that Ian had been to the Coroner's office enquiring about the circumstances of her death.

Ian remembers Brian (now deceased) as a most unusual gentleman who had told everyone that he had spent the war in Britain in the air force.

In 2005 Ian sent off for his family's war records—including his uncle Brian's. They came back with the surprising information that Brian Gray had served in the army—not the air force as Gray had told everyone. More intriguing still, Gray's records were designated 'Classified' and were unavailable for viewing.

Over forty years after the event, all that Ian is left with today is a sense of murkiness about the whole thing and a sense of disquiet. The full truth of his mother's bashing and untimely death will likely never be known.

Regardless of the true course of events, however, what is clear and most significant to Ian Gawler's story is the profound impact the death of his mother had upon him—just as it would have on any twelve-year-old child. But there were two further events immediately after her death that only intensified the indelible impression on his already tender psyche.

First, Ian remembers comforting himself immediately after his mother's passing with the knowledge that, whatever had happened, he still enjoyed the loyalty and unquestioning companionship of Bimbo, his dog.

His father, it seems, as well as not talking of what had happened, had not hugged him once to console him around this time. The Gawler family, true to their Victorian antecedents, were firmly of the non-touching type. Also his sister and he (although later they would become very good friends) did not have a very good relationship at the time.

Bimbo was his best friend.

A week after his mother died, Bimbo went missing. Several days went by and then riding his bike home from school, Ian found him lying stiff on the side of the street. Bimbo had been hit by a car and killed.

Then to compound matters more, another week after Bimbo's death, while away on a school religious camp, he awoke in the middle of the night to discover one of the teachers 'lying next to me and rubbing up against me'. Totally confused, utterly ignorant of homosexuality, Ian lay motionless for some time, working out what to do. He said nothing, but sat suddenly up in bed and the teacher 'just went out of the room,' he remembers. The next morning he told two prefects what had happened. He never heard any more about it and he told no-one else about it. Not his father. Not his sister. No-one.

In the weeks and months after his wife's death, Alan Gawler carried on as a single parent to the very best of his abilities. A succession of housekeepers kept the home running smoothly and Ian and Susan have fond memories of their father taking them on a number of weekend trips away camping, to the beach and to the Snowy Mountains to ski. And then in 1963 Alan fell in love with a young engineer's secretary named Glenyss Lock.

The couple were soon spending a lot of time together until Alan was transferred to Melbourne to take up an even more senior position with Rocla. Hefty phone bills were racked up and Alan headed back to Adelaide as often as he could until—as he writes in the family history—his two children finally said: 'What's wrong with you, Dad? Why don't you get on with it?'

Alan and Glenyss were married in April 1964 and Glenyss moved to Melbourne directly after their honeymoon. Alan Gawler was 42 and Glenyss 29. It was two years after Billie's death.

While the newly married couple were away on their honeymoon, Ian and Susan had been looked after by their grandparents, Oswald and Doris. To greet the newlyweds upon their return Ian, now fourteen, had organised what he believed would surely be a pleasant surprise for his new stepmother—a lizard he had caught in the garden and was keeping in a shoebox in his bedroom.

'Grandma—bless her cotton socks—had managed to leave the lid off the box so that the lizard could escape,' says Glenyss. 'She had thought the new bride wouldn't be all that thrilled to be presented with this big lizard.'

Glenyss' memory of Ian as a young teenager was that he was 'grubby and untidy and late. He had no idea of time and had a great talent for losing things.' He was also very small for his age. By contrast, when twelve, Ian had been tall for his age and had excelled in athletics, particularly his chosen sport, high jump. After his mother's death his growth seemed to stall for several years.

By all accounts Ian was an intelligent lad, who did not have to put very much effort into his schoolwork to do well; much to his sister's chagrin. Moreover, 'If something came along that interested him, he became totally involved,' says Glenyss. 'He had a huge amount of enthusiasm and perseverance. He was a funny little boy actually, but he had lots of very good qualities.'

During one period, the family was thrown into chaos when Glenyss became bedridden for a few days with an illness. One day Ian burst through the bedroom door with a glorious fan-shaped display of flowers for his stepmother. 'I can see it to this day,' she says. 'He'd picked the flowers out of the garden and it must have taken him forever to put [the arrangement] together. He had a very sensitive side to him.'

Sister Susan also remembers him as a very bright child—although she was not quite so well acquainted with his more caring side on account of the fact that in those earlier years the pair used to often squabble, much like most siblings do. Susan remembers that when he was younger she used to get the better of him by sitting on him. But then came the day when he got big enough to shove her off and the power base shifted.

Thinking back, Susan reflects that it must have been very difficult for Glenyss having to come in and deal with a teenage girl and a teenage boy who were not her own. 'Imagine trying to be newly married and romantic and have two young teenagers. It must have been shocking,' she says. 'We were shocking.'

Glenyss, for her part, reckons she 'must have been mad taking them on. But you'll do anything for love.'

Still, her instant family did prove very useful. Susan and Ian could babysit their stepsister, Helen, born to Alan and Glenyss in 1966.

'One night we were babysitting and I couldn't get her to settle down,' says Susan. 'It made me really mad because Ian picked her up, soothed her immediately and she went straight to sleep. Helen adored Ian.'

Later, when Ian was old enough to own and ride a motorbike Glenyss remembers him taking Helen out, as a toddler, around the block on the back of it. 'She loved it,' says Glenyss. 'He was very good with her.'

Ian was attending the University of Melbourne at the time, studying veterinary science, just as he had planned to from the tender age of twelve. It was the ambition from which he had never wavered.

Ian had sat the matriculation exam at the Melbourne Church of England Grammar School in 1966, the year before he was finally admitted to the University of Melbourne. Although he gained admittance to veterinary science that first year, being only sixteen his parents and teachers had decided he was too young for university, so he repeated his final year of secondary school. These were the days before gap years.

At school Ian indulged his passion for all sport, particularly athletics, and had a long-held ambition to win a place in the Victorian team. In the early days he was a very good athlete and in 1963 he won the Inter Schools high jump for his age. As his secondary school years went on and his contemporaries outgrew him, he was no longer as competitive as he used to be. Ian remained determined to find a place in the state team.

'By that stage I'd worked out that I wasn't good enough in an individual event to do it,' he says, adding that in Year 12 he discovered there was an event called the decathlon 'and you could do a bit of everything. So I took that up.'

The decathlon consists of ten events contested over two days. On the first day athletes compete in the 100 metres sprint, then the long jump, shot put and high jump and the 400 metres. The following day they contest the 110-metre hurdles, throw a discus and javelin, compete in the pole vault and finally run 1500 metres.

Points are awarded for the performance achieved in each event and the person with the highest number of points is the winner. Not surprisingly, decathletes are considered to be the best all-round athletes in the world.

At the time Ian was training with Franz Stampfl, a well-known coach and tough taskmaster who had trained Ralph Doubell to win the 800-metre gold medal at the 1968 Mexico Olympics. Stampfl had a 'real disdain for anyone other than elite athletes and it took me an unduly long time to realise he was not a very good coach for me,' says Ian.

Nevertheless, Ian trained for two or three hours a day and sometimes worked so hard he would vomit. 'I had a terribly low pain tolerance,' says Ian, explaining that to be competitive in the 400 metres and the 1500 metres required that athletes pushed themselves right up to, and beyond, the pain barrier. 'I could train hard and push myself through 400 metres but I couldn't do the 1500 very well at all—like most decathletes.'

Ian maintains he was 'reasonable' at all of the ten decathlon events, which gave him an edge over his competitors. His training and perseverance paid off and he was selected for the Victorian team, going on to represent his state at the annual national championships three times. Discus was his worst event, 'but even then I could do that reasonably,' he says, adding that other athletes might well be very good at nine events, but if they were very poor at even one, say, the pole vault, then they were out of contention.

Decathlon is all about consistency, adaptability, and the capacity for both rapid recovery and endurance—which were all skills that Ian would later use to save his own life.

Repeating his final year at secondary school, having won a reserved place at the vet school, Ian took the opportunity to indulge his long-held interest in both literature and art. While academically he had concentrated on science throughout his senior years, at the same time he read voraciously. He regularly got through two or three books a week, being drawn to the classics as well as twentieth-century greats like Somerset Maugham, Hemingway, Steinbeck, Camus and Sartre.

One of his teachers in his second Year 12 was Ron Miller, who became a particular mentor. An art critic and an artist, Miller also knew enough about the history of art and adolescent boys to figure that if you included nude women in your lessons then you could capture the attention of your class.

'He also organised a series of life drawing classes at Melbourne Grammar,' says Ian, 'with a naked female model—which was a cause for some excitement throughout the school, as you can imagine.' They were held in a second-floor room, at night, so that no-one who was not directly involved could peer in.

For the first session Ian's class trooped into the room with a great hum of nervous excitement. One classmate, a keen artist who had great plans to make a career of art, took prime position near the front of the class with a specially-prepared and very fancy wooden drawing board. His drawing paper was held on by big rubber bands. The life model entered the room, took off all her clothes and assumed a pose.

'It was quite a while before things settled,' says Ian. And then just as the room had almost completely quietened down, one of the straining rubber bands on the keen young artist's board broke 'and it hurtled off the board and hit the woman square in the chest.'

The class erupted into hysterical laughter. 'It was hopeless. *Everyone* lost the plot,' laughs Ian. Miller could not regain order, the evening was abandoned and everyone went home. 'We came back again the following week and tried again.' Ian continued to draw and paint throughout his life.

When he matriculated from Melbourne Grammar for the second time, at the end of 1967, he did manage a pass in art but also won a first-class honour in English literature. Along with most others, he was quite surprised and deeply delighted by the result. It was an important milestone for Ian because up until that time, although he had a passion for reading, he had thought of himself as a student of the sciences. It instilled in him a determination to pursue his own writing; he went on to edit the student magazine while at the vet school and, eventually, gained the confidence to pen his own books.

It also made him aware of the gap that existed between the arts and sciences. Later Ian would champion an inclusive, holistic approach to medicine, but in these years he felt a broader, more inclusive approach was needed in his own veterinary studies. More specifically he actively agitated for an arts subject to be included in the veterinary science curriculum. Although he managed to have the idea formally accepted by the student body, it never went any further with the powers-that-be. 'Actually, in those days, I think it was taken as heresy,' he says.

During the early days at university Ian used to get around on a 125cc Kawasaki (motorbikes had been an ongoing obsession with him ever since he had been old enough to have a licence), which a year later he swapped for a substantially more powerful 350cc machine.

'I hated that motorbike, I can tell you,' says Glenyss, with a concern that is still palpable after all these years. Her worry was well founded.

'I had delighted in its power,' wrote Ian in a journal. 'The ever imminent danger involved in riding it fast, put many a problem into proper perspective. What was past was unalterable. What was in the future would go better if I concentrated fully on what I was doing at the time.'

Once as a student, riding from the vet school to the main campus of the university to visit friends, he swept into a curve near Melbourne zoo, misjudging it badly. 'I came hurtling around the corner and was met by a solid concrete barrier on the median strip in the middle of the road,' he says.

'It's funny what your mind does when faced with impending disaster, but as soon I saw this median strip I knew I was going to hit it. The image that came to me was the scene from *The Great Escape* where Steve McQueen jumps one barbed-wire fence and then crashes into the second,' he says. Ian remembered McQueen standing up on his bike to make the jumps and did likewise—just as the front wheel hit the concrete. He was sent 'off like a rocket'.

Motorbike and rider arced spectacularly through the air and then landed with a sickening thud in the middle of the other side of the road. The bike bounced, slid, and slammed into a parked car. Ian meanwhile, although having landed awkwardly, had little but a sore toe, a deep gouge out of his helmet and impressive scratches down the back of his heavy leather riding jacket to show for his unexpected flight and sudden encounter with the bitumen.

As Ian was picking up the bike, its front forks bent, dusting himself off and thanking his good fortune that there had not been any oncoming traffic, a man darted out of the building adjacent. 'That was the most amazing thing I have ever seen. You must have been 20 feet in the air at least,' he exclaimed, adding almost as an afterthought that it was his car that had stopped Ian's bouncing bike. Ian apologised profusely, gave the startled man his details and asked him to send a bill for the damage to his car. 'He never did,' he says. 'But he got his money's worth, I reckon.' Ian later went back and measured his flight from take-off to landing: around 21 metres.

That bike was repaired but then sold at the end of Ian's third year at university to help pay his way. It was not until fifth year that he had saved enough for another motorbike.

This next one was arranged for him by his father and specially imported from the UK—a handsome old-style 500cc Velocette Venom. 'I rode it for a while and then decided to restore it. The only place to keep it was in my bedroom at Bacchus Marsh,' Ian says. 'I used to start it up from time to time and it used to make the whole house rattle. Kathy would go nuts. Gail too thought me crazy to have a bike in the bedroom.' The throb and roar of the bike's powerful engine would send visible little waves rippling across the surface of their waterbed.

Ian never really had the time to fully restore the bike, as it transpired, and fed up with not having one to ride—and making good money with the thriving veterinary practice—he bought the expensive and powerful 750cc MV Agusta only weeks before his visit to Mr Doyle.

As for pursuits of the mind, Ian had maintained his interest in the arts and literature throughout his university years by reading widely in addition to his studies. But now as well as the classic and contemporary novels and assorted non-fiction, he began to read books related to his fast-emerging interest in more esoteric matters.

Of all the reading during those years, one book that had a lasting impact was *The Imprisoned Splendour* by Raynor Johnson. Published in the 1950s, and now out of print, it was subtitled 'an approach to reality based upon the significance of data drawn from the fields of natural science, psychical research and mystical experience'.

Dr Raynor Johnson had been the master at the Methodist Queen's College at the University of Melbourne. He hailed from the UK, had a PhD in physics and had taught the subject in London and Belfast before coming to Australia in 1934. In later years he had also become interested in investigating matters of a psychic and mystical nature, and in this study he continued to apply the rigorous scientific method which, as a physicist, he was well versed in. Raynor came to the vet school at rural Werribee in 1971, when Ian's class was in residence, and gave a series of lectures on his beliefs and theosophy.

The lectures were a very significant experience for Ian because they introduced him to many eastern concepts such as karma and reincarnation and the idea 'that man is a spirit inhabiting a body, rather than that man is a body that happens to have a spirit.' Johnson, although a local pioneer in his field, later had his reputation destroyed when he became involved with a Melbourne-based cult called The Family, led by Anne Hamilton-Byrne.

Regardless of his unfortunate later associations, the concepts that Johnson presented came as a revelation for Ian. 'They opened me up to a whole new way of looking at life which both appealed to me logically and on a gut level.' It sparked an interest in the metaphysical, beyond his own Christian upbringing and was the genesis of Ian's own critical investigations into the connections between body and mind.

After one of the lectures, Ian approached him to find out more. He was desperate to find out something, anything, of the specifics of meditation. Many of the esoteric books that he had been reading had mentioned the word meditation. It seemed to be given great importance as a key technique on the spiritual path, yet Ian had found little that explained what meditation actually was, let alone how to do it. So he began by asking Johnson directly if he meditated himself, unaware that this might be a fairly personal question to ask a friend, let alone a perfect stranger. Johnson was 'a little taken aback by the directness of the question', says Ian and did not answer it in explicit terms. Instead he gently suggested to the young vet that he could use a mantra. Unsure of what a mantra was, Ian then asked Johnson if 'that was what he did'. Johnson remained coy, but volunteered a begrudging 'sometimes'. Ian pressed him again on what Johnson used, what he did. 'I was quite in his face and I wasn't going to take no for an answer,' he says, despite the fact that the academic was patently reluctant to spell out any personal details. In the end, perhaps exhausted by Ian's interrogation, Johnson suggested to him that he could use The Lord's Prayer as a mantra—a point of focus for one's attention, quietly spoken in repetition—to still the mind.

Ian was part of a group of students that were 'really fired up' by what Johnson had to say. One friend who was particularly enamoured was Anne Neville—who had in fact arranged for Johnson to visit the vet school. 'She was more inspired and motivated to pursue his concepts and techniques than I was,' says Ian. 'And in fact she kept on goading me over the next few years after I graduated by sending me books, telling me more about these things and stimulating me.'

Anne Neville was a friend. A female friend. Ian maintains he had many female friends as a youth and young man and that many of these were platonic friendships. Non-sexual relationships came easily for Ian. He would often go out with attractive women, having developed what was simply a good friendship. As for sexual relationships, Ian says that he was 'always very shy, very slow to make advances.'

Perhaps this stemmed from his non-demonstrative upbringing or the early trauma of the mild sexual abuse he experienced as a twelve-year-old; perhaps it related to a difficulty with intimacy itself. Remembering his feelings of abandonment when his mother died suddenly and mysteriously, how each of his girlfriends ended those fledgling relationships and then how his first real love left him too, it is easy to understand how Ian had developed an emotionally defensive attitude towards women in general—and then to Gail in particular. In fact it is also easy to understand why, when he became ill, he assumed Gail would leave him, much as had all the other key women in his life.

But Ian would be proved wrong. Gail stuck solidly by him from the very first diagnosis—a diagnosis that had arrived so suddenly and so shockingly into their young lives.

4

Second Life

It was early morning, fourteen days after the operation, when Ian realised that he had to give himself over to the grief of losing his leg. The previous night had been a fitful one punctuated by a dark and disturbing dream. One nightmare layered inside another, wrapped inside another. Like a Russian babushka doll.

Ian woke up gagging on his tongue, fighting for breath and desperately ringing for the night nurse. Nobody came for what seemed like forever.

Even when nursing staff did finally come they dashed around in panic not knowing quite what to do.

But this too was part of the dream and Ian drifted off into unknowing again . . . only to wake up properly—or at least he thought he had—equally panicked.

He pressed the night bell. Nothing happened. He pressed it again. Nothing. And again. And again. Still nothing.

Now quite breathless, I realised I was still dreaming and forced myself to find the real thing. It seemed to require a superhuman effort to struggle out of the dream and find the actual buzzer. In touching its cold metal surface, I awoke with a start, jolted back into reality. I have never been so scared in all my life.

His terrible loss, lodged deep in his psyche, was beginning to surface.

Twelve days earlier, two days after the operation, Susan and her husband Ross had helped him get out of bed and take a first, tentative lap of his room. Apart from these beginnings to get mobile again, those first couple of days only offered pain, extreme fatigue and introspection—often still taking the form in his journal of a personal rebuke for reverting to old patterns and for giving scant consideration to his spiritual wellbeing.

All thought is centring on where and what work I shall do, where and in what I shall live, and what exercise etc. I will do. Obviously I must reorganise my priorities.

In those first days it was the pain, the grinding pain that was a constant. It was stifling any real chance of establishing any stability.

The physical and emotional effect pain has on me never ceases to amaze me. The type I get is low grade, although it stems from quite a large area and is continuous. You can concentrate and block it out for a while but as soon as you relax, back it comes, usually with a little extra. The end result is that the pain and discomfort dominate the senses, the mind pitches and tosses in despair and it becomes increasingly difficult to maintain stability. How people managed before modern analgesics, or what it is like once they become inadequate, I hate to imagine. The courage of pioneering types and the suffering inflicted in war is just too horrible to conceive.

By Friday 17 January—nine days after the operation—Ian also began to feel the tedium of hospital life bite. He also wondered if it was the barrage of drugs he was taking to dull the pain that was also dulling his mind. Always in the back of his mind was the fear, he wrote, that the drop in 'initiative or desire to improve will precipitate secondaries'.

He was certain that ensuring the cancer did not return—something his doctors secretly believed was inevitable—was, in other words, ultimately dependent on his own state of mind and motivation. It was a pivotal time for the young man. He was experiencing both serious pain and drug-based strategies for its primary management, but he was also in no doubt of the crucial importance of nurturing and maintaining clarity on the long path back to health and wellbeing. It would prove to be a cornerstone of the foundation of his recovery and future work.

By day 11—19 January—Ian had been venturing out into the corridors on crutches, although he was finding that remaining vertical for too long soon became painful around his right pelvis and the area where his leg had been.

Two days later the bad dreams came to him even in waking hours. Ian remembers half sleeping and 'having depressing imaginations much like nightmares'. In one he saw himself being flattened by a huge, malevolent truck. In another he was painting with a brush on canvas, but his strokes became ever more violent, until deep, savage imprints covered the canvas as well as the air around it. 'I had to open my eyes to settle my mind,' he says. Like ripples on the surface of water, these were the inevitable mental responses to major surgery and the manifestations of his underlying physical and emotional disquiet. Indeed when surgeon John Doyle visited the emotional floodgates had opened.

'It was the only time I remember him breaking down,' says Doyle.

Doyle and Ian Gawler had developed a strong bond. More than that though, as Ian admits, Doyle provided the only tangible professional support he received at the time.

'The thing that really came across was that Mr Doyle cared,' says Ian, 'and I think that was a very significant thing in its own right. Other professional people that I saw would put a barrier up. It was as if all I was going through was too painful for them. You could tell that they did not want to get involved with me. It was too hard.' Ian admired Doyle for being someone who was 'enough of a person' to express his care.

The retired surgeon is clearly touched to this day by Ian's assessment. 'It's kind of him to say so,' says Doyle, adding that he had an enormous amount of respect and admiration for how courageously his young patient had handled such a mammoth crisis. 'He was extraordinarily calm,' he repeats—until the inevitable, and as Doyle deemed it necessary, breakdown.

So on the morning of 21 January, as Ian tried to explain his nightmare to the surgeon, he sobbed uncontrollably while his body heaved in fits of grief and anguish. Doyle had been expecting the explosion of Ian's emotional agony for a while. He asked Ian if he knew what was going on; if he knew what was happening to him. He could only manage a simple 'no'. Doyle explained he was finally letting go of all the bottled-up feelings he had held on to all through the horrors of the previous weeks.

This simple, perhaps obvious explanation, came as a great relief to Ian. And he soon realised that the emotional outpouring also related to a letting go of his old life.

Ian remembers looking down what seemed to be two very clear but different possible roads to a future life. One would involve dwelling on what he had lost and what he could no longer do. Along that road, he knew, lay bitterness, misery and perhaps even madness. The second path promised a life lived in the present moment; where a concentration on the inner, rather than the outer, would hold sway.

With the benefit of hindsight it is probably easier to make sense of such a radical shift. At the time Ian made what seemed to be a conscious choice that rapidly moved him out of feeling adrift in such profound psychic, emotional and spiritual upheaval, into a much more peaceful and stable state.

Nevertheless, there came the emotional anguish and waking nightmares, followed by the sense that 'I had made a dramatic change, but I am not sure to what,' wrote Ian. 'My mind seems like a void.'

Ian remembers that as that day went on, he began to feel like he had lost all contact with reality. He was aware of his body, and even of talking to nurses, but he felt completely disconnected from his physical reality. He believed himself to be dying. Or felt sure he was experiencing how it must feel. Yet at the same time he experienced a profound feeling of warmth and oneness.

At one stage I closed my eyes and had a vision of moving through a long tunnel of light and of beginning to pass out the other end. It was like being a part of a stream of water moving down a hose, then bursting up and out of the nozzle, into a shower of light reflecting droplets that radiated out to form a crown of glorious splendour. I wanted to flow with it and to be a part of it; but it was too much . . .

Ian remembers being aware that he had a very clear choice to go with the flow of all this, but that if he did he would reach a point of no return and die. 'It seemed very much like a conscious choice. It was as if I stuck my head out of this pipe, this tunnel as it were, had a glimpse of another extraordinary and beautiful world and said "No thanks, not yet." '

I retreated back down to the tangible world. There I found the presence of the nurse to talk to was enough to root me in the physical until this strange period passed.

'It was like being out into the middle of space. A vast, empty, but immanent, luminous space,' he says. 'Not being aware of such things back in those days, I am sure that . . . was a near-death experience. And it left me feeling comfortable about death as a process, and dying as a process and death itself. I lost my fear of dying.' As he wrote in his journal:

A hallucination perhaps, but it was such a real experience for me that it has left me convinced of life's continuity after death and that there is no need to fear death itself. I am convinced by what I read and by what I have experienced that death involves only a change in consciousness. We do continue, but in a different bodily state, operating in a different frame of reference.

Another time he was lying with his eyes closed and opened them to discover a little old lady standing at the end of the bed. 'She had quite a saintly air about her,' he says, 'and I presumed she was just one of the little old nuns that was doing her rounds or something.' She said nothing and went out through the door. Ian was wearing a hospital smock, it was a hot day and he realised he had it 'up around my ears to cool off and I didn't have any undies on,' he says, 'so I presumed that what she saw must have impressed her enough to take her voice away!' She appeared again the next day, and once again said nothing. Ian asked the nurses who she was, but to his dismay nobody else had seen her, nobody knew her. 'To this day I don't know if she was real or I imagined her.'

Ian had plenty to contend with on both the psychological and the physical levels, given the cold reality of his wounded and battered body. In fact, immediately following his terrifying layered nightmare came the realisation that he had to actually grieve for the loss of his leg.

Indeed, he came to the strong realisation that he had spent the two weeks since the operation so obsessed with a need to process the spiritual aspects of his situation, that he had not actually come to terms with the physical reality of his loss.

> I think a lot of the pain is due to the same thing. The impulses that still want to pass down the leg but there is nowhere to go. I look down the bed and see the outlines of one knee and one foot. That is all. There is no more.

On top of that, the powerful painkillers he was taking were also making him feel like he was losing his mind. He tried facing the pain without them for a day.

Needless to say it was a long and torturous day. By the end of it, when Gail visited, he reached out for comfort from her for the very first time since the operation.

> I felt a lot better for it, and I think that she, despite her grief and concern for my condition, was happy to feel me admit my need.

It was yet another of the countless incremental steps on the road to recovery.

The next major step forward came the next day when an American nurse showed Ian how to help manage his pain using progressive muscle relaxation. She showed him how he could gradually relax his entire body to get some relief.

She told him to tense his toes and then relax them, then do the same with the calf muscle. Tighten and relax. Then she told him to do the same with his thigh, pelvis, abdomen, back, hands, forearms, upper arms, shoulders, neck, jaw, mouth, eyes and forehead.

Ian was amazed to discover how such a simple technique could provide some effective pain relief. It was a very welcome development because a couple of days earlier he had stopped his tentative practice of meditation in an effort to end the fearsome images that entered his mind the moment he tried to settle it. Giving himself over to sleep and, now, progressively relaxing his muscles, he found to be more effective ways of handling his current demons. That said, very soon he was heading home, a place where he hoped there would be more time and space for introspection and meditation.

Ian likened returning home to the farmhouse at Melton to be like leaping into a void. Nevertheless, after the confines and relative security of the hospital, Kippen Ross and its wide, open verandas were literally a breath of fresh air.

Although already determined not to indulge in any feelings of self-pity or dwell on what he had lost, he returned home having been told bluntly, as he remembers it, that he only had a 5 per cent chance of being alive in five years. 'I found it pretty easy to identify with the 5 per cent,' he explains. He felt that recovery and rehabilitation rested squarely in his own hands. 'I felt that if I made the right changes in my life then I ought to be okay.'

At home he stood on a set of scales for the first time after the amputation to discover that he had lost around a quarter of his body weight. Despite the loss, there came a dramatic realisation. Even while still balancing on the scales it hit him. He realised that he felt like the same person he had been before the operation. 'Obviously there was more to me than just my body,' he remembers thinking.

In other words, we might ordinarily experience our identity, our character, our very being as indivisible from our whole physical self, yet Ian had discovered that he felt as if he was exactly the same person he was before, despite having lost 'a quarter of my body. Less body. Same person. Clearly that is to do with the spiritual aspect of who we really are.'

Also, it was really helpful for Ian that Gail, right from the very moment she first saw him after the operation, treated him exactly as she had before. 'At no stage did she make me feel like I was any different. There was no pity. No sympathy. Curiously, we have never spoken about what grief she may have felt, but she treated me as the same person,' he says, 'and you know in retrospect I think that really was an extraordinary gift . . . she still regarded me as the same person.'

Not only did Gail accept Ian's new body shape, but for him, her response seemed to him to be clear evidence that she loved him. Unconditionally. Gail puts her attitude down to a 'pragmatic view of life. If you have a bit missing it doesn't really matter, the person is the same,' she says.

Back at Kippen Ross, pain continued to be Ian's constant companion, as were the mind-numbing effects of the analgesics. Gradually he decided again that to ride out the pain was preferable to the side effects of the drugs he had been prescribed. Without them the discomfort would ebb and flow, but with a clear, relatively drug-free mind, he found that he could meditate better and that everything seemed much brighter.

A few days later he wrote that a sharp acute pain, whose origin was hard to track down, arrived as soon as he relaxed in bed at night. He found it hard to sleep and went back to having a nightly shot of morphine.

It was a source of unending frustration to Ian that he could not get on top of the pain. John Doyle had told him that he thought he had a very low pain tolerance. In fact, just taking Ian's stitches out had been an excruciating experience. Mr Doyle observed that he regarded Ian as being in the top few per cent of people most sensitive to pain that he had experienced. Whatever his pain threshold, Ian recorded with a sense of despair that the pain 'manifests as intense and I cannot turn off to it or relax out of it'.

He redoubled his efforts to meditate, writing in his journal, 'It seems obvious that meditation is a vital step and one that must be pursued.' At six o'clock every evening, he sat in the lotus position in his big, high-ceilinged bedroom. For half an hour he would settle with his back leaning up against a wardrobe for support, his left ankle drawn up to his groin.

> I hold my arms out straight, one resting on my knee, the other on my boot, which I take off for the occasion. The fingers are extended except for the forefingers which curl around the tips of my thumbs.

At the same time, Ian continued to read the book by Chogyam Trungpa, *Meditation in Action*. Trungpa was a Tibetan Buddhist master instrumental in bringing to the West teachings that had hitherto been locked away beyond the Himalayan mountains in Tibet. Trungpa's book was, as Ian admits, 'a bit beyond him at the time' and he had difficulty understanding much of what he had to say. Far from offering an introduction to the mechanics of meditation as he had hoped, Trungpa's *Meditation in Action* presupposes a fair deal of existing knowledge and concerns itself with the profound; the deeper and complex concerns of developing generosity, patience and wisdom through meditation.

However, there were some practical guidelines in the book, such as the importance of keeping the back straight:

> ... so that there is no strain on the breathing ... trying to become one with the feeling of the breath'. [Try to see] the translucent nature of thoughts. One should not try to suppress thoughts in meditation ... one should not become involved in them, nor reject them, but simply observe them and then come back to the awareness of the breathing.

Ian concentrated on the flow of his breath in an attempt to quieten his mind. Distracted by thoughts, he would bring his attention back to the breathing again and again. Gradually his mind would still.

> Usually I end this phase by trying to repeat the mantra three times, more if possible, without diverging into thought. Clearing my mind and just repeating the mantra. I try to fix my gaze and concentration where the tip of my nose is. I then do more breathing exercises, before bringing out my thoughts in prayer form, in the Christian tradition, addressed to God and asking for His guidance.

On the more practical side of rehabilitation, Ian felt enormously fortunate to have found himself with the funds to support a long and meditative road back, without money worries. The fact was that Ian had won the chance to ponder his physical and spiritual wellbeing—rather than fret how Gail could possibly support them both in the short to medium term—thanks to a little good fortune that came his way just before he fell sick.

Since university days Ian had sought advice on financial matters from his friend Tony Bongiorno. Bongiorno also owned a horse stud, so the pair of them had developed a special relationship: Ian looked after Bongiorno's horses and, in return, Bongiorno looked after the young vet's finances and tax. Three months before he fell ill, Ian went to Bongiorno to have his tax return completed. 'Every time I went to get my finances sorted out he would have another insurance that he felt I should take out,' Ian remembers. 'It always seemed reasonable and sensible so I would always go along with it.'

This particular visit Bongiorno advised Ian to take out sickness and accident insurance. For once Ian did not think it was such a good idea. 'I said: Tony, you have got to be kidding. I'm going to be running for the state in the decathlon again in a few months, why would I want sickness insurance?'

'You never know what might happen,' was Bongiorno's reply. 'What happens if you get injured?'

Glenyss also remembers standing in the family kitchen and asking her stepson if he had insurance to cover illness or loss of income, just before he was to take over the Bacchus Marsh practice. 'Why would I need that when I'm perfectly healthy?' she remembers him saying.

Perhaps Glenyss' concern had lodged somewhere in the back of Ian's mind, perhaps he needed to hear it from someone other than his stepmum, but Bongiorno's advice changed his mind. He signed on the dotted line.

Three months later, desperately ill and recovering from major surgery, he was drawing more money from the insurance than he had been from working an 80-hour week. The policy lasted two years.

The other canny thing Tony Bongiorno had done for Ian early on in his working life was to organise a personal loan—which he used as the deposit on his 40-acre block above Bacchus Marsh. When the insurance money ran out after those initial two years, Ian sold the block for double what he had paid.

As for his relationship with Gail, before he became ill and during the first year of the illness, Ian admits that there were periods 'where we could easily have broken up'. In fact, had he not been diagnosed with cancer, he believes they probably would have.

From Ian's point of view Gail seemed head-over-heels in love, yet he did not share anything of the same intensity of feeling. At least at the start.

'I actually became more loving as time went by,' he says. Whereas Gail 'went the other way to some degree. The flow of love between us . . . never seemed to be really equitable. Physically our relationship was a very good one,' he says, 'but what it lacked was real emotional intimacy.'

There were, nonetheless, some comical moments. One day in March, two months after the operation, he convinced Gail to come out with him for a final ride on his MV motorbike. He had put the bike up for sale and a prospective purchaser was to visit later that day. The first problem of course was that Ian was unable to change gears with his right foot, because he did not have one. Gail would have to do that sitting behind, while Ian worked the clutch, accelerator and front brake with his hands; the back brake with his left foot.

The next problem was that Gail had determined never to travel on the superbike after the fateful and, for her, terrifying ride to Hanging Rock on New Year's Day. So Ian had to use all his powers of persuasion to coerce her onto the bike, for what he imagined to be this last time. He explained to her that what she needed to do was quite simple. When he said 'put your foot up', she was to lift the gear lever with her right foot and the bike would change gear. When he said 'put your foot down', she was to push the gear lever down and the bike would change down a gear. Gail was persuaded.

Just as they roared off up the long drive of the house to join the road, they saw another bike coming the other way quite fast. It had to be the possible buyer. 'But had he seen us and would he stop?' says Ian, who immediately decided to slow down. As the bike slowed he instructed Gail to change down the gears with her foot. 'Put your foot down,' and down went the gears again. By now they were nearly stationary.

Now, a stationary bike needs two legs on the ground to keep it upright. Ian only had one. Unfortunately in the excitement Ian lost the plot a little. Just as they were about to come to a complete halt he shouted with some urgency for Gail to 'put your foot down'. Gail, not surprisingly interpreted this as another instruction to continue to change down the gears rather than to place her foot on the road. Clunk went the gears. 'Put your foot down,' yelled Ian with mounting urgency. Clunk again. 'Put you foot down,' he screamed. Clunk again.

The bike came to a complete stop and over they went, in comical slow motion.

There we were lying on the side of the road, me roaring with laughter, Gail roaring and swearing, the bike just roaring. Once we got reorganised, I asked the chap if he would like to take me for a ride. Judging by the rate at which he disappeared into the sunset, I do not expect him to buy the bike. He did not even stop to help us lift the bike up again.

The days and weeks drifted on. In mid-March Ian was booked in for more x-rays—a prospect that 'causes more apprehension than the initial surgery,' he noted in his journal. His efforts at meditation had lately not been as successful as he had hoped—too often he would find himself drifting off to sleep.

He felt frustrated to be doing very little, especially given that Gail was doing everything for him unquestioningly. He was all too aware he could be a demanding and ungrateful companion. But the X-ray proved clear and he felt 'more confidence to go on, perhaps not so desperate, and certainly joyous'. His meditation improved, as did his relationship with Gail.

The wound at his hip had fully healed and he had become expert at getting around on crutches. In the earlier hospital days, Ian had tried wearing pants again. But his sense of aesthetic, harmony and balance was deeply upset by rolling the empty trouser leg up and into his waist. Gail had bought Ian a red kaftan, with a huge red dragon on its front and presented it to him while he was still in hospital. His first reaction was blunt and unkind. But seeing the need to try something different, he put it on. It hung loose and free and put no pressure on his stump. Ian saw no reason to ever return to trousers with one of the legs rolled up.

As he began venturing out into society again, he noticed that children were fascinated by a kaftan-wearing man on crutches and with one leg.

> I try to act normally, attempting to set their minds at rest when
> they say the obvious: 'Look mummy, that man's only got one leg.'
> I have to accept that I am now different, and obviously so. Perhaps
> if everyone's problems were so obvious, we could all be more open
> with each other.

His energy had returned, the pain had gone, but his mind was filled with developing a philosophy with which to carry on. The struggle between the spiritual and the secular paths also remained an on-going one—the self-confessed causes of his illness notwithstanding. He began to wonder how he could reconcile his fate with the 'transgressions' he was aware of in this life.

Surely others who continued to walk and to run had committed bigger transgressions? ... I have now swung around to feel that my situation almost certainly is a matter of karma; that I have a lesson to learn or a situation to cope with as a result of transgressions in a previous life ... Regardless of the cause of my situation the effect has been to increase my interest in religious subjects. My future is still imminently uncertain. Just tonight, I pause to wonder if one should not make uses of the time available to get the greatest immediate dividend of enjoyment from this life. Should I dive into material pleasures and grab them while I can?

Ian was a man struggling to find both his spiritual and his temporal bearings. He spent the evening of 19 March by an open fire on the couple's waterbed, propped up with pillows. Gail was out, watching television had been giving him a headache lately, he felt too lazy to continue work on an antique chair he had started to upholster. The light was too dim to read by.

I have no ambition. There is nothing in this physical world I really want to do. I succeeded moderately in most fields; athletics, football, my practice and the myriads of mundane events that masquerade as life. I am content with my lot but it seems likely to get more boring as time goes on. Imagine at 25 having no ambition. Nothing you want to do, to achieve, to attack.

I have been reading existential literature and this has increased my torpor. I still have great enthusiasm and zeal for spiritual pursuits but it is difficult to carry this over towards a total lifestyle ... jaded is how I feel. Yet I am happy and content and do not wish for anything else. I have no desire for travel, no desire for work, no desire for anything. I am content with jaded! Yet there must be more.

I am the supreme optimist.

During April and May of that first year after the amputation Ian and Gail began to attend furniture auctions. This became more regular and they bought many pieces to furnish the grand living rooms of their rented colonial homestead. Being healthy enough to be out and about was a great satisfaction, but returning to the consumer society stirred ever more questioning.

It seems difficult to avoid coveting items and not to gloat over apparent bargains. I am enjoying it as an interest, however, and it seems good financial sense to invest in antiques at this time. Is it morally sound though? I hear my conscience say no, but it cannot be denied that it is a material world that we live in.

More than that though, Ian was acutely aware that he might be running out of time. 'Fancy spending a tenuous present going to auctions,' he wrote.

May 1975 was also marked by another trauma—the disappearance of the couple's dogs: Ian's Saluki, Sara, and Gail's Afghan, Mr Dog. Gail had let them out the front door for a run one morning and they disappeared. They suspected the dogs had been stolen and offered a substantial reward for their return. Soon after someone called looking to extort money. After several misadventures the extortionist was caught by the police, but the dogs were never seen again.

Ian's working future remained unclear. Jo and Kevin Bell had decided to sell the veterinary practice and move to Perth. Ian still was not sure if he could or wanted to work as a veterinarian. The days were typically spent wondering about work, his spiritual direction, his future with Gail, watching television and reading very little. When Ian first returned home from the hospital he had painted a series of landscapes in oils with much enthusiasm and joy. Now even painting was beginning to feel like a chore. 'My life is non-directional,' Ian recorded in his journal at this time.

The couple decided a road trip might shake Ian out of his indolence. With winter approaching, they hitched a caravan to their new car, now a Saab Combi Coupe, Ian's thrashing of the rotary Mazda having twice burnt out its motor. They headed for the heart of South Australia—or more particularly Lake Eyre and the Birdsville Track, one of the harshest dirt roads on the continent.

The eight-week adventure proved to be one of the happiest of their lives. They camped under river red gums in the Flinders

Ranges and saw water in Lake Eyre. The previous year had been a very wet summer and the dry lake had filled up with water for the first time in 200 years. They managed to negotiate the unforgiving Birdsville Track but then, the next evening, heading east from Birdsville on the most rugged and rudimentary of roads, they became bogged at a place called Betoota. The two of them ended up having to bash through the bush on foot, and swim and wade through the Diamantina River in an attempt to get help at a homestead they had spotted way off in the distance.

Four hours later, in the pitch dark, they reached the isolated home. Ian remembers a young mother coming to the door, with a small child on her hip. She was completely taken aback by the sight of the two of them, one on crutches, wearing a red kaftan emblazoned with a dragon, and with only one leg. Both Ian and Gail were covered in mud and soaked in smelly, brackish water. The woman said nothing, simply backed away from the door open-mouthed, and disappeared. After a while her husband came to the door. Incredulous, he finally took in what had happened and where they had come from. They were given a shower, clean clothes, a meal and a bed for the night.

The next morning, the managers of the cattle station, a place called Durrie, a property of 4000 square miles and 4000 head of cattle—pulled Ian and Gail's car and caravan out of the mud with chains attached to their four-wheel drives.

It was a very memorable trip and they returned home, refreshed and invigorated. 'Living in the close confines of the caravan had welded us closer together,' says Ian. He was now ready to work—at least once an artificial leg was fitted.

The only device possible for Ian to use was called the Canadian Hip. It had a fibreglass girdle that wrapped around his waist with a wooden leg that was jointed at the hip and knee. The idea was to swing the thing forward from the hip like a pendulum to simulate the movement of an ordinary leg. Ian was sent off to a rehabilitation centre to learn how to use it.

It was not a success. Firstly Ian was appalled by the condescending attitude of the 'nice ladies' charged with the job of teaching him, and secondly he found that the prosthesis severely restricted his mobility.

'I don't know what it was with those women,' he says. 'I don't know whether they had a difficulty in relating to a young guy on one leg who had cancer . . . there was a distancing and a falseness about it that I didn't like. Besides, I had been a serious athlete who was used to being trained by coaches who shared a common goal, gave clear instruction and functioned with mutual respect. They left me feeling very frustrated and very angry.'

In any case, Ian by then had become adept and comfortable using crutches despite the fact that he found it difficult to carry anything because of them.

Through meeting his son at university, Ian came to know the great Australian war hero Sir Edward 'Weary' Dunlop. Ian remembers Weary relating to him how he knew the English air ace Douglas Bader. 'One evening Weary and Bader were at a grand function in London. Both in tuxedos, they were walking down a sweeping, theatrical flight of stairs when Bader tripped and went sprawling down the stairs. Weary, a big man, bent down to pick him up.' Ian recalls that Weary told him that 'Bader was so insulted that he actually took a swing at me.'

'This always seemed absurd to me. I became very comfortable with what I could and I could not do on one leg,' says Ian, 'and comfortable with asking for, in fact welcoming, help when I need it.'

Ian spent a couple of days at the rehabilitation centre, only to come home furious; ranting and raving about how the leg would only slow him down and how he had nearly gelded himself with the contraption when he had tried to sit down. Gail thought it very funny, and Ian—his keen sense of humour never far from the surface —soon did too. The wooden leg was consigned to a wardrobe.

Another area of experimentation for Ian at the time was with his attitude to food. This manifested in the fortunes of a young Murray Grey steer affectionately named Nelson by Ian. Nelson was one of a small herd that Ian had kept on the block of land at Bacchus Marsh and was earmarked as a fine animal for the table.

Ian's readings in Eastern philosophy were leading him to consider vegetarianism as an option but he had also become aware that 'eating any food involves another organism giving up its energies, its life force, for me to carry on'. Ian believed that food should be recognised for what it was—once a living, breathing creature—and honoured for the life it gave by losing its own.

> I am sure that the modern food industry with its processing plants, far removed from the sight and thoughts of the average consumer, have aided in further alienating man and nature. I have no moral objections to meat eating, as long as the diners are willing to accompany their meal from the field, through the abattoirs to their table. How many people relate the lamb gambolling in the paddock with the Sunday roast?

And so Nelson was dispatched to the slaughterhouse, and the local butcher dressed the carcass, delivering it to the local fish and chip shop to store the meat in their freezer until it was needed. Nelson's light-brown hide meanwhile was tanned and found its place on the floor in Kippen Ross's impressive dining room, where the couple would host what were to become 'rather bizarre dinner parties'.

Ian, Gail and their guests would sit around their big old mahogany table (a prized find at one of the auctions they had been to earlier in the year), roast beef would be served and guests inevitably would compliment their hosts on the freshness and tastiness of the meal. At which point Ian would tell them that they were eating a handsome young steer called Nelson and then—pointing to the new cow skin lying beside the table—he would say, 'and there's his hide on the floor'.

'I thought it was good for them to connect the dots,' he laughs. 'Needless to say the dinner parties thinned out pretty quickly. They didn't seem to feel the need to know that they were eating something that had actually been walking around on the grass a little while earlier.'

Gail, having only relatively recently resumed eating meat, took it all with remarkably good humour. She was coping not only with the physical and emotional reality of looking after a partner who had just lost a leg to cancer, but also with keeping up with a man who was constantly questioning, introspective and clearly undergoing some sort of metamorphosis.

By October, meanwhile, Ian was becoming less communicative again and had disappeared even further into solitary and quiet reflection. He had what he thought was a new lump growing inside his pelvis. He did not tell Gail and the pair planned another road trip to clear the air. This time they hitched a trailer to their car and drove across the Nullarbor to the south coast of Western Australia, camping all the way.

'We came up the coast to Perth,' says Ian, 'and by then things had deteriorated further and we were arguing big time.' The couple hit the city at rush-hour one evening late in November and were driving down the main street in heavy traffic having a 'big brawl,' he says. Gail remembers that Ian had been silent virtually the entire way from Adelaide, 2700 kilometres away, and it was driving her crazy.

'It was more than just the silence,' she says, 'there was something else he wasn't telling me'—so in the heat of the argument, she jumped out of the car at the next traffic lights right in the heart of the city.

'She'd really lost the plot,' says Ian. 'It was one of those pivotal moments. I could have just shut the door and left her and God knows what would have happened then. But I just stayed there and all the traffic was tooting their horns, she's on the footpath and I'm refusing to move.'

Eventually Gail got back into the car and they drove off, in profound silence. The underlying reason for the tension, it seems, was that Ian still had not told Gail that he could feel a lump inside his pelvis and was starting to suspect the worst. His silent but growing anxiety had been creating ever more distance between the two of them for weeks. The couple would typically argue, the argument would become heated and they would reach an 'unhappy impasse,' he says. 'By the time we got back to Melbourne things were pretty tricky.'

'If someone had given me two cents to walk the other way I would have,' says Gail. 'But it was a conscience thing. How could you walk away?'

Once back in Melbourne, Ian shared his suspicions with Gail, phoned John Doyle and was sent to a cancer clinic for tests. Ian knew, if secondary cancer were diagnosed, that his life expectancy would shrink to a meagre three to six months. But first the tests.

Ian remembers that they were carried out painfully, in callous indifference, in a dreary and depressing clinic that seemed to him— as he wrote at the time—to be like a 'production line, geared to producing a filled coffin as an end product'.

The results confirmed that Ian had indeed developed secondary cancers, or more precisely there was 'osteogenic development inside my pelvis and chest'. The future looked very bleak indeed.

5

'God be with You and Good Luck'

Not long prior to the Nullarbor trip, and before secondary cancer had taken its invidious hold, Ian had decided it was time to go back to work. He had thought it the only way to snap out of the deep malaise and sense of uselessness that would come and go in those long months of recuperation and repair at Kippen Ross. Ian considered a range of possibilities. He settled on an offer to work with one of his old mentors, Dr Jim Gannon, who specialised in greyhounds. He was to begin just as soon as he and Gail had made their return from Perth.

Now, with the crushing diagnosis of new cancers in his lymph nodes, Ian had to ring Jim and decline. Meanwhile a familiar nagging feeling gnawed inside him. For most of the previous year, resolute as he thought he was to tread an inner path, the uncomfortable truth was that he had let himself fall into old patterns and old ways.

And then Ian remembered that in the time leading up to the trip across the Nullarbor, an article in Melbourne's daily broadsheet *The Age* had caught his eye. For the first time this article formally linked his interest in meditation with cancer. Ian had cut it out planning to follow it up later, but had not actually got around to doing so. It seems Ian had become swept up in the plans to return to veterinary practice as well as the torpor that had coloured those last months of 1975.

Now with a prognosis of three to six months to live, and with the understanding that there was little or nothing conventional medicine could do for him, Ian's hand was drawn. Ironically, the cancer's spread was precisely what Ian needed to sting him back into action. He had always thrived on a challenge. The bigger the better.

Ian rummaged through a drawer, found the clipping and re-read it with an urgent, renewed and burning attention.

Meditation Theory in Control of Cancer
Melbourne psychiatrist Dr Ainslie Meares is seeking volunteers to test a theory that cancer may be controlled by an intensive program of meditation.

Dr Meares has asked doctors to refer to him cancer patients who are prepared to undertake instruction in meditation for several months and to practise for two to three hours every day.

He specifies that the patients must know they have cancer and be aware of their 'gloomy prognosis'.

Dr Meares, 65, who is now retired, is regarded as an authority on hypnosis and meditation.

Writing in the Medical Journal of Australia, the official organ of the AMA, he explains the theory: 'I believe there is evidence to suggest that some cancers are influenced by immunological reactions.'

Ian immediately picked up the phone and told his story to Ainslie Meares' assistant, Mrs Vere Langley. He vividly remembers the powerful impact of her words. After listening to Ian describe his situation and his background interest in meditation, she told him that it sounded like he was 'just the sort of person who would do well in this.' Her skilful choice of words really stuck in his mind and 'set the tone' for the whole experience. An appointment was set for 12 December.

Ian was already aware that Ainslie Meares had been a respected psychiatrist for over 30 years. Dr Meares was an author of a number of scholarly texts, as well as commercially successful books and he had latterly become a world-recognised authority on hypnosis. He was president of the International Society for Clinical and

Experimental Hypnosis and was an expert on meditation and mental relaxation.

'He had achieved great success in showing people a simple method which they could use to relieve tension and anxiety,' says Ian. In so doing, Dr Meares had successfully treated everything from insomnia, phobias, asthma and speech difficulties, to nervous rashes, sexual problems, smoking and nail-biting—all conditions with stress and anxiety at their core. One of the spin-offs of the technique was also a great deal of relief from pain and much of Meares' time became devoted to pain management. It was his deep understanding of psychiatry and a possible link between cancer and stress that led Meares to wondering if intensive meditation and relaxation could possibly have an effect on cancer.

From what he already knew, Ian expected 'something significant' at his first meeting with the great man. In his journal he noted:

> It is good when meeting someone to try and be open to their influence, to gain an initial impression. As Dr Meares shook my hand and began talking to me, I felt my awareness being sharply focused and drawn towards him. I drew back into myself, satisfied that the man can have a powerful hypnotic effect.

Ian found Meares to be a lean and fit man with intense eyes, a restrained air of intellectual superiority and a gift for offering his undivided attention to whomever he was speaking. He was always turned out in a suit, he had huge bushy grey eyebrows and swept back silver-hair.

Dr Meares talked with Ian for an hour at that first meeting to familiarise himself with all the details of his medical history and to gauge a sense of Ian's state of mind.

Ian told him that he had been influenced by Dr Raynor Johnson's ideas and of his efforts to meditate over the preceding year. Ian wondered aloud if his meditation had been the reason why the cancer had spread to only two lymph nodes rather than through his lungs, as normally occurs with osteogenic sarcoma.

Meares didn't answer, but instead asked Ian what his biggest wish would be.

Ian laughed and later recorded the details of the conversation in his journal.

> It probably seems silly. I really want to do the right thing for this particular life, at this particular time. I want to advance more positively. I can see that the experience of disease, even dying, could be very positive, but I would prefer to live.

Meares also asked Ian what he thought was the biggest problem in life.

'Finding direction.'

'Do you have any big regrets?'

'Not really. It was a pity to have become so involved with work. To have turned my back on my own development.'

Meares gave another of his characteristically sage and non-committal nods and went on to explain his methods. He also instructed Ian to find copies of his books *Relief without Drugs* and *Strange Places and Simple Truths* and told Ian to read them before the first meditation session.

Ian's meditation sessions were scheduled for every weekday morning and would take up most of those mornings. Meares' method was uncomplicated; consisting fundamentally of first progressively relaxing the body and then sitting quietly and letting thoughts come and go 'like ships in the night'. The hope was that gradually, given enough practice, one could deepen one's relaxation to the point of completely letting go and entering a simple inner silence beyond thought. To this end Ian was expected to commit to three hours of meditation per day. In fact he was so keen and feeling so much benefit from this meditation style that he was soon meditating for five one-hour sessions each day.

The consultations were to be free but Dr Meares, on that first visit, had him sign a form absolving himself from any responsibility for treating him. Ian remembers being taken aback by the form but realised that trying a new treatment for cancer is 'like walking the razor's edge,' he wrote.

One slip and to one side lies condemnation by the profession; to the other, the ire and law suits of not-so-keen relatives. He could be cut in half by either.

Dr Meares began each meditation session by greeting each person individually in his waiting room. Little was said but he made physical contact with his subjects, usually with a reassuring hand on the shoulder or arm. Then he would lead each person into his meditation room and sit them down in one of two rows of well-worn wingback leather chairs he devoted to the sessions. There would be up to fifteen people in a session. 'The chairs weren't very good for your posture at all,' remembers Ian, 'and I think it might have been part of what led to the difficulties with my back.'

Ainslie's meditation room was decorated with assorted devotional icons and marble statues, including a magnificent pair representing Kuan Yin, the Chinese Buddhist goddess of compassion. There were major Australian landscape paintings and a number of old, exquisitely-bound copies of the Bible, the Koran and other great works of spiritual import.

Dr Meares had become so convinced by the power of meditation that he decided to devote the final years of his professional life to treating people using little else. When it came to cancer, he believed that meditation inhibited the body's production of cortisol, thereby bolstering the immune system and its ability to destroy cancer cells. 'Cortisol inhibits the immune system,' he explained in a documentary from the time. 'Anxiety, tension, worry, stress, nervousness, all this sort of thing increases the level of cortisol and so reduces the effectiveness of the immune system. What I'm trying to do is have people meditate. Less tension, less anxiety, less cortisol and the immune system is freer to work.'

Meares led and taught meditation in order that the 'logical, rational part of our mind is in abeyance,' adding that it was then that the 'more simple aspect of our mind is functioning. And it's when this more simple aspect of our mind is functioning it has this profound effect of reducing our anxiety and its consequent effect on cortisol and the immune system. It is just purely a stillness of the mind, not asleep, not unconscious, not drowsy, quite clear, but just a stillness.'

Meares was deeply interested in Eastern religion and philosophy, had travelled to India and Nepal and had reportedly been taught his simple meditation techniques in Nepal by Shivapuri Baba, a mystic who was reputedly aged 137 when he died. Nevertheless, Meares chose not to talk much about his own teachers.

There is no doubt that Meares himself was 'a very spiritual man' says Ian, 'but he was very averse to talking about it.' Personally Meares was a paradox, he adds, being 'very conservative in his manner and dress . . . yet clearly he was mystical and other worldly and there's no doubt that he had a healing gift.'

Dr Meares guided Ian through progressive muscle relaxation, much as the American nurse had in hospital, although with more depth and nuance in his words and voice. He slowly, steadily worked through every part of the body for twenty minutes or more, suggesting Ian contract the muscle—the calf as an example—then let it go. 'It is a good feeling,' he would say. 'Say it to yourself. It's a letting go. A good feeling. Natural. So natural. We feel it all through us.' And then on to the next muscle, Meares' voice guiding him expertly into a deep feeling of relaxation. Meares then turned to the mind and thoughts, suggesting Ian let them come and go. 'Let them go. It is a good feeling.'

Part of Meares' routine—which was captured in the 1970s ABC-TV documentary, *Healers, Quacks or Mystics?*, presented by the long-haired and bearded Nevill Drury an author specialising in the fields of shamanism and spirtuality—was typically to first touch his patients on the shoulders and loosen their clothing to help them relax. He would also typically slide his hand onto the chest of the patients, to make contact with the skin. 'I like to have physical contact,' said Meares. 'Physical contact is a way of communicating.'

Gail went for one session with Meares and remembers being sat down in silence as Meares made a 'low, grumbling, guttural sound'. Later in the session he came up behind her and 'the next moment there was a hand down my shirt and I just kind of leapt to the roof,' she says. 'But what he did to me was apparently the norm in there.

It was some kind of Freudian thing. I wasn't going back after that. I was fixed on that. I thought the meditation was a reasonable thing, but I could not abide by that and a lot of people had trouble with it.'

Ian, on the other hand, had no objection to Meares' techniques and found them enormously practical and useful.

Ian was also, it turns out, applying the same passionate, intense application to getting well that he had to his veterinary practice and to his athletic training. 'Even the meditation itself, I could not leave simple. I used the technique but kept the mantra. I kept the mind active. Relaxed yes, but active. Not just alert, and relaxed,' he says. 'I was still preoccupied with the spiritual aspect of the thing. I had yet to realise, that to achieve a physical result, this very simple technique was all that was required. Different need, different technique.'

Unknowingly Ian was creating more tension.

That said, after six weeks of learning with Meares, at a time when his tumours were expected to double in size every month, they did not grow at all—although it was not only meditation that was clearly having a powerful effect. Ian had also radically changed his diet.

By coincidence, the very same day that Ian had re-read the newspaper clipping about Ainslie Meares, a woman named Pat Coleby had rung the Gawlers. She had heard through mutual friends of Ian's predicament. Coleby was successfully treating her son—who had Hodgkin's disease—using natural methods, including diet, and she suggested Ian accompany her to a cancer group meeting offering advice along similar lines. Ian might have been inspired by the idea of learning meditation with Dr Meares, but he was less than keen on a public cancer meeting—and not so politely declined.

'I don't want to go to a bloody AA meeting for cancer patients,' he remembers mouthing at Gail when she first related Pat's invitation. Ian reflected for a moment. Gail was keen. He knew he needed to do everything he could, and so in the end he agreed.

At the meeting when Ian found himself being addressed by a man that looked and talked 'just like' comedian Paul Hogan—then relatively new to Australian television—Ian's initial apprehensions and expectations quickly dissolved.

Hogan's real-life double, Steve Henzler, told the story of his wife Annette's battle with cancer. The group presenting the meeting was called the International Association of Cancer Victims and Friends, or the IACVF for short.

Steve told of how Annette, a young nurse, had been diagnosed with inoperable cancer in her ovaries and abdomen. Doctors told them there was nothing they could do for her and she was given six weeks to live.

Unwilling to merely watch his wife die without doing anything, they decided to head for the Philippines—immediately—where a friend had told them that so-called psychic surgeons could operate on the sick and the dying with their bare hands, without scalpels or any surgical instruments, plunging their fingers deep into their patients to remove diseased tissue, leaving no scars and sometimes engineering miracle cures. They flew there with nothing to lose.

They returned having seen and experienced amazing things they could not explain. That said, Annette's physical condition was little improved. Nevertheless, she was in a much more positive frame of mind *and* it instilled in them a determination that there were things that could be—had to be—tried that were outside the bounds of conventional medicine. As was the case for Ian, the conventional medicine of the day offered someone in Annette's position no hope at all.

Next the Henzlers headed to California to visit Charlotte Gerson Straus, who ran a clinic following the ideas of her deceased father, Dr Max Gerson. Gerson had stumbled onto his radical diet in 1928 as a result of trying to manage the migraine headaches he had habitually suffered as a young doctor in Germany. By trial and error he added and subtracted various foods from his diet. When he began to only eat apples, Gerson discovered that his migraines ceased. Then he found he could add some foods and the migraines stayed away. But when he added certain other foods to his diet the migraines would return within fifteen minutes. So by using the headaches as a sort of measuring device for dietary dos and don'ts, he came up with a diet that kept him migraine-free. Next he tried to treat others with migraines. Somewhat to his surprise, but no doubt to his patients' delight, it worked for them too. But better still, he claimed it also worked to cure patients with the skin disease Lupus, and even TB. Later on, what was now becoming known as the Gerson Diet or Gerson Therapy was tried on twelve cancer patients. Seven would remain free of symptoms for up to seven years.

Gerson's ideas can be boiled down into five basic principles, according to Ian. In his own 1984 book *You Can Conquer Cancer* he lists these as:

1) That the body should be detoxified;
2) Any vitamin and mineral imbalances need to be corrected;
3) The digestion should be restored and flooded with fresh, vital, pure and suitably prepared food;
4) The patient needs to develop and maintain a positive attitude both in a general sense and towards their diet in particular;
5) Regard the diet as an integral and key component in an overall plan.

Gail was already tuned in to the importance of diet and embraced the ideas presented by Steve immediately and with enthusiasm. Ian, more analytical by nature, was taken with the idea but bought one of the copies of Gerson's book *A Cancer Therapy: Results of Fifty Cases* so that he could investigate further. He was soon convinced by what seemed to him to be the logic in Gerson's arguments.

It should be made very clear, nonetheless, that by the time of the release of Ian's book in 1984—and in all subsequent editions to the present day—Ian *does not* recommend the Gerson diet for others. 'It is much more of a therapy than a diet. It is very demanding to follow at home and very few would find it appropriate, taking into account their total situation.'

At the meeting Steve had made the offer that if anyone was keen enough to come to their home in Sydney and learn more of the diet, they were welcome. Ian and Gail were on the plane the next weekend. There they were further convinced and from then on took Gerson's theories as gospel and applied them to healing with fervour.

THE DRAGON'S BLESSING

'It seemed better to try and stimulate the body to do the healing itself, rather than trying to batter it into submission with radiation and drugs. Particularly when there were no curative medical treatments available to me anyway.'

Ian realised that as a veterinarian he had been mixing up special diets including vitamins and minerals to improve the performance of his clients' greyhounds and horses, yet he himself—a busy vet and athlete in training—had been 'running around living on steak sandwiches, pies, cream buns, a high-meat diet, missed meals and high stress,' says Gail. 'That night was a real "ah-ha" for him.'

But now, to follow Gerson's regime, organic fruit and vegetables had to be bought in prodigious amounts.

To this end they found a man named Angelo, the only supplier of organic and bio-dynamic food in Melbourne at the time. 'A portly, happy Italian, he and his family had a magnificent shop,' says Ian. Gail and he would travel one and half hours across town once a week and then arrange to have Angelo forward more produce midweek via train. The couple would also supplement the shop-bought produce with some from their own vegie garden at Kippen Ross. Ian began to put a lot of effort into building up the vegie garden.

The diet fundamentally consisted of organically grown fresh fruit and vegetables. 'He recommended that most, if not all, be eaten raw,' says Ian. 'What was cooked should be either steamed, baked or simmered in its own juices using stainless steel or iron pots.' Grains were also recommended in the form of porridge, without milk, and wholemeal bread.

Gerson also suggested that no protein (apart from liquified raw liver) at all be digested in those first six weeks and oils and fats were to be removed from the diet altogether. Also to be avoided were white sugar, alcohol, nicotine, salt and processed food.

Juices were also part of the program. Lots of juices. For the first six weeks, making twelve juices per day with a hand-juicer lent to them by Steve was literally a full-time job for Gail. An automatic juicer, sent from America and organised by Ian's father, eased the load after those difficult first weeks. The dozen juices included orange (one per day), apple and carrot (five), green leaf juices (four) plus two made from the raw liver, chased down with a little lemon to make them palatable.

And then there were supplements to be taken. These included: a special water-based solution of potassium gluconate, phosphate and acetate taken ten times daily by the teaspoon; a few drops of iodine solution was added to the juices; there was a stomach acid supplement called acidol pepsin and pancreatic enzymes; Ian took niacin to aid blood flow as well as thyroid tablets; and Gail injected him with liver extract and vitamin B12 twice a week.

But the *pièce de résistance* was regular coffee enemas. In Sydney, Steve had shown Ian how to self-administer them using an enema bag.

For some reason Ian seems somewhat reluctant to describe in detail what it was like to be given a coffee enema by Paul Hogan's double. It would seem fair enough to say it must have been quite hilarious.

The actual technique goes like this. Essentially a 'long black', says Ian, is put into the enema bag and suspended higher than the patient who lies on their right side, knees drawn up. Attached to the bag is a tube and a nozzle which is inserted through the anus into the rectum and a clamp on the tube is released. The enema then runs in and is retained in the body for ten to fifteen minutes. 'The secret is to relax,' says Ian, 'then it is no trouble to hold it. Laughter is definitely not recommended.'

Gerson maintained that by introducing coffee into the rectum the caffeine would be absorbed and go directly along the portal veins into the liver. Gerson regarded the liver as the 'major organ of elimination and vital in the regeneration of the body ... There it stimulates bile flow,' says Ian. 'Bile is a major means of eliminating toxic material from the body.' It is also now well known that the lower bowel produces many hormones.

'Having a coffee enema produces an endorphin-like rush which relieves pain and generates a sense of wellbeing,' he adds. 'It may well be that something in the coffee, the caffeine or something which as yet we do not know about, stimulates Peyers Patches [lymphoid nodules] in the large bowel. They then produce these endorphins which are released into the bloodstream to very positive effect.'

Ian used coffee enemas typically three times per day, and, once used to the strangeness of the procedure, found them to help lessen dramatically the sciatic pain he had begun to develop in his back and down his left leg.

Gerson's overall cancer theory was that the body's immune system could be maximised by restoring a mineral balance and good nutrition (not to mention the strategic use of a little coffee).

'While the coffee seemed so weird at first, as did a few of the other things, as I studied Gerson's book in more detail, his ideas appealed to me as being logical and natural,' says Ian. What also appealed to the veterinary scientist was that Gerson's diet was more than a theory and had been thoroughly researched and clinically trialled by Gerson.

Excited by Steve's story and his reading, Ian took Gerson's book to one of his cancer specialists. 'I was really excited. I thought it offered me some real hope. The specialist listened for a brief moment, took one look at the book and said: "That won't do you any good. Just go home and have a good steak." I was amazed,' says Ian. 'He obviously did not know of the book, he did know I was a veterinarian, he did know I was desperate, yet he just attempted to debunk what I was clinging to without any evidence. Gail and I went home even more determined.'

That said, it was also a radical change of direction for a body used to an utterly different diet.

'Three days after beginning the diet in full, I awoke in the early hours of the morning with tremendous colic pains,' says Ian. 'My head felt like an axe had been sunk into it. I began to vomit and produce diarrhoea.' In the middle of the night, distressed and desperate, Ian rang his GP.

'He had the good sense not to answer the phone and so I tried Maurice Finkel's number.' Maurice was a naturopath who had been recommended by Pat Coleby.

At 3 am Ian rang him for the first time.

Finkel answered the phone, listened patiently and then explained that he felt sure Ian was having a healing reaction. He recommended cleaning out his colon with water enemas, to drink peppermint tea to 'flush the bile and toxins through' and then have another coffee enema. It worked and Ian felt 'much improved', although as Gerson had warned, the headaches and the vomiting returned every seven days, gradually becoming less intense, until they disappeared after six weeks.

It was a tough six weeks for both Ian and Gail. Ian's body gradually came to grips with the radical new diet—all the while Gail was working full time to administer it with extraordinary dedication.

Another problem loomed when it became clear that the new diet was low in proteins and carbohydrates and that there was not enough to fuel the cracking pace Ian was setting. He began to lose weight and then with all the physical exertion, sciatic pains developed to the point that he could not even sit upright in the car. The couple needed to drive from the farmhouse at Melton to the organic fruit and vegetable shop in Box Hill and to visit Dr Ainslie Meares in Melbourne for meditation. So now, to get to Dr Meares or the vegie shop, with the back seats of their Saab station wagon folded down, Ian would lie on an old mattress in the back while Gail drove him around. Ian remembers Angelo, the owner of the shop, packing all the laden boxes around him.

He laughs at the memory now, but his sister Sue says it was an enormously difficult time. Visiting their home one day she remembers having to help Gail put him into the back of the car 'and he was in so much pain,' she says. 'To get him into that station wagon was just awful.'

Ian apparently bore the pain quietly and stoically, but Sue said you could see the magnitude of the pain was 'shocking'. Not only was there acute lower back pain but the sciatic pains were creeping down Ian's left leg, as he described it, 'like a sizzling stream of molten metal'. Meditation became more and more difficult.

He tried a number of strategies to relieve it. First he went to a chiropractor knowing that if his spine was affected by cancer (it was not clear at that stage if it was) then there was a chance it could collapse and he would be crippled.

'As the vertebra cracked, nothing gave out and some relief came,' he said. But still the pain was intense.

He tried mega-vitamin therapy—huge doses of vitamins and mineral and enzyme supplements—126 pills per day. 'I learnt to take 30 pills in one swallow,' he remembers. And then it dawned on him that all the vitamins he needed were already contained in the Gerson diet he was following anyway. Ian cut back to supplementing his diet only with high doses of vitamin C—5 to 10 grams daily.

The most effective relief from pain Ian was getting at the time, particularly at night, were coffee enemas, taken every two hours. 'Gail would get up regularly through the night to make them,' he says.

And then a friend suggested he try acupuncture. Ian had no knowledge or even understanding of what acupuncture was but it sounded interesting and he was keen to try anything that might work and did not involve going back into narcotics again. He made the suggestion to Ainslie Meares that he would like to try the technique.

Meares' response was that he was of the opinion that if Ian could just endure the pain while meditating for the next one or two weeks he would come out the other side feeling better. He was also of the opinion that acupuncture would be of no use. In fact he believed it would actively interfere with the meditation. He gave Ian an ultimatum: If Ian was to choose acupuncture, then he would not be welcome to come back to the sessions.

Quite taken aback by Dr Meares' direction and uncompromising stance, Ian made his way downstairs to where Gail was waiting for him with the car. In the lift he was joined by Fiona [name changed]. Fiona was the only other person with advanced cancer undergoing intensive meditation with Ainslie Meares. She too was reaching a crisis point and the pair decided to sit in the café underneath Meares' rooms and discuss their options.

First Ian went over to Gail to explain what was happening. She already had the hatch of the car up so that Ian could climb onto the mattress. At the same time a parking officer appeared around the corner. Gail was close to the corner and was parked in a No Parking zone. The parking officer approached Gail at the back of the car just as Ian arrived.

'You can't park there, love, you'll have to move on.'

Ian's response was short, direct and intense.

'F★&% off!'

The parking officer promptly did.

Back in the café, Ian and Fiona shared their difficulties.

Fiona was one of three people who had responded to Ainslie Meares' call for cancer volunteers. The third person who responded was really ill and had died not long after. Ian had never met him.

Fiona and Ian meanwhile would often be at Meares' Melbourne offices at the same time. There were up to fifteen meditating in the groups Meares was holding at the time, but Ian and Fiona 'quickly worked out we were in the same boat'. They had a lot in common and would often to talk about their situations before and after the sessions. They soon got to know each other well. Fiona had breast cancer with secondaries in her liver and had a great deal of fluid buildup in her abdomen. 'She had to go off to hospital a couple of times and get it drained and she was having quite a bit of pain,' says Ian.

In the café Ian told Fiona that Dr Meares had just given him an ultimatum: choose acupuncture and he could not return. He also asked how she was coping with her own pain and if she had ever considered other approaches to manage it.

Fiona, as it turns out, had been to a Mexico clinic offering nutritional therapies much like the Gerson approach, but her cancer had advanced regardless. Conventional medicine offered her nothing and now she told Ian it felt like she had exhausted all her options. 'Her words were: it is Ainslie or nothing. If Ainslie can't fix me then that is the end of it. I'm prepared to make my stand with Ainslie.'

For Ian, though, the pain had become so bad, he told Fiona, he simply could not meditate and had decided to head off and try acupuncture.

'And that's where we parted,' says Ian. 'But Fiona's story is very interesting because very quickly she became a good deal worse. She went into hospital a couple of times and had the abdomen drained.' But Fiona stuck with Meares and continued intensive meditation.

'And then the whole thing swung around for her. She had a full recovery and she went into full remission.'

Meares subsequently reported Fiona's amazing recovery in the *Medical Journal of Australia*, the mainstream press got wind of it, and Fiona soon became a *cause célèbre* in the local press. On the other hand, this attention from the media was too much for her, she became tired, stressed, her condition worsened and the cancer returned.

Fiona returned to intensive meditation, around three hours per day, with Ainslie Meares' guidance and the cancer cleared up again.

In January 1977, Meares went on holidays for a month and by the time he returned, so had Fiona's secondaries.

'She got back into the intensive meditation with Ainslie once more,' says Ian, 'and the cancer went away a third time.'

Finally however—as Ainslie Meares later recounted to Ian— Fiona became influenced by another patient who urged her to attend the controversial Milan Brich. Fiona became confused about which way to turn, lost faith in Meares and her meditation, the cancer returned one final time and she died.

Ian and Fiona were the first two intensive meditators who had followed Ainslie Meares' techniques to combat their cancers and, with their two quite varied paths, had enjoyed remarkable success. Where they fundamentally differed, however, was that Fiona eventually dropped the meditation and died; Ian meanwhile became utterly committed to meditation in the long term and battled on with his fight for health.

But for now the pain was intolerable. He chose acupuncture and said goodbye to Dr Meares.

Trained in Western medicine and acupuncture, respected surgeon Tim Lo believed that acupuncture could be of enormous benefit for general back problems, but that if the sciatic pains Ian was experiencing were related to a tumour it would be of little use at all. Having looked at his own x-rays, Ian felt the pain could well be related to his lack of weight, the strain of being on one leg and possibly disc damage. There was no sign of cancer anywhere near the spine.

So Ian began the acupuncture treatment in early February 1976 at a time when his back and leg were 'completely wasted,' he says. 'The muscles were thin and light, strung tight between protruding bones.' Lo placed needles in his lower spine and into his leg. The treatment gave him about four hours of relief and returning the next day, a follow-up course of needles provided even longer relief.

It was also around this time that Ian and Gail reassessed the Gerson therapy, realising that although it had worked well to ease his body's load and detoxify it, Ian had not been eating the recommended amount of carbohydrates. In fact he had not had any carbohydrates for two months on account of the fact that organic grains were impossible to buy in Australia at that time. Also Gail's attempt to bake 'pure bread' had failed and they hadn't substituted it with any rice or oats as an alternative.

So, as they seemed to do whenever there was a setback, the couple looked for whatever else might be helpful. Now they decided to augment Ian's diet with some of the suggestions outlined in a book by Dr William Kelly, a dental surgeon from Texas.

Kelly had treated his own terminal cancer by taking some of Gerson's ideas and adding some of his own. Kelly's method included taking tablets containing pancreatic enzymes after each meal to aid digestion and for what he regarded to be their anti-cancer properties; he suggested both coffee and yoghurt enemas (the yoghurt to introduce—by direct means—the healthy organisms the intestines need for general wellbeing); and he advised a mix of purging and fasting to aid recovery. The purge consisted of drinking a gallon of fresh lemon, grapefruit and orange juice mixed with distilled water for a day or two; a fast—drinking only carrot juice and distilled water—followed for the next three days.

Ian could not understand the rationale behind the purge and felt that there was no merit in it, but took up a few of Kelly's other dietary recommendations. These included eating around ten almonds at breakfast for protein, as well as alfalfa, mung beans and ground apricot kernels for the vitamin B17 they contain. Also, Gail began to rub his body with equal parts of castor and olive oil before Ian would hop into a hot bath for fifteen minutes. Kelly's idea was that if he were to cover himself up in bed for an hour immediately following the bath, his body would sweat out toxins directly through the skin. This was to be repeated every four hours.

Ian and Gail were willing to literally try anything if they thought it might help. Ian found the dietary changes useful and they continued; but after a few days experimenting with the body sweats, they were dropped.

The next idea that inspired and influenced Ian at this time came from the book *Hatha Yoga* by Yogi Ramachakra. It outlined a number of breathing exercises calculated to improve the energy flow around the body. Drawing on ancient Hindu philosophy, Ramachakra argued that the body's vitality and its functions depend upon a subtle energy, or 'prana', that flows within it. It is almost like the prana provides a blueprint for the structure and function of the body. Just as in the West we know we have blood circulating around our bodies, in much of the Orient there is the understanding that this subtle energy also flows around the body. In a healthy body the prana is balanced and as a result all the body's functions and requirements are automatically nourished and maintained. In times of illness, Ian read, the prana can be drawn upon via a number of breathing techniques to aid healing.

For Ian, these concepts reinforced the hints he remembered from Raynor Johnson's lectures and other reading over the years. Ramachakra wrote in such a clear and evocative way that Ian was both moved and excited by the prospects.

When it came to the exercises, Ramachakra's book reintroduced Ian to the type of breathing we all naturally do as infants—that is, using the whole of the lungs, rather than the more shallow 'high' breathing (using only the top of the lungs) that our stressful modern lives can habituate. But also, he was given the technique to begin to work with these more subtle healing energies. Ian applied himself with real enthusiasm and a fresh sense of hope.

Sitting in an upright position, his back against the wardrobe as he did to meditate, Ian relearnt how to fill the whole of his lungs with mindful breaths. He performed the 'cleansing breath'—a full, deep breath held for a few seconds, and then forcefully exhaled. As Ian described at the time, 'It sounds like a steam train in motion. It is very refreshing.'

Ian also practised rhythmic breathing, a more complicated technique that requires checking your pulse and then, by counting, familiarising yourself with the beat of your heart. Ramachakra's instructions in *Hatha Yoga* were to complete one breath in for each six beats of the heart, hold it for three beats and exhale for another six beats. In his journal, Ian described the technique thus:

> Lie out flat with your hands resting over the solar plexus, just below the ribs. Begin rhythmical breathing. Then, as you inhale, will prana to flow into your lungs from the universal supply. It can be visualised as a vital, white light. It flows in with the breath and collects at the solar plexus. Then, as you exhale, will the prana to spread over your entire body, sending energy, strength and vitality. It does not take effort. No forcible use of will is required, just calm command.

From the rhythmical breathing Ian graduated to another technique which used the rhythmical breathing as its foundation but expanded into visualising waves of prana flowing in and out of the body; as well as, finally, being directed to the tumour in his pelvis as a healing 'beam of prana'.

Ian embraced the technique with gusto and he had a particular breakthrough one Saturday night after Tim Lo had administered his second acupuncture treatment.

> I did the breathing and imagined the prana flowing into me as if there was a great cosmic funnel through which it poured into my body. Then I imagined it flowing out through my fingers. As I put my fingers onto the tumour inside my pelvis, I felt as if it would almost break down on the spot. ... I had never felt such energy and I had little sleep.

Next morning he felt surprisingly refreshed, although the pain remained in his back and leg. Furthermore he was thrilled to discover that there was a significant change in the lump inside his pelvis. 'Up to this point it had always been firmly attached, now it moved!' It was a small and very welcome victory.

His excitement was short-lived. The following day came more bad news via a phone call from the cancer clinic: recent x-rays had revealed a fresh growth in his spine.

As cancer was now linked directly with his back pain, Ian suspended the acupuncture on the advice of Dr Lo. Feeling to be in an ever more precarious position he returned to John Doyle, his surgeon, to discuss his medical options once again. He embarked on a short but intense course of radiotherapy, hoping to treat the new growth and rid himself of the sciatic pain that had been incapacitating him and making it difficult to meditate. Perhaps, if nothing else, it could buy him more time.

Ian lay down in the back of the car as Gail—nurse, cook, companion and chauffeur—drove him to his first radiotherapy appointment in Melbourne.

By now Gail was spending every waking moment uncomplainingly, lovingly, looking after her partner. But this was a situation that made Ian deeply uncomfortable. When he had first become ill the pair of them had become very much 'a team with the goal of healing', as he puts it. They had become fully committed to the tasks at hand and it worked really well. But then more recently, with the onset of secondaries, Ian had become very ill, thin and weak and was utterly dependent on Gail. 'I actually felt that the balance of giving was lopsided,' he explains. 'She was doing all this stuff for me and there wasn't anything I was doing for her and in a sense of real affection, gratitude and genuine appreciation, I offered to marry her.'

And so it was, on the way to a cancer clinic in Melbourne for that first session of radiotherapy, just as they were coming off the freeway that led into the city, Ian suddenly sat up and completely out of the blue said very simply, 'I think we ought to get married.'

Gail thought Ian was delirious. But he said it again, she paused for a moment and agreed. It was 10 February 1976 and the wedding was set for Saturday the twenty-eighth.

The radiotherapy was completed in three intensive sessions. Each time Ian went under the huge machine, he imagined the radiotherapy much like the prana he had been experimenting with. But this time he imagined a destructive beam of light from the radiotherapy machine, going through the cancers in his pelvis and spine. He also tried to imagine the healthy tissues withstanding the damaging treatment and being filled with life-giving prana and recovering quickly.

But then a few days after completing the treatment, the hospital rang and reported that Ian's x-rays had been re-examined and now they did not believe he had cancer in his spine.

This news was quite devastating to both Ian and Gail. By now the radiotherapy was complete and it was clear that it was making little impact on the pain. They were beginning to feel as if all their options were used up.

While there was no sense of giving up, what to do next? It was time to see Dr Warren Hastings.

Hastings was a GP offering alternative therapies to people affected by cancer and at the time was considered an enormously controversial, if not downright heretical figure by the medical establishment.

'He was the first GP that I was aware of who was considering other possibilities,' says Ian. 'He was sticking his neck out a fair way in terms of how he was likely to be treated by his colleagues.'

What Hastings was coming to realise—and experiment with— was that some alternative therapies were showing some encouraging results for people for whom conventional medicine offered no hope at all. For Ian's sciatica he suggested using Plenisol, an extract from mistletoe that was unavailable legally in Australia but that could be bought on the black market. It needed to be injected into Ian's skin for his sciatica and back problems and Ian agreed to try it.

Hastings also floated the idea of giving him Bacille Calmette-Guerin (BCG) vaccine. BCG is used to vaccinate against tuberculosis (TB) and, in the 1970s, researchers in Japan had discovered that people with TB were less likely to get cancer. They had also discovered that BCG vaccinations had caused some cancers to regress. Ian liked the idea and was keen to try it as it was another way to work with and boost the immune system. This vaccine did not come through the usual channels either.

The plan was that Hastings would give the initial injections and then Gail, familiar with administering injections from her days as a vet nurse, would continue the treatment in the coming days, gradually increasing the dosage. Ian agreed.

On Ian's second visit to Hastings' clinic, Hastings' colleague Dr John Piesse was on duty. Ian already knew him—John was an old friend from university. It was yet another synchronicity in the many that blessed Ian's extraordinary journey. Although very happy with Hastings' work, Ian was delighted for John to take over his case from that point on.

'The Plenisol really made a rapid difference,' says Ian. 'It really was a saviour.' But then just as the pain in his back ebbed and as the tumour in his pelvis began to seem a little smaller, Ian developed an obstruction in his kidney.

Every time something positive seemed to come his way, another new challenge would rise up to swamp it.

By now he was jaundiced and he was still in constant pain. While the Plenisol had helped, the pain was really beginning to wear him down and so reluctantly Ian began taking three or four painkillers a day. He weighed a mere 41 kilograms, or six and a half stone. He was skin and bone.

Ian asked surgeon John Doyle if anything could be done for his partially blocked and swelling kidney. Doyle replied that it was not worth operating. 'I think that was code for, "You're not going to live very long and I don't want to operate because you would probably die on the table,"' says Ian.

And then came the night sweats. Profuse night sweats.

In response, the couple set up a bed on a wooden slat for Ian.

He would lie down every night wearing a t-shirt and a night shirt, with a towel underneath him and a towel on top of him. 'I'd sleep for a while and then I'd take the t-shirt off because it was soaked and replace the night shirt,' he says. Then it would come off, once it was soaked. Then the towels, once sopping, would be removed. Once the sheets were wet through, he would move to the other side of the bed and proceed to soak the sheets there too. Then he would wake up Gail for fresh bedclothes, sheets and towels and the whole rigmarole would begin again. 'I'd do two rounds of the bed every night,' he says.

Meanwhile, there was a wedding to celebrate. The question was, would the groom be able to stand up for the occasion. Actually, the real question was would the groom be alive, but it seemed no-one wanted to talk about that.

The wedding was held in the garden at Kippen Ross, on its expansive lawns under the shade of the property's huge trees. The weather was warm and clear and the service was led by a young Anglican minister—a friend of Ian's sister Susan. It was a blissfully happy day for the young couple, although from the gloomy looks on their guests' faces pictured on the day, they appeared to hold little confidence that the groom would get to spend very much time at all with his new bride.

On the evidence of Ian's physical state, it would have been hard not to draw that conclusion. Photos from the day show a young man who was painfully thin and drawn-looking, big eyes dominating a jaundiced face that was framed by collar-length hair cut page-boy style. It was only three days after the wedding that Ian's right kidney became completely blocked and the kidney became swollen with a condition called hydronephrosis. To make matters worse, three new cancerous, bony lumps were visibly beginning to grow on Ian's breastbone. It was time for some radical intervention.

The couple remembered Steve Henzler's talk about the psychic surgeons of the Philippines. Ian rang and discussed the possibilities again. Steve provided the addresses of a couple of healers in the town of Baguio as well as the contact details for a young boy who had helped the Henzlers during their trip.

Again, without hesitating and with a sense of real hope and anticipation, Ian booked their flights for Thursday 13 March, only a matter of days away. Ian was drawn by the possibility of a 'miraculous' cure, but also by the possibility of witnessing something 'miraculous'. As he wrote in his journal:

> The possibility is there that some of my physical problems will be relieved in some way. Perhaps clearing of the kidney and some lumps removed. Just as importantly, the spiritual possibilities appeal greatly. I believe such things are undoubtedly possible. To experience such a thing could affirm many things.

It was an incredibly upbeat outlook for a man that Gail said looked like a 'walking coathanger' and was not expected to live more than a couple of weeks.

Aunt Pat remembers visiting Kippen Ross around that time and says she found him 'absolutely yellow and he couldn't lift his head from the pillow. I really thought that would be the last time I would be seeing him.'

When approached by Gail, John Doyle refused the authority they needed him to sign to enable Ian to fly. Doyle felt sure his patient would return home in a 'pine box' and told Gail he 'didn't want her to go through that'.

'He was being compassionate,' she says, adding that she then begged him to sign it because they had 'nowhere else to go. We've got to do it,' she had implored.

Doyle 'begrudgingly' handed the letter to Gail saying simply: 'God be with you and good luck.'

6

Bare-hand Surgery

Ian and Gail Gawler were fortunate enough to have a whole central row of seats to themselves on the Philippine Airlines 747 bound for Manila.

By now, sitting up for more than a few minutes seemed almost impossible for the desperately ill Ian, who by anybody's measure looked close to death. Lying down provided much-needed relief for the acute pains in his back. Weighing only 41 kilograms and his face the colour of 'dark custard' with severe jaundice, sitting up for take-off and landing was, he says, 'probably the most difficult part of the whole affair'.

Arriving at dusk they struggled from the jet into the hot, steamy evening with their four pieces of hand baggage: one held their hand juicer; another bag was packed tight with personal effects and papers; another brimful with various pills; and the last was filled with yoghurt and organic raisins, oranges and apples. Ian was pushed across the tarmac to the main terminal in a wheelchair, Gail in tow, just as two jumbo-loads of Japanese tourists joined the tide. The groups merged in a single stream and surged in through the doors in the sort of numbers the couple had not seen since the races at Hanging Rock.

At Customs, at the front of the crowd, they were appalled to see a Filipino official insisting on vaccinating everyone in the arriving horde who did not have a certificate for smallpox. He was plunging a 'multi-pronged metal thing into this obnoxious little pad' and then stabbing it into each passenger's upper arm.

That Ian was so averse to this particular unplanned and less-than-sterile procedure is entirely understandable, but he also had an aversion to vaccinations at the best of times. In fact Ian's condition was so dire, they were genuinely worried that the vaccination might be the end of him.

Ian suggested to Gail they just walk straight past without looking at the Customs official—which they did. 'He was yelling and carrying on,' says Ian, 'but we just kept on walking and we got through.' Gail attributes the fact that she got 'really stroppy' as the reason for their passage. Whatever the exact course of events, the two of them successfully slipped through without a multi-pronged jabbing.

A week later the couple bumped into a passenger who had been just in front of them in the queue at the airport—and who had grudgingly acquiesced to the vaccination. 'His arm was quite severely swollen and infected by the time we saw it,' says Ian. 'I reckon it would have killed me if I'd had that.'

Passing through Customs, they were then confronted by so many people and so much confusion that they bundled into the first taxi they could and checked in to a different hotel to the one that they had pre-booked. The hotel manager was called, took one look at Ian, assessed the situation and then let them stay—without charge.

Once in their room, Ian went into the bathroom and caught sight of himself in the mirror.

'I actually gave myself a real fright,' he says. 'My face was so gaunt, so haggard, my eyes were sunken back in their sockets, my skin so yellow with jaundice, my hair oily and matted from the flight and the sweating. It really scared me. I think that was my lowest point. It was probably the only moment when I really thought I would die and wondered how I could survive. I knew we had to drive to Baguio in a day's time, a six- to eight-hour trip and that probably I would have to sit up; and for a moment I just could not imagine how I could do it.'

But some food, a coffee enema, a long sleep and next day Ian's energy was back. He insisted on going out with Gail to buy a Super 8 movie camera.

'I was really putting a lot of hope in the psychic surgery but I did not want to be tricked,' says Ian. 'If it was a trick, I wanted to know. If it was not a trick, I was probably even keener to know.' He hoped to record any sleight of hand, as well as being able to discount the possibility of hypnotic effects being responsible for any apparently miraculous goings-on.

Ian and Gail stayed the night and the following day in the capital and then caught a tourist bus which delivered them, at white-knuckle speeds, across the plains and up the narrow, winding roads to the mountains and their final destination.

It was a hellish and, for Ian, an excruciatingly painful ride. They were both tired and grumpy, and Gail remembers the rigours of the whole journey had left her husband in a foul mood. 'It had got so bad that stuff really needed to come out,' she says. 'But it was good he was getting angry—at least he was talking.' Up until that moment he had, she says, been bearing his illness with more of his long periods of silence. At last, thought Gail, he was opening up to his wife.

Baguio City is the summer capital of the Philippines and a health resort town at 1500 metres above sea level with a population of around 110,000 at the time of the Gawlers' visit in 1976 (an earthquake devastated the city in 1990, killing over 1000 of the residents, but it has since been rebuilt).

Baguio is best known to foreigners for the group of individuals known collectively as faith healers. Many of them claim to directly channel the will of God to cure their patients' ills; others practise darker arts. There are purveyors of countless unexplained miracles as well as sleight-of-hand artists, scammers and frauds. The most sought-after, the most impressive and the group that the Gawlers had come specifically to see, though, were the so-called 'psychic surgeons'—shamans who practised bare-hand surgery, or appeared to push their fingers deep inside their patient's body to retrieve diseased tissue and mysteriously fix ailments.

Formally trained in veterinary science, Ian was cautiously sceptical of the procedure but he was open to the experience and the hope that the procedure might trigger his recovery.

Checking in at the Pines, a large Western hotel in Baguio, Ian rested for a couple of hours and then in the afternoon they headed out to find Alan, their young Filipino guide. Without Alan they would have little hope of sifting through the multitude of faith healers in the hope of finding the genuine article.

Alan was small, being only fourteen years old, but was enormously friendly and spoke good English. He had been lined up through friends Steve and Annette back in Australia to take them to a few of the most highly-thought-of psychic surgeons in the area. First, though, he took them to the local markets to buy some supplies. Then he suggested they move to a more friendly and cheaper family-run hotel. Alan had a 'lovely manner and a great deal of wisdom about him,' says Ian. 'And he knew quite a lot of the healers, having had an interest—a personal interest—in them.'

The following day the group headed off in a hire car in the hope of seeing a venerable old healer named Eleuterio Terte.

Ian lay in the back, still unable to sit up without experiencing insufferable pain.

Terte had been one of the stars of a 1959 book written by Ron Ormond and Ormond McGill, *Into the Strange Unknown*. The book had introduced the technique Ormond and McGill had first described as 'psychic surgery' to a wide and incredulous audience. In it they described Terte's work as 'fourth dimensional operations' and had observed Terte's hands apparently sinking directly into a patient's flesh and removing a gallstone. 'Either that man is working miracles or he's the greatest magician that ever lived,' they wrote.

Since the 1940s Mr Terte, as he was respectfully known by everybody, had been performing psychic surgery in the area. He was reportedly the very first to have been noticed doing so in the modern era. The practice stretches back hundreds of years and actually began, most likely, around the time when Catholicism was introduced into the Philippines by Portuguese explorer Magellan in the sixteenth century.

In light of this, visiting Mr Terte was an auspicious way to start their Baguio adventure.

Gail—leaving Ian in the car to mount the steep stairs of the building where the old healer was said to be—bumped into another Australian, Norma Pelic, a confident woman in her thirties with piercing blue eyes and long silver hair.

'Norma came up to me and said, "Are you a healer?",' says Gail, unsure of exactly what Norma meant. Gail then quickly gave Norma an abridged version of Ian's story. Norma suggested she could help, indicating she was something of a psychic and healer herself, that she lived permanently in Baguio, and had been learning healing from the old Filipino surgeons as well as supporting and actually providing healing for them. Mr Terte was her main mentor and they had a close relationship.

Norma remembers Gail's 'bright auburn hair styled in a fashionable cut' and that they chatted about Ian, about horses and about the Gawlers' land at Kippen Ross. Mr Terte was not in that day, she went on to explain to Gail, although he did regularly travel there by bus from his own church which was down in the lowlands, near the sea at a place called Pangasinan.

In town Mr Terte consulted from a single tiny room in the home of Arsenia, his daughter. The room was only big enough for 'a bed and two chairs,' says Norma. On any other day there would have been people packing the home—not to mention crowding outside, where Norma and Gail then stood talking—waiting for healing.

The two parted. Norma neglected to give Gail her address.

A day or two later, thanks to Alan, a touch of intuition and some amateur detective work, the Gawlers tracked the Australian healer down to Sun Flower Cottage. It was perched up the top of another run of steep stone steps cut into the side of the hill. Ian struggled up the stairs and Norma remembers seeing his 'two wide open eyes,' she says—and being struck by the depth of the obvious pain he was in. 'I looked into a soul that had been startled from life into an existence of pain, suffering and loss.'

As she got to know them over the ensuing weeks Norma never ceased to be amazed and impressed with what Ian could do on one leg, despite his distress. 'Ian would set his mind, switch on his will, you could virtually hear it click into place, and off he would go like a mountain goat.'

Gail meanwhile was 'always the faithful support person,' she says. 'I learnt to respect Gail as I did Ian and felt myself blessed for their friendship and presence in my life.'

All of the healers Ian visited over those weeks shared a 'deep spirituality,' says Ian, 'and they were very compassionate.' They varied widely in age and experience from Mr Supnet who was in his late seventies, to Josephine Sisson, in her mid-thirties. The first healer Ian visited, however, was a diminutive gentleman ('only five feet in his bare feet') named Placido.

Waiting in the wood-lined living room-cum-kitchen of Placido's home Ian and Gail chatted to another Australian, from Sydney, on his second visit for treatment for abdominal cancer. He professed to be feeling much better for the experience—although he stressed the need to accompany healing with meditation. One of Placido's aides took a $22 donation for the treatment. It seemed like a very modest fee to them. Ian was then ushered into a small, adjoining room with a flat table inside.

Placido, small, petite and shy, was flanked by two assistants only slightly taller than himself. Ian was the second patient for the day but he caught a glimpse of the blood-stained water in one bucket and then bloody cotton wool and a few pieces of nondescript tissue in another.

Ian was keen to explain his situation to Placido but he ignored him. Instead he seemed to stare at Ian's body, through his clothes, in a somewhat unfocused way.

'He then described my symptoms; the fact that I had my appendix removed and where my tumours were. I was impressed by this apparently psychic diagnosis and started to immediately try to figure out how he did it.'

Ian was instructed very directly to strip to his undies, lie back on the table and pray.

'Given all the circumstances, this seemed like pretty good advice at the time,' he says. 'I lay down, closed my eyes and did my best.'

Placido immediately appeared to plunge his fingers into Ian's skin just above his hip, in the region of his old appendix scar. Ian says he felt a sensation like 'a pop, like if you get a rubber balloon and stretch it out and poke your finger through it ... I felt a numb sort of feeling like you would with a local anaesthetic and it felt like there was something crawling around underneath the skin.' Ian could feel Placido's hands on his pelvis and then on his chest.

Gail was standing next to him observing the whole thing while Alan shot the footage with the newly-acquired movie camera. Gail recalls clearly watching in amazement as Placido operated using his bare hands without any anaesthetic or instruments. Blood appeared to flow and he apparently removed bits of tissue from Ian's insides. When Placido had finished he simply cleaned up the blood that was there and there was no scar. Placido had gone straight to Ian's kidney, says Gail, and had 'pulled out a long piece of tissue and then said, "Oh, that should be okay, come back tomorrow if you want to." '

It was all over very quickly. One of the assistants advised Ian not to have cold drinks, coffee or a shower for 24 hours. 'Go back to your hotel, lie down and have a good rest.'

Back in their taxi, Ian was now quite excited. He asked his wife what she had seen.

Gail said she saw Placido's fingers disappear into Ian's abdomen and then, when he pulled his fingers apart, 'I saw the top of the tumour with my own eyes. They could not have known what that tumour looked like so they couldn't have reproduced that. But I could actually see a bony growth. Placido massaged and massaged and actually peeled it [the skin] apart and I could see some of the structure down inside the pelvis.' Gail had been present at countless, if more conventional, operations on animals. It looked utterly authentic and real and was over in less than two minutes.

Gail was amazed by what she had just witnessed and was thoroughly convinced of its veracity. Ian remained less sure, at least initially—'I suppose I'd had a much more thorough conditioning process in my training'—and had been unable to watch the process as easily as Gail, being as it was that his eyes were closed and he was preoccupied with his attempts to pray.

Watching the footage today, as old and grainy as it now is, it is difficult to say you can see fingers going directly into Ian's skin. Given that the procedure is so far outside the bounds of ordinary experience, not to mention modern physics, it is also something you would frankly have to see for yourself to really believe and verify. At times it very much looks as if fingers have gone in as deep as to the second knuckle, but on the evidence of this version of the film (transferred to DVD and poor quality) it is difficult to be sure. The surgeons used a technique whereby the fingers are bent in and away from view and the possibility of sleight of hand—as the technique's critics have long maintained the psychic surgeons habitually use— seems possible. All that said, Ian and Gail are both adamant they saw fingers plunge directly into skin, on many occasions, with their own eyes.

Another psychic surgeon Ian visited on the trip, Blanche, had a technique whereby he made an incision without a knife, instead using the finger of a bystander hovering at least a hand's span away from the patient's skin. When it came to treating Ian, Blanche took Gail's finger in his hand, and moving it in a cutting motion 10 centi- metres above Ian's skin, a 3-centimetre incision appeared—as if spontaneously—in Ian's upper chest. The footage does not show the incision being made, but it does show what followed. With the cut clearly visible, Blanche placed a small glass cup on the area, with a lighted taper inside. Blood was slowly drawn from the wound. Afterwards, on camera, Blanche clearly pulls a 10-centimetre piece of dark tissue from the open wound. There is no suggestion of sleight of hand. The footage records the procedure in tight close-up. Ian still has the scars from that procedure on his chest to this day.

After their first visit to Placido the couple returned to the hotel. Ian was both excited and animated; certainly less preoccupied with his pain after their extraordinary outing. Nonetheless, doing as he was told, he lay down and almost immediately he fell into a deep sleep, 'the heaviest sleep I think I've ever experienced,' he says. Gail was feeling quite emotionally exhausted and keen for some fresh air. So while Ian slept on into the afternoon, Alan and Gail took off for a horse ride.

When he awoke, Ian was alone. His stomach and joints ached, he was nauseous, his head was spinning and he felt like he was generally 'falling apart at the seams'. In fact the gravely ill Ian once again was genuinely concerned that he was on the way out. He became highly distressed and broke down in tears, sobbing for some time before the riders returned. Gail comforted him and Alan assured him that what Ian was experiencing was a 'healing crisis'. Yet another healing crisis.

Outside of some of the novels he had read as a student and young vet interested in classic literature, a healing crisis was not something Ian was particularly familiar with. Then again, before the advent of painkillers and paracetamol, the world—particularly the literary world—was full of them. Typically a healing crisis involves a terrible fever. Often there is pain and whatever other symptoms have been occurring seem to become more acute, more severe. The body is in crisis and at worst everyone wonders if the patient will live or die. If all goes well there is a resolution, a crucial turning point in the patient's physical state.

Ian's healing crisis lasted all that afternoon, but by the evening it reached a peak and turned quite rapidly. He began to feel extraordinarily better. He ate dinner, slept a long and peaceful night and woke up radically improved.

A couple of days later they returned to Placido for a followup treatment. No donation was required this time—apparently you only paid for the first visit—although Placido himself was not present. Instead his assistants, Jimmy and Marcellino, performed a 'magnetic healing'.

Ian was told that the idea was to 'spread the spirit' in order for it to work more effectively. Indeed, Ian felt much the better for it. Also, as he received the magnetic healing, he found his heart was really racing far more rapidly than normal. This effect continued for around an hour afterwards and then his heart rate dropped suddenly back to normal.

Magnetic healing was a technique Norma Pelic had learnt from Mr Terte. Norma later introduced the technique to Gail, she tried it and then panicked, remembers Ian. 'She said it was all too much for her and she could not do it. I had to reassure her that she could, that I needed her to do it and persuaded her to give it another go.' Gail persevered and soon became progressively more enthused and adept. At the time she said it was like something she innately knew but had almost forgotten. It was like 'a remembering', more than a learning process.

'In my view we all have the capacity to heal like this to some degree,' says Ian. 'Gail had it very strongly and Norma was the catalyst that reawakened it in her.'

Later that afternoon, the group headed for the town of Pangasinan to see another healer, Josephine Sisson.

In a landscape of banana and mango trees and rice paddies, Josephine Sisson worked from a small concrete shed with a sign saying 'Healer In' on the wall. A larger sign intoned: 'GOD does the work and I am only HIS instrument. PLEASE PRAY.'

Inside were five rows of benches separated by metre-high partitions. Again there were a number of buckets on the floor containing bloodied water or various bits of human tissue or bloodied cotton wool from recent procedures.

Ian remembers Josephine as a jovial and plump woman in her thirties with twinkling eyes and a palpable compassion. She began her work by scribbling on a piece of paper and alternately looking up at Ian with great concentration and intent.

This 'automatic writing' was Josephine's way of carrying out a psychic diagnosis. Ian was then instructed to lie on his stomach on the nearest bench. Ian then heard 'mumbled prayers' and then Josephine 'went down both sides of my spine with her fingers,' he says, 'sort of opening the skin up and closing it as she went. It felt very much like something being done under anaesthetic'. Ian says the sensation was again much like something crawling under the skin, with no pain. Josephine then worked on Ian's leg.

Once finished this treatment, she refused a small donation and then advised him that he should be worked on only one more time—either by herself or by another healer.

The next day Placido operated on him and he was left feeling much better than he had for some time. Conversely, he admitted to being very puzzled by the whole experience—it falling so far beyond the realms of known science and contemporary thought. 'I saw a lot of blood, a lot of fresh blood,' adds Gail. 'I saw people with nothing in their hands and nothing up their sleeves, just putting a few drops of water on the skin and then actually massaging the skin and appearing as if they actually went through the skin.'

By now Ian's kidney pain had miraculously vanished. 'It was never a problem after that,' says Ian. 'Never has been.'

In his own book *You Can Conquer Cancer* Ian writes that he felt sure that the sudden pain relief he felt at the time was due to 'both a physical and psychological benefit' from Placido and Josephine Sisson's treatments. 'The healers are very aware of the psychological impact of this visually dramatic procedure,' he says. 'They recognise that if a patient believes that the disease which they have is normally considered to be terminal, then it takes something quite out of the normal to change that belief system and replace it with positive healing thoughts.'

In conventional medical terms this psychological aspect of the phenomenon falls under the umbrella of the placebo effect. That is, if a patient truly *believes* they are receiving treatment or medication that has a curative effect then—even if they are not—a significant number will actually be cured.

The faith healers of the Philippines have an 'exceptional capacity to radiate healing energy,' adds Ian. 'These people have a healing gift, there's no doubt about that.' The Filipino healers have the capacity to heal without the psychic surgery, in other words, but the bare-hand surgery and the blood and gore reinforces the procedure to dramatic effect. 'It's similar to the effect of a drug in the Western sense,' says Ian. The drug has its own benefit, but the total effect is substantially heightened by a patient's belief in its power. 'The psychic surgery is almost like an accessory after the fact, but for many people it does strengthen the experience. The more you believe in it, the more likely it is to work.'

This would mean that even if the particular faith healer was a 'fraud' and was performing psychic surgery by sleight of hand, it could very likely, especially given the apparently radical nature of the intervention, aid some positive improvement or even a cure.

Indeed, researcher Harvey Martin, in his essay *Unravelling the Enigma of Psychic Surgery,* wonders if this could in fact be the intent of many faith healers. Martin discovered references to the therapeutic use of sleight of hand in the Philippines dating back to 1565.

Martin quotes Spanish explorer Pedro Chirino:

> He [the sorcerer] placed one end of the hollow bamboo upon the affected part while through the other end he sucked up the air; then, he let fall some pebbles from his mouth pretending they had been extracted from the affected spot . . . In times of sickness, these men were at their best, because in times of sickness they (the patients) were ready to venerate anyone who could give or at least promise to obtain a remedy for them.

Ian, on the evidence of his own experience and noticeable improvement, remained open to all possibilities. In fact his critical, scientific mind was soon mulling over the multitude of possibilities given that clearly 'something happened' in his own body (and, most importantly, the films they took of the procedures showed some remarkable things). As far as he and Gail had observed, the surgeons had gone into his body with their fingers, he had bled, tissue had been removed, yet there was no apparent scar.

In *You Can Conquer Cancer* Ian writes:

> If just once a healer's hand, even a finger, had gone through my skin under these conditions, then my view of reality, my knowledge of physics and how surgery was possible, was quite inadequate to explain it.

Ian says he spent a lot of time watching psychic surgery at close hand 'and they really do something that challenges our conventional understanding of matter. I think that they are doing true magic, as opposed to illusion.' True magic, he maintains, 'is where you can either manifest matter or de-manifest matter. It is where you actually change the physical nature of matter. It is almost like changing phase as in steam changing to water and water changing to ice.' Challenging stuff. For a Western mind the only way to make any sense of it at all is perhaps to think of the process in the context of quantum physics. Contemporary physicists are quite clear that matter is not solid. Instead, at least when you look at particles at a sub-atomic level, everything is merely made of energy. There is nothing 'solid' there. Perhaps, by some inscrutable process, the psychic surgeons are able to change the phase of human tissue—turn it from ice into water as it were—somehow tapping into the non-solid energy-based fundamental nature of all matter, and plunge their fingers 'through' the skin. It is a lot to get your head around.

Whatever the explanation, the plain facts were that after a few days in the Philippines, Ian no longer felt the need for much of the medication he had been on and the painkillers were ceremoniously flushed down the toilet. He could now walk and sit comfortably, whereas so recently he could only lie down. When he had left Australia he had literally been at death's door; now they could look to the immediate future with some hope. His tumours were the same size but his general feeling of health and vitality was 100 per cent improved.

Another contributing factor since their arrival was the fact that Ian had been following a much more relaxed diet than he had been up until he left for the Philippines—and felt much better for it. As he wrote in his journal,

Gail is concerned with the relaxation of the diet and I am wary, but it seems to me it was not being successful up to now.

As it was, he admits to becoming 'miserable and disinterested' in food before leaving Australia—mainly on account of the fact that much of what he was eating under the Gerson diet was raw.

I feel if we maintain a rudimentary diet—salt-free and avoid meat, I may build up my body to where it can fight the cancer better.

Ian was rested and in good spirits; his kidney problem had vanished. While the pains in his lower back and pelvis remained, they were of a much lower intensity than before and quite manageable. He was gaining weight and his lungs were gradually becoming less congested.

It also helped that everyone they met in the Philippines seemed in no doubt that he would recover. This was in stark contrast to the situation he had left in Australia where virtually all his visitors had seemed in no doubt that they were in the company of a man on his death bed. As Norma Pelic puts it, 'It is fair to say, after working in the Philippines with the psychic surgeons, what seems very important and real in Western society loses its grandeur there.'

But now it was time to visit the old and venerable healer they had first planned to see, Mr Terte. He was back in Baguio and this time Ian was able to negotiate the steep stairs at his daughter's place, something that had been an almost impossible proposition when he had first arrived.

At the top of the stairs they entered a small room—a chapel, living room, dining room and bar combined. A painting of Christ in a rural setting dominated the space, together with a series of brightly coloured statuettes, a table, a kitchenette and a bar groaning with gin, brandy and bottles of assorted spirits. Met by Arsenia they were ushered into a small adjoining room where her father, Mr Terte, then 74, was reclining on a bed. He was chewing tobacco and introduced himself with a handshake. They were instructed to buy two Bibles and Terte arranged an appointment at his own home in Pangasinan for later that afternoon.

Mr Terte conducted business in a concrete chapel decorated with religious murals. Later that day, with an audience of around twelve locals looking on, Alan explained Ian's condition and mentioned that they had seen Placido.

Mr Terte, who had trained Placido, became visibly agitated and criticised at length his ex-student for requesting money. Mr Terte, in contrast, asked for nothing in return for his efforts.

To begin he blessed Ian's Bibles by uttering a prayer and passing his hands over them. Then, flicking the pages open apparently at random, he blew on the book. Next came a further small ceremony that appeared to be a combination of diagnosis and ritual. It involved the use of a small wooden wheel-like contraption with a pointer that was waved at various parts of Ian's body. Next Ian was instructed to lie on the bare table.

Mr Terte appeared to go inside Ian's abdomen and remove various pieces of bloodied tissue and a hard object—two centimetres across—which he had progressively worked up from his chest to his neck. The procedure was over in a matter of minutes and after he was finished he gave Ian instructions that once he was home he should regularly read and contemplate some verses from Ephesians in the Bible.

Mr Terte suggested he would then, upon Ian's return to Australia, be able to continue to work on him with 'absent healing'. The old healer suggested that if Ian felt the need to, that he place the Bible anywhere on his body where he should feel any pain and he, Mr Terte, would send him healing and relief.

He told Ian that he would cure him and advised him not to visit 'healers who heal by black magic', charge money or are 'led by greed'. According to Mr Terte, Placido was 'abusing his powers and now he is losing them'.

(Thirteen years later, in 1989, Placido Palatayan was arrested in Washington. A United States publication *CA, A Cancer Journal for Clinicians* reports that 'he was scheduled to see about 130 clients in two days at \$75 each' at the time of his arrest. Placido was charged with theft and unlicensed practice of medicine. A bucket containing tissue from a 'bovine animal' was removed from his premises.)

On another visit to Mr Terte, Ian asked him how he had become a healer. He explained that his own abilities came when he was young, very sick and close to death. Ian jotted down his words at the time. 'I pray very hard and one night two little angels come to me. They were beautiful,' he said. 'They tell me if I accept the healing power and are willing to help my brothers for the sake of all humanity, then I will be cured. I agree and wake next morning healed, but very weak. Next night they come again and give me authority to heal, in the name of the Holy Spirit, using magnetic healing or laying on of hands. I heal many people.'

Mr Terte told them that after the Second World War, 'the Spirit' told him to do spiritual operations. 'I use knife first, but doctors charge me with illegal operation. So Spirit tells me not to use knife anymore, just hands.' He was the first to use this apparently miraculous technique in the modern era.

But it was more than just the spiritual and psychic healing that helped Ian return to the road to good health. The Gawlers were also touched by the warmth and generosity of the Filipino people they met. At their little hotel, the staff took over the responsibility for making Ian's juices. 'The chef said don't worry, I will make him juices,' says Gail. 'So they went out and bought extra stuff, and that man stood in the kitchen and put all his care and his love into carrot juices and beetroot juices and anything they had in their garden.'

If they did not have it in their garden they bought it. 'They didn't ask for extra money,' she adds. 'They gave and they gave and they gave. The healers did not ask for money. Placido was the only healer we ever paid money to.'

'Also,' adds Ian, 'it was only as we were leaving that we found out most of the hotel staff, after they finished work, stopped in at church on their way home and prayed for me.'

The couple returned to Australia, having received more care and support than they had ever imagined. It was also a quantum leap in the long road to recovery.

'After the Philippines I had experienced a remarkable and generalised healing boost,' he writes in *You Can Conquer Cancer*.

> Yet the tumours kept growing, although slowly. It was obvious to me that I had not made the necessary changes in myself . . . There still remained the ongoing process which faces each one of us, that of developing a system in which to maximise our potentials, correct our shortcomings, and live in accord with our principles.

'It's very rare to get an instantaneous, miraculous cure,' he says today, adding that it is better to consider the process as 'another way of stimulating your immune system.' For Ian this meant that the trip totally relieved his kidney blockage, substantially eased his back pain and set him on the road to better general all-round health and weight gain. In his experience 'a lot of people who went would have that initial healing boost, and feel a lot better, and minor symptoms would disappear,' he adds. But then, if they did not make significant lifestyle changes 'within three months, most commonly, up to about six months, either that initial condition would reoccur, or there would be a relapse. Sometimes even a whole new disease would appear.'

Clearly, for Ian, the road ahead meant a lot more changes, some more subtle than others.

7

Chemo, Faith and Sai Baba

Returning home after an astonishing month away, Ian and Gail Gawler fully expected friends and family to be gripped by the details of Ian's story of survival. Instead everyone was utterly thrilled to have him home alive and looking so much better, but few had any interest in the specifics of how the couple had managed to miraculously pull it off.

'I thought that people were going to be really excited about this,' says Gail, 'but they could not accommodate the thinking. A lot of people said goodbye to him before we left and thought we were off chasing rainbows.'

When the couple mentioned they had films of the surgery, friends mostly 'changed the subject'.

John Doyle, meanwhile, like most people, had imagined Ian would 'come back in a pine box'. He had realistically estimated that before he left Australia Ian Gawler's life expectancy would be about two or three weeks.

Indeed, anyone who saw the shockingly scrawny and jaundiced Ian before he left, a man looking like a concentration camp inmate, unable to even sit up, would have been forgiven for thinking his surgeon was erring on the side of optimism giving him even a couple of weeks to live.

Against all odds and expectations, Ian returned home jaundice-free, happier and 6 kilos heavier, tipping the scales at 47 kilos (or seven and a half stone). His weight fully fit, just before the ampu-tation, had been a few grams shy of 80 kilos. Now at least he could sit up and get around on his crutches—where before only lying down provided any relief from constant pain. Perhaps most inexplicably—at least as far as conventional medicine was concerned—was that his blocked and swollen kidney, for which his doctors had told him nothing could be done, was no longer painful.

Before they headed overseas Ian was at his sickest, he admits. 'I had a real sense that I was close to death.'

John Doyle was accordingly 'quite perplexed', adds Ian, at his living-and-breathing triumphant return. 'He said that he couldn't understand it and that there was no medical explanation for how much I'd improved. He was just delighted that it had happened.'

Something mystifying and wonderful had clearly happened. Something had eased. 'Ian had a belief in his own ability to heal,' explains Gail, but there was patently lots more work to be done.

'It was funny but I had this almost overriding sense that I wasn't going to die, yet a real knowing that I could die and real doubt about how I was going to get well.'

The next six months was a period of great uncertainty and experi-mentation. The couple spent all of their time trying to make sure the long process of healing—which they felt had really turned around in the Philippines—could gather momentum.

During this period of Ian's healing, they used 27 different techniques in all—from surgery and radiotherapy, to acupuncture, iridology, psychic surgery and magnetic healing massage. Many of these approaches, novel for their day, were directed, as Ian explains, 'at looking at ways of stimulating the immune system and getting the body's healing process to work as it should'.

If living underwater for weeks at a time had been suggested as a possible therapy, the couple would have found a way to do it.

Before leaving the country Gail had already been massaging her husband for 'three hours per day in separate one-hour sessions,' she says. Now back in Australia she continued performing long sessions of 'hands-on healing', or the magnetic healing technique that Norma had taught her in the Philippines. 'It's a matter of working off the body,' explains Gail. 'Ian could actually feel my hands while they were off the body, feel the heat.' For Ian it felt like iron fillings were being drawn to a magnet. 'I was told that this was going to have to be continually done for a very long time after he left [the Philippines] to help build up his energy again.'

All through Ian's illness after visiting the Philippines the couple remained in contact with Norma by post and Norma herself remained 'tuned in' to his physical and spiritual needs.

Some of her suggestions to meet those needs were more extraordinary than others.

In one letter she recommended Ian visit two ladies, Mrs Curl and Miss Jessie, who were respected and renowned for their psychic healing abilities, so he dutifully rang them up—figuring he had nothing to lose by the experience—and made an appointment for the following Saturday afternoon. As it happened, a total eclipse of the sun was also due that afternoon and this only conspired to add more than a little extra frisson to the occasion.

Arriving at the home of the ladies, a gothic-style mini mansion in a suburb on the foreshore of Port Phillip Bay, the Gawlers knocked on the door. Mrs Curl, around 70 years old and sporting a bright red wig that looked as if it had been hastily pulled onto her head and was 'about 15 degrees off square' opened the door. She was wearing a dress 'with various remnants of about a week's worth of food down the front of it,' adds Ian.

After a conversation at the door about spirit guides—apparently Ian was accompanied by an unseen Greek gentleman and a Native American warrior—they were invited in and met the younger of the psychic pair, Miss Jessie. 'She was in her fifties and had the same meals down her front too,' laughs Ian. 'They were delightful, but were living on another plane entirely.'

The conversation continued about spirit beings, all of whom had, they were told, constant and insistent messages to impart to Gail and Ian.

And then it came time for the eclipse, whereupon Mrs Curl drew the curtains and instructed the Gawlers to bend over, with their heads between their knees, and press their clenched fists tightly to their eyes.

The eclipse came and went without incident. Mrs Curl then asked Ian if he would like a 'healing'. Ian, thinking he had done 'sillier things' in his time, agreed.

A chair was placed in the middle of the room and Ian was instructed to sit upright in the chair, while Mrs Curl put one hand on his shoulder and one hand supposedly on his hip.

'I don't know if she was unaware of the anatomy of somebody who has had their leg amputated through the hip,' says Ian, but she placed her hand on a more intimate place that left him looking and feeling 'quite startled'.

'And I looked down and she was kneading quite hard at it, healing her heart out.'

Gail meanwhile was busily fending off the affections of the ladies' dog and trying her level best not to dissolve into complete hysterics.

But it was not only her more eccentric contacts that Norma put them in touch with. She had also, it transpired, sent a telegram to her friend Peter Hoddle, a yoga teacher, suggesting that it was imperative that he made his way to help Ian. The only problem was that Hoddle lived right across the other side of the country—over 3000 kilometres away—in Perth.

Ian's health was still going up and down. He had times of relative lack of pain and good movement; at others he became desperately weak and bedridden. That winter in the old and draughty Kippen Ross homestead, Ian's health had hit a particular trough—and Norma became concerned enough to send this urgent SOS to Hoddle.

Peter Hoddle remembers receiving the telegram from his psychic friend and put himself on the first available plane, at his own cost, to help a man he had never met. 'I try to work with my intuition,' he explains of his sudden selfless act. 'When somebody suggests something I just get a feeling of yea or nay, really. So I didn't even question it. I just dropped everything and went.'

Hoddle arrived on the overnight plane to Melbourne in the pre-dawn morning and was met by Gail at the airport. She briefed him of Ian's full story on the way back to Melton. When they arrived he found Ian 'couldn't get out of bed, he couldn't move, he was really weak,' he says, adding that he was 'cranky and grumpy and was snarling at Gail. She was getting really hurt and upset. He was okay with me, but he was throwing everything at her, which is what you tend to do when you're crook, you throw it all at the person you're closest to.'

Hoddle remembers being struck by the extraordinarily tireless work Gail was doing under very difficult conditions. 'I remember having one conversation with her and her saying, "Well, who helps the helper?" All the focus was on Ian and no-one really considered her . . . she carried a huge load. Had he not had Gail beside him he would never have got through it. She was the one when he was in the pits who held him up.'

Over the next week to ten days Hoddle talked at length to Ian, did some massage and taught him some yoga and breathing exercises. 'I really tried to gee him up,' he says. Within a couple of days Ian could get up and 'could walk around a bit' again.

Hoddle also got in touch with Perth-based Christian mystic Reverend Mario Schoenmaker, who happened to be in Melbourne giving lectures at the time. Schoenmaker was the head of the metaphysical college where Hoddle was studying and Ian had previously been in contact with Schoenmaker. Peter Hoddle hoped Schoenmaker 'could gee him up as well' and the reverend turned up and talked to Ian for two or three hours.

As he was leaving, Schoenmaker told Hoddle on the quiet: 'I don't like his chances. He's pretty bad.' Hoddle could not have disagreed more. 'I always knew he'd get better,' he says. 'The moment I saw him I didn't have the slightest doubt he'd get better, that was my inner belief and I tried to convey it to him.'

What did concern Hoddle, however, was the effect the cold and bleak homestead was having on Ian. 'The weather wasn't very kind and it was a dull and dismal place,' he says. 'The energy just wasn't good in the house. It just wasn't helping him. It was obviously creating this heaviness.'

That same week a letter from Norma arrived saying she thought that Ian might be susceptible to the subtle energy effects of underground streams. By coincidence Ian's friend Annie Neville from university days phoned to say hello (Neville was the one who had organised the Raynor Johnson lectures). 'She was always interested in this sort of stuff,' says Ian, so he mentioned the underground stream issue to her. Annie knew just who to contact, she said: next door to her parents in one of Melbourne's well-to-do suburbs, Brighton, lived a man called Dick Molesworth (aka Dick the Dowser).

Dick Molesworth, it seems, had owned a farm in the Western District of Victoria during a particularly long and protracted drought. So bad was the drought, and so desperate were the farmers to find water for their crops, that his neighbours had resorted to using the services of a dowser to discover if there were any underground supplies. Dick was very sceptical but was intrigued to observe the man his neighbours had employed hunting for water armed with nothing more hi-tech than a forked stick. The man wandered around holding the dowsing stick above the ground and when it dipped—as if by itself—he suggested that they dig and that they would find water.

So intrigued was Dick that he gave it a go on his own property. He asked one of his farmhands to blindfold him and he wandered around the paddock with a stick as he had been instructed. Every time he came to a spot where the professional dowser had suggested they would find water, the stick would dip. They dug down and there was an underground stream.

Dick Molesworth had the gift, although he was soon to discover that he could be far more effective using a mini-crowbar than a dowsing stick. Indeed, so effective was Molesworth that he was soon making his living finding water for people and became known as 'Dick the Dowser'.

Ian rang Dick and arranged for him and Annie to visit the following weekend—with his crowbar.

When he arrived Dick got started straight away and wandered around the property holding the crowbar horizontally in his hand. He told the Gawlers that when the tip dipped, there water would be found. Once he had ascertained the location of the water, Dick's method was to hold the bar horizontally, click a stop watch 'and depending on how long it took for the tip to hit the ground,' says Ian, 'he'd tell you how far down the water was.'

Sure enough, Dick found water. In fact he found two sources of it that met directly underneath the house. Dick decided from the dip of the crowbar that there were two underground streams that went under the structure, one coming in from the front and one from the side. One was 36.5 metres below the ground and one was 38 metres below the ground and they met 'straight under my bed where I'd been sleeping,' says Ian.

'It's interesting because Gail and I had been feeling increasingly uncomfortable with the house. We thought there was really something wrong with it. And then Peter had too,' he says. 'It was a lovely house in its layout and its location. In so many ways it was a good place for us, but we had begun to feel quite strongly that something wasn't right.'

'You didn't need to be a genius to know the place was damp,' adds Glenyss, his stepmother. 'Heavens above.'

Glenyss remembers being horrified that Ian was living in an old damp farmhouse in his condition and had been trying to persuade him to shift to their heated beach house at Torquay. 'He wouldn't be convinced that the house was damp just because mother said that the house was damp,' she says.

'But that's how his mind works, you see—you find out, you don't assume—you find somebody who comes with his stick and says, "Oh yes, there's a stream under here, this is not a healthy place to be." '

And so it was that they came to move to the beach house at Torquay—although Ian's father Alan insisted they paid rent. Ian explains: 'At the time I thought fair enough,' adding that it might seem a bit mean looking from the outside.

Ian was still receiving money from the health protection scheme but once that ran out—which happened while they were staying at Torquay—he had to transfer to a disability pension.

While monetary support did not come from his father, a different kind of support came to Ian in a most remarkable way. A couple of weeks after they had moved down to the seaside, Ian wrote and posted Norma a letter listing six, quite specific, questions he hoped she would answer.

That same afternoon a letter arrived from Norma—faster than a jumbo jet could fly a quarter of the return distance to her home in the Philippines—with all the answers in it.

'We'd get letters from her saying: "Oh you know that part down there that you were massaging on Ian's back,"' says Gail. '"I'd like you to try doing this and this because I think it will work better."' Gail never gave Norma any precise information of the massaging she was doing but she was also never in any doubt of exactly what Norma meant. 'The advice never failed.'

While living at Torquay, another of the more remarkable happenings was that the Gawlers had been put in touch with a man called Ralph Thomas. Thomas had a special gift.

Ian had sent him a floor plan of the house, giving true north, in the hope that he would let them know if their home—unlike Kippen Ross—was conducive to Ian's return to health. Thomas was apparently an expert on geomancy—now more commonly referred to by its Chinese name, feng shui.

Simply put, Thomas could reputedly assess the earth's energy flows at a particular location and how these might affect the people living there.

A few days later a letter came back, saying that the house was not too bad, but contained within the letter was a pebble to sort out the minor problems Thomas had detected.

'What I was instructed to do,' says Ian, 'was to go to the north-west corner of the house, measure 8 feet up from the floor and stick the pebble on the wall.

'It was another of those things where I thought, well I've done sillier things than that, so off I went and stuck the pebble on the wall.'

He thought no more about it and there seemed to be no obvious effect. Until spring came around. Then the wattle bushes just outside the back door of the house came into their full golden bloom. As Ian explains, in those days Gail suffered a very strong allergy to wattle pollen. However, this particular year a couple of weeks went by before they were amazed to realise that she was suffering no allergic reaction. No itchy eyes, no sneezing, no runny nose.

A couple of days later the couple visited Ian's parents in Melbourne, who also had a wattle bush in bloom in their front garden. Gail's hay fever began almost as soon as she got there.

Returning to Torquay, the symptoms vanished.

All of this was so out of the ordinary that when a few days later she began sneezing and Gail's hay fever returned with full force it seemed almost normal again. He then decided to check on the pebble. 'Sure enough, it had fallen off the wall. So I picked it up, stuck it on the wall and within half an hour, Gail's [hay fever] symptoms were gone. I never noticed any difference in my own health from the pebble, but that was the last year Gail ever had hay fever.'

As for Ian's health, while he was much improved physically and had 'a much better peace of mind,' the tumours were slowly getting bigger.

During this period Ian tried a whole raft of alternative and complementary therapies—some more esoteric than others. He was in no doubt that most of them worked in theory. Nevertheless, he was having trouble applying these therapies to his own situation. 'I did have a lot of difficulty in thinking that they would work for *me*,' he says. He was all too aware that he was still suffering from a very 'subtle obscuration' that prevented him from taking the next step in the healing process.

'Part of my problem was that in my mind I was still thinking like a vet who had been trained in Western medicine. I was having a lot of difficulty believing that something like meditation and diet, let alone the extraordinary forms of healing we had been experimenting with, could overcome something as potent as osteogenic sarcoma.' So it was back to the surgeon once more. He asked John Doyle what other conventional treatments might be on offer.

Doyle suggested chemotherapy and referred him to Dr Ivon Burns.

Burns offered a two-year course of a newly introduced, experimental cytotoxic chemotherapy. He pulled no punches on the likely side effects or the fact that it was completely experimental.

What Burns was able to tell Ian and Gail was that the treatment would most likely make him violently ill for anything between a few hours and a few days immediately after treatment. Ian would also temporarily lose all his hair, there was a good chance it would affect his eyesight—perhaps even make him blind—it could severely weaken his heart muscle, and it would almost surely make him sterile.

Perhaps not surprisingly, Ian told Burns that he would like to think about it.

He decided to intensify his efforts with meditation, diet, massage—everything—for two weeks, in the hope of the tumours decreasing. If so, he would defer the chemo. If there was no change, or things got worse, he would start the chemo. In fact, after two weeks there was no discernible change. Ian agreed to begin the treatment.

It is often said of Ian that he must have had real faith in the psychic surgeons to fly while he was at death's door to the Philippines, but the way he sees it—especially after the scant recommendation given to him about the experimental chemotherapy—he must have had a powerful sense of faith in the chemotherapy, too, to go through with it.

The two-year course, instead of the shorter course more commonly offered now, was the conventional wisdom. 'We now know that with sensitive cancers short periods of treatment are all that is necessary,' Burns says. World champion cyclist Lance Armstrong, for instance, when suffering with metastatic testicular cancer in 1996, received four cycles of chemotherapy. These were far shorter intensive bursts compared to the two-year course suggested for Ian twenty years before.

'In those days [1976] it was early days for medical oncology,' says Burns. 'There were very few people in Australia who were treated for solid tumours with chemotherapy.' Ian Gawler was a guinea pig—and knew it. There was no evidence at all, unlike Lance Armstrong's treatment, that it would be curative.

Gail used to drive him into Melbourne for the treatments, which consisted of being hooked up to an intravenous drip for about an hour, by which time he was 'already feeling like he was about to throw up.'

Torquay was around one and a half hours away by car. On the way home they would make sure they had a plentiful supply of plastic bags. 'I used to roar like a lion,' says Ian. 'Vomiting like this is a violent business. It really feels like you are throwing up from the tips of your toes. It is quite an involuntary thing. So we used to drive home through the morning traffic, with Gail driving and me throwing up.'

One day, not long after they had left the clinic at about 10.30 in the morning, Ian remembers pulling up at a set of traffic lights in inner Melbourne. A big interstate transport truck pulled up beside them. 'There was this huge truckie sitting behind the wheel, tattoos all down his arms. A really big tough-looking dude. And then he looked down at me . . . we made this really good eye contact . . . and in the same moment . . . I threw up.'

A moment later the lights changed and Gail drove off. 'We got about 100 metres on and I thought to look back and the truck hadn't moved. Poor bloke. We were still laughing by the time we got home.'

Once home, after each treatment Ian would suffer violent bouts of uncontrollable vomiting for the next three or four hours. Then it would pass and he would rest, exhausted, for the rest of the afternoon. His long hair, meanwhile, dropped out in handfuls and he rapidly became bald.

By the end of two and a half months of the program Ian developed a deep inner sense that it was time to end the chemo. This proved to be very much against the advice of Dr Ivon Burns, who was of the opinion that to do so then might cause the tumours to grow more vigorously. As it was, there was little evidence of the lumps reducing. Burns said that if Ian stopped treatment then the tumours would 'grow quickly because chemotherapy tends to drop your natural immune system.' Ian again took time to contemplate what to do. 'We really felt that I had had enough of this treatment and got whatever benefit was available from it,' he says. 'Also, my mind had had enough of a jolt now that something physical had happened.'

Burns' observations of the episode were that he saw 'definite evidence of response while he was on chemotherapy' and wanted Ian to continue with the treatment. Ian, as well as keeping a journal, was taking monthly photos of his chest throughout the period. While the tumours on his chest clearly increased in size regularly up to the commencement of the chemo, and they did stop growing at that point, there was no discernible decrease.

And so while the tumours were still very much in evidence, Ian says his own reasons for having chemotherapy in the first place were satisfied. He had sought a treatment within the Western medical paradigm that would hopefully help in a direct physical way. Yet he was also hoping that the chemo was going to help his 'mind swing around'. In fact, at this time it was Ian's main aim in deciding to accept the chemotherapy.

He says that he wanted to do something that 'actually justified me getting well. I really felt afterwards that I got more benefit for my mind from the chemotherapy than I did for my body.

'With chemotherapy, it's such a bloody tough treatment, that you almost feel that if you have gone through that, then you justify getting well,' he says. 'If you have any thoughts lurking at the back of your mind that illness is a punishment, chemotherapy is a great way to purge it.'

Ian might not have thought of his osteogenic sarcoma as a punishment, but he was of the mind that his disease was some kind of radical wake-up call for having taken an outer, material-based path rather than charting an inner, spiritual one.

It was late 1976 when Ian decided to prematurely end his chemo-therapy course. He decided that the best course of action was to head straight back to the Philippines in the hope of affecting the same sort of radical shift they had enjoyed on the previous trip.

Also this time, with Ian's general health much improved, he and Gail hoped to study and learn more about the faith healers and how they worked. They intended staying longer and decided to rent a house in Baguio, hoping to stay for three months. From there they would head on to Europe via Egypt and come back through India.

They left Australia in January 1977.

Ian's tumours were still large but 'weren't affecting me at all,' he says. On this second trip they saw fifteen healers in all, talking to each at length and taking more footage of their experiences. All of this only confirmed the couple's strongly-held sense that the psychic surgery was genuine.

'A lot of those healers were seeing 40 people a day at least,' says Ian, adding that he found it hard to believe that anyone could be under that sort of pressure and work with 'conjuring and dishonesty. I just don't think many people could maintain this kind of charade for so long, with such sick people and not crack up. Also, if they did have the strength to do that, surely they would find a better way of making a dishonest dollar, or even an honest one!'

The most 'extraordinary' healer they met on the second trip was a man named Flores. Ian went to see him for a 'hardening' in the centre of his abdomen and a feeling of indigestion that seemed to accompany it, something that had puzzled his Australian doctors. At the back of Ian's mind was another unspoken concern. Perhaps this was another bony secondary cancer.

Flores' healing sanctuary was a concrete building similar to Mr Terte's. There were the religious murals on the walls, rows of pews much as you would find in a conventional church, and a wooden operating table in place of an altar. It had a very 'spiritual, peaceful, natural sort of air,' says Ian—as opposed to the pagan, sacrificial atmosphere such an image might conjure.

Flores began Ian's 'surgery' as usual—by asking him to lie on his back and pray. This time Ian was feeling better and a little more confident, so he kept his eyes open and watched—at very close range.

Flores 'stuck his fingers in through the skin ... just below my solar plexus and pulled out a loop of small intestine,' says Ian, adding that the intestine looked very 'fresh and viable'—Ian was certainly in a position to assess this, having seen countless intestines during his own surgical work at his veterinary practice. Importantly, too, the temperature inside Flores' concrete healing chapel was over 32°C, estimates Ian, and 'well over' 90 per cent humidity.

'Having operated in the field on many animals I know that as soon as you pull intestines out of animals in those sort of conditions, the intestines start to dry off, they start to desiccate really quickly,' he says, adding that it was clearly a genuine small intestine and the 'right sort of size that I would expect to come out of my own tummy.'

In those conditions, if it was an animal intestine, produced by sleight of hand, then it would have had to have been removed from an animal very recently killed. Flores and all his helpers had been in the building, in clear sight for about two hours.

But then Flores reached over and grabbed a rusty pair of old scissors, took the intestine that Ian could plainly see resting on his stomach, and cut it in half. Flores held one end of the intestine. To Ian's utter amazement, the other end retracted back into his stomach and disappeared from view.

'Well, a basic principle of abdominal surgery,' he says, 'is that if you have a loose bit of open intestine then you have one helluva big problem.'

Undeterred, Flores took the half of the intestine that he was holding, then squeezed a pus-like liquid from it. He did so like you might try to 'squeeze the stuffing of a sausage out from its casing'. He then filled the intestine with methylated spirits to 'clean it out'. The sensation of this procedure, says Ian, was much like someone had tied a piece of string around his spine and was pulling it from the front. There was no actual pain, just a weird tugging sensation.

Flores flushed the intestine out with the methylated spirits a couple more times and then plunged his fingers back into Ian's abdomen to retrieve the other end of the intestine. It miraculously appeared and he began to roll the two bits together. 'It was just like watching healing taking place instantaneously,' he says. 'It was just like the two pieces melted back together again.'

Flores stuffed the loop back into Ian's stomach and squeezed it shut with so much force that it was excruciating. Nevertheless, almost immediately, the indigestion disappeared and so had the mysterious hardening that had been there previously.

Neither ever returned.

The great pity, though, is that Flores is the only healer who would not let Ian film or take photographs. Ian supposed this was because he was not keen on publicity but was keen to keep his healing gift very low-key. A rice farmer by choice, unlike many of the healers he would only operate twice a week on around half a dozen people per day.

Flores also had a theatrical flair. One day Ian observed Flores remove a huge tapeworm from a woman's abdomen and then wind it around her husband's neck as he stood alongside. Flores thought that this was very funny! The husband was aghast. At other times he would splash observers of the operations with blood if they came too close. He would also 'flip in and out of personalities at a great rate,' says Ian. 'One minute he'd be involved in an operation, and the next minute he'd fling himself back against a wall exhausted like he couldn't go on. And the next minute he would be back laughing and carrying on and full of energy.'

Other healers were less flamboyant. Some restricted themselves to a few specialities. Ian sought out those who could work on his pelvis and his chest—particularly to work on the three small tumours that had appeared on his chest where the ribs meet the sternum.

They also revisited Mr Terte again, although from a journal entry dated 5 February 1977 it is clear that, as with all the healers, Ian's critical mind had a great deal of difficulty believing what he was apparently seeing. Doubts lingered about the authenticity of his technique. 'Is he faking?' he wrote.

On one visit Ian joined eight other cancer patients and was first up onto the bench. Mr Terte removed a length of tissue from Ian's solar plexus and then performed magnetic healing on his hip. Ian then observed the others.

Each time he precedes a materialisation by putting his right hand under his table and appears to grope for something. His right fingers are then curled and only his forefinger is directed into the patient. It then is impossible to tell where the mass comes from as he manipulates his fingers and extrudes it, apparently from the skin.

Ian's doubts are very real, yet . . .

I know the benefits from his healing. This is all very confusing, a test to faith developed . . . Norma says when Mr Terte is grumpy and working fast he is healing well. He must be at full power today.

During this time, as in the first trip, there was little visible change in the tumours. Again for Ian it was another turning point in recovery and repair, rather than a cure.

He was already aware that after an initial healing boost, significant life changes had to be made to effect any lasting improvement—and to the Gawlers' way of thinking this meant 'that someone's physical situation, their emotional, mental and spiritual state' had to be taken into account.

What the psychic surgery did offer was the psychological benefits of seeing something happening. 'It's very good in helping you to build an expectation that you are going to get well.'

On the opposite of this equation is the fact that at that time in the West, as a patient with terminal cancer, the medical establishment commonly underlined the expectation that you are going to die. Ian likens this to 'pointing the bone'.

In Australia an Aboriginal shaman, known as a kurdaitcha man, points a special sharpened killing bone, or kundela, at the intended victim. In Aboriginal law, this is a traditional, ancient and highly effective form of ritual execution for anyone condemned for a capital crime by his tribe. Within days or weeks the condemned man, terrified and utterly convinced that the curse is real and inescapable, is dead. Yet no-one has laid a finger on him.

Likewise modern society has its own shaman, in our case a doctor dressed up in a white coat and carrying a stethoscope. As Ian points out, the medico has the capacity to deliver their prediction in 'a ritual type atmosphere', only instead of pointing a sharpened bone with the authority of the spiritual mastery of the kurdaitcha man, he invokes the imprimatur of his medical training and the weight of statistical evidence. 'You have cancer and you only have six months to live.' Or even if a specific survival period is not stipulated, the patient often reinforces any expectation of their survival prospects for themselves in accordance with whatever is the accepted wisdom. In our society this can be a ritual experience, every bit as powerful as pointing the bone.

Fundamentally, says Ian, giving bad news in this way commonly leads to a patient believing themselves to be a dying person as opposed to a living person.

The Filipino faith healers, on the other hand, can act as a sort of psychological circuit breaker in this process—regardless of whether they actually plunge their bare hands into a person's body or not. The important point is that the healers represent an authority figure suggesting that you can get better. They can help to change people's perceptions of where their lives and their illnesses are going.

And it was the same for Ian, although he describes his problem at this point in his healing journey to be one where he realised that he had a particular mental block that was the 'remaining obstacle to me getting well'. Physically he was on the mend, he was told this by the faith healers, but his mind still had to make a fundamental shift. Ian was fully prepared to go through the motions of changing his lifestyle, attitudes and belief system if that was what it took to effect a cure, but—as healer after healer told him at the time—he had yet to *believe* on a very subtle and deep level that he would get well.

And then fortuitously, one day during a lunch break at Flores' place, in another of those remarkable 'coincidental' meetings, they met Hari, from India, and his wife, Pamela, from New Zealand.

Hari was utterly amazed by Flores' miraculous techniques but in the same breath told Ian that he thought that for matters of the mind 'the Indian holy men had all the answers'.

The Gawlers had already heard of a man named Sai Baba, to whom Christ-like miracles had been attributed. They had intended to seek him out on their travels, but only on their way home after

Europe. Hari insisted they come and stay with him and Pamela at their home in the Indian city of Pune straight away. Also he suggested that his sister could put them up in Bombay when they first arrived. The Gawlers rearranged their travel plans.

The city of Pune, inland from the west coast of India in the state of Maharashtra, was also where Bhagwan Shree Rajneesh (later known as Osho) had an ashram on 2.5 hectares of land. It was literally around the corner from Hari's place in the well-to-do suburb of Koregaon Park.

Rajneesh's followers, commonly then known as the Orange People, numbered 200,000 around the world at the time, wore red/orange robes and a wooden beaded necklace around their neck containing a picture of their spiritual master Rajneesh. His teachings synthesised aspects of Hinduism, Jainism, Buddhism, Taoism and Christianity.

Walking through the large grounds of Rajneesh's ashram 'filled with drifting orange-clad figures' Ian's initial impression was that it felt like a sanitorium and it was vibrant with 'tensions and complexities being worked out. There are few happy faces, most are earnest or intent,' he wrote. They found the ashram was full of mainly Americans, casualties of overindulgence in the free drug and sex culture of the previous decade.

'A lot of them were pretty scrambled up,' says Ian, 'and yet were together enough to know that they were in trouble and were looking for a way out.'

No way was it the right scene for a young Australian vet, a man who had led a relatively sheltered upbringing, and was fundamentally looking to get well via some quiet introspection and spiritual practice.

I would prefer controlled inward endeavour leading to a physical manifestation of the inner peace.

While Ian came to have a lot of respect for the benefits he witnessed in people who spent time at the Pune ashram, on this occasion it made him feel physically ill. He and Gail left immediately.

On 31 March they flew to Bangalore and then on to the hill station of Ooty, one of the homes of the important religious leader Sathya Sai Baba.

The following day Ian and Gail found themselves in a crowd of 300 blissfully expectant devotees patiently waiting to see a man revered by millions.

Born in 1926 in a small Indian village called Puttaparthi, Sathya Sai Baba was the son of a poor farmer. The legends vary but he was an ordinary boy, by all accounts, with no apparent great gifts, until he was stung by a scorpion in early March 1940. He immediately fell into unconsciousness until the following morning.

From that day on the boy regularly fell into a trance, spouting philosophy, reciting poetry and songs of realisation. In May the same year he left school and he reportedly began to perform the miracles that would later become a daily occurrence.

Sai Baba's fame gradually grew, increasing numbers were drawn to him, and by the time the Gawlers met him his devotees already numbered in the millions.

Ian and Gail sat on a lawn outside the ashram, an impressive two-storey colonial house with a large olive tree out the front. Behind were terraces of tea bushes rising steeply up to a granite peak. It was strikingly beautiful and completely inspiring for the couple, offering an atmosphere of 'calm reverence' that neither of them had ever struck before. The only negative, at least to Gail's very strong feminist sensibilities, was that men and women were segregated into two separate areas.

After some time Baba emerged from the building and walked around, acknowledging a few of his devotees, some of whom, wrote Ian, 'worship him as a God'. Ian managed to catch his eye and Sai Baba asked briefly where he was from and then continued wandering among the crowd.

A little later he returned and, incredibly, asked Ian to come with him for a personal interview, along with a rich Indian man and his family, a young Indian couple and their young child and a man of eighteen or nineteen, on his own.

Ian asked if Gail, sitting some distance away, could come with him and Baba agreed. 'Now my body is tingling all over and after a short wait we are ushered in by Baba,' he wrote of his experiences later that day.

For the first couple, the Gawlers saw Sai Baba materialise some of the healing ash called vibhuti, for which Baba is famous. He spontaneously produced, or manifested, this ash by rubbing his second finger and thumb together 'in a steady, gentle manner'.

For Ian and Gail, after all their time amongst the healers in the Philippines, that Sai Baba could do this seemed 'almost perfectly normal. It took us a while to realise that other Westerners were awed by Baba's "miracles". We almost expected them.'

After Sai Baba had talked to the first couple for a while, he then turned to the Gawlers and talked about 'avoiding differences between two of us', wrote Ian.

> He radiates joy and love and talks to us like a dear friend. I listen eagerly. Then he throws me by asking if I had an accident. I reply no, I have cancer and he says not to worry, it is alright.

Baba then told Ian and Gail he would give them some vibhuti to be taken after lunch and dinner in a little water. They were instructed to wait in the hall and were ushered out.

Outside Baba gave them a handful of packets of the healing ash and Gail was told to take it too. Speaking to Gail, he said 'Your health is not good, too much tension and anger,' reads Ian's journal. 'We laugh and I call out and say that it is better now and he is gone.'

After their own first audience with Sai Baba, the Gawlers soon found themselves crowded by devotees wanting to know what Baba had said and to share in their good fortune at having been blessed with such a rare private meeting.

A traditional Indian holy man, or saddhu, approached. Dressed in an orange robe and with a red dot on his forehead—perfectly round and applied expertly with vermilion powder with a finger—he told them of his complete faith in Baba and assured Ian of his good health. He told them of the vibhuti's power to produce 'anything that the taker believed in with undivided faith. In other words, the healing is within.'

They also struck up a conversation with three Americans, Ed, Jay and Mike, who had been there for four months. Ed, the 'most grounded' of the trio, told the Gawlers that 'Baba is a gradual process, with rarely any fireworks'. He also told them that it is not uncommon for people to come to see Baba and wait a year before they have had barely a glimpse. Remarkably, the Gawlers had spoken to him—and received Sai Baba's blessing—on their very first day.

In the following week, Ian and Gail joined the crowds anxious to catch a moment, a glance, possibly a word with Sai Baba at dashan—the vigil held morning and evening—much as the first day. Baba would 'come out and he would walk around among us. He might say hello to a couple of people, and ask people to come in for an interview, and he would quite often produce his healing ash.'

People dived at his feet, hoping to touch him. Sai Baba routinely materialised vibhuti and put it on people's foreheads or instructed them to put it on affected parts of the body or take it with water, as he had for the Gawlers that first day.

Ian swiftly came to realise that his very first meeting with Baba was the most important breakthrough in his entire recovery. There had been no blinding light. No mystical out-of-body experience. No sudden insight.

Baba had simply told him 'You are already healed, don't worry.'

Ian came to believe. Completely. The great man had catalysed precisely the subtle shift for which Ian had been searching, but had not known where to find.

Sai Baba's influence and compassion helped Ian to realise that he had a clear and profound choice. Either he could stay in a 'half state of doubt and concern about what the future might hold,' he says, or he could shift from that to a 'certainty that I could recover.'

As Ian puts it these days: 'That's the role of a true healer, to help people to change in a really fundamental and obviously significant way. If you do see disease as a process as I do, then if you've been going through a particular life pattern that has brought you to a point where you have an illness, if you're going to truly recover you need to change that direction. And, while it is possible to make that sort of change on your own, very often I think you need a catalyst to help. That's where the true healer comes in. They can either show you or help you through that change, that transition, and help you to move off in a different direction.'

On the most fundamental and subtle level Ian was now healed— a fact that seeped deeper and deeper into his being as time went by. On a more practical level there were still countless trials to face and problems to solve.

8

Abundance

It was a real struggle for Ian to make his way to into the King's Chamber in the heart of the Great Pyramid. 'Those ancient Egyptians must have been a good deal shorter than me. I had to half hop, half crawl and I was a bit exhausted once we made it into the chamber.'

Leaving India in early May 1977, Ian and Gail had flown direct to Cairo.

The couple had become fascinated by Egyptology and having read widely on the esoterics of pyramids, were keen to experience them in real life. Their idea of 'experience' was a little different than that of your average visitor to the mystical and monolithic last resting places of Ancient Egypt's kings.

The Gawlers' plan was to sit quietly and meditate in the King's Chamber; to feel the power and the presence of the place and perhaps to experience something numinous and profound.

'We were just settling in, cross-legged beside the empty sarcophagus, when a sea of American tourists burst into the chamber. They were archetypal tourists, so excited, so anxious, that one fell over and several others toppled over her,' says Ian. 'They picked each other up, babbled incoherently and took photographs of each other. One man came up beside Gail and asked her in a deep Southern drawl, "You're not meditating are ya, honey?" '

In the next moment they were all gone, leaving Ian and Gail totally bemused. The moment was gone.

There was nothing to do but to struggle out of the pyramid, ride a camel and travel onward.

Arriving in London they made a shock discovery. Their bank account was empty, the funds all used up during the three months they had spent in the Philippines. Fortunately they met up with Ian's grandmother, Doris, who was also in the UK on holiday. The trio had planned to travel on from England to Europe together.

When she heard of her grandson's monetary plight Doris agreed to fund the rest of the trip—apart from the travel that Ian and Gail had already paid for.

Gratefully the couple headed north to the Findhorn community without delay.

Findhorn is a seaside village way up in the north-east of Scotland, at the end of a small peninsula, south of the Moray Firth. There was not much to distinguish Findhorn from any of the other myriad little communities clinging to the coast of the British Isles. The townsfolk quietly got on with their lives in their windswept, often bitterly cold but peaceful little corner of Scotland, supported by shipbuilding, fishing and trade with countries at other corners of the North Sea.

And then the Caddys arrived.

At the beginning of the 1960s Peter and Eileen Caddy and their three sons had moved there to manage a country hotel in the area, but had lost their jobs and had been forced to move into a caravan. The couple had long been interested in spirituality and had studied with noted spiritual teacher Sheena Govan. By 1962 the Caddys, together with their friend Dorothy Maclean, who ending up living with the couple in an adjoining annex, had established a spiritual community nearby bearing the name of the Scottish village.

The family had little money and were forced to grow their own vegetables. The climate might have been forbidding, the soil sandy and barren and woefully ill-suited to horticulture, but it mattered little to Maclean when she discovered she could contact the 'spirits of the plants' or devas, as she called them. The devas gave her careful instructions on how to grow and nurture each type of plant. Soon there was an extraordinary, and abundantly healthy, array of organic vegetables, flowers, herbs and—most famously—cabbages that weighed in at 18 kilograms (or 40 pounds in the old measure).

News of the trio's astonishing green-thumbed abilities soon spread. Conventional horticulturalists who visited were utterly dumbfounded by their successes. And it was not long before other spiritually-minded people had settled with the Caddys.

Over the years, Findhorn grew into a thriving community committed to pursuing a spiritual path in peaceful accord with nature.

By the time the Gawlers visited the community it had become a registered Scottish charity, had changed its name to The Findhorn Foundation and had bought Cluny Hill Hotel (where the Caddys had worked and subsequently lost their jobs). Renamed Cluny Hill College, it was an ideal venue to hold courses and accommodate spiritual seekers.

Although they could afford to stay only a couple of weeks, for Ian and Gail Findhorn was an important affirmation of their own ideals. Their time there helped confirm and strengthen their own relationship with 'manifestation' and 'abundance'.

In the early days of his illness Ian had been struck by how many coincidences seem to occur around him. 'Steve Henzler, Norma, Peter Hoddle and Dick the Dowser—so many people appeared and so many things happened at those critical moments when I needed them,' says Ian. 'The coincidence rate was unbelievable. I repeatedly found myself saying, "What a coincidence that was."'

When Ian heard of the Law of Manifestation, 'it all seemed to make sense. It really is as they say in the Bible: "Ask and you will receive, seek and you will find, knock and the door will be opened."'

For Ian, again his scientifically-based scepticism battled with all of this. On the other hand, he was yearning to believe it to be true. The harder, more pragmatic side of his nature debated it fiercely.

One evening back in Torquay, the principle had been put to the test. During one particular intense period of the chemotherapy treatment Ian describes 'waking up one day and realising there was no fun in what he was doing. It was all so intense, so serious, so humourless.'

Determined to go out and be entertained, Ian scanned the local paper. Two Bill Cosby films were on at the drive-in—but it was pouring with rain. Over dinner Gail attempted to talk Ian out of the outing. 'I don't want to sit in the car with the windscreen wipers going all night,' she said. Ian was adamant. 'We will go and it will stop raining.'

On the way to the car, Gail gathered the rubbish and was intent on putting the rubbish bin out for collection the next morning. Reaching the door, she tripped, spilling the rubbish onto their shag pile carpet. Cursing, the two knelt down to pick the rubbish up but in the process found Gail's engagement ring. In the hurry to leave it must have been swept off the bench along with the rubbish and without the 'accident' it would have been lost forever.

But there was more. As they left the garage and moved onto the street, the rain stopped. They sat through two films, dark clouds billowing all around, but not a drop of rain. The windscreen wipers remained motionless.

Returning home, Ian and Gail pulled into their garage and stepped out. Right on cue, the rain poured down again; continuing throughout the night.

'It was beyond remarkable,' says Ian. 'It was almost as if we were being told—"See, do you believe it now." Manifestation was real and it was almost like the more we acknowledged it, the more grateful we were for it, the more we expected it; the more reliable it became. We really trusted it.'

To those of more cynical, materialist sensibilities, manifestation might seem just like simple coincidence at work, 'like very romantic, new age esoterics,' Ian admits, 'but it worked for me. All through my illness it was not just a theory, it was happening,' he says. 'And here was a place [in Findhorn] where they were putting those theories of manifestation into practice.'

Over the years Findhorn has found itself in dire financial straits from time to time but always depended on divine guidance to manifest the necessary funds.

'Guidance has always been core to the community's decision-making processes,' says current resident Jonathan Dawson, quoted in the *New Statesman*. 'This has led us to many merry adventures that we would have been most unlikely to have embarked upon had we been governed by left-brain rationality and economic logic alone.' Findhorn's faith-based approach to life has indeed been so central to the community's philosophy, that at one point in the 1970s some senior members of the community left in disgust when a bank loan was taken out to buy Cluny Hill Hotel.

The other thing that appealed to Ian about Findhorn was that it represented a working community, based on spiritual lines. It was run with the sort of open, compassionate and believing attitude that he dreamed might one day form the philosophical basis for the couple's own work—whatever form that might take.

Leaving Findhorn, the Gawlers travelled across Scotland to briefly visit Iona, a small island off the mainland in the Inner Hebrides. Iona has been considered a deeply sacred place, first by Irish druids and then by Christians. Saint Columba was exiled to the island in 563 AD and had established a monastery there. It is a holy island, a place of great spiritual power and a number of kings of Scotland, Ireland and Norway were buried on the tiny, isolated isle (which measures a mere 5 kilometres in length and 2.4 kilometres in width).

Before they left Ian sought out Saint Columba's cell, a circle of stones now the only remnant of where he was believed to have often meditated. Ian sat there for some time in solitary meditation and contemplation.

The trip through the Philippines, India, Egypt and finally to Scotland had been long, but physically and spiritually nourishing. Now it was time for the Gawlers to head home and figure out what they were going to do with the rest of their lives.

There was every reason to be optimistic: the tumours had begun to recede and Ian had started coughing up small pieces of bone as the cancer began to break down in his diseased lung (his cancer, osteogenic sarcoma, resulted in the growing of new bone where it should not be—in Ian's case on his chest, pelvis and the inside of his left lung).

On the way home from Europe they stopped off in Perth and in Adelaide, visiting friends and investigating possible places to settle and start again.

And then, while in Perth on the way back from their recent overseas travels, Ian and Gail had a 'big discussion' about children. It was a long and animated dialogue that lasted—on and off—for the best part of a week. 'Gail had been pretty strong that she didn't want them,' says Ian. 'She'd never held a baby before she had her own and she didn't even like being around little children.'

From there they went to stay with Ian's cousin Glen and his wife Sophie and had another chat about the relative merits of starting a family (they had not been using contraception the previous year, incidentally, assuming the chemotherapy had left the couple unable to conceive).

'And we had this fateful day where she had a major turnaround and said, "Okay, let's do it",' he says. Gail had had a radical and sudden change of heart.

Intention can be a mighty powerful thing. That night they made love and afterwards Ian remembers Gail telling him she had had this 'most amazing experience'. She had an 'image of a big egg floating in space and this little red worm-like thing swimming along and going into the egg,' he remembers. 'Then the whole thing exploded like cosmic fireworks. And it was really quite funny because at the time she didn't know what it meant.' Ian felt sure Gail was pregnant.

They returned to Torquay with no definite plans, apart from the continuing obsession with Ian's getting well.

The next few months drifted by and, despite some strong physical signs that he was on the mend, Ian began to feel himself to be 'a confused spectator' to his inner journey.

> I feel my higher self is really trying to exert itself over my lower
> self and that the conflict is getting rather desperate. I really am
> tiring of the old bad habits and wanting to choose the right path at
> every opportunity. At times its seems almost wilful as I continue to
> eat second rate foods, argue with Gail, not do yoga. Each incident
> becomes a major test, a battle. I am losing less but often my lack of
> will power amazes me.

The months between their return from India in the middle of the
year to December in 1977 marked another period of torpor, despite
the extraordinarily rewarding and meaningful time away. Ian felt
spiritually becalmed.

And then in a journal entry from December that year, Ian berates
himself for letting 'grumpiness and frustration' get on top of him,
although he adds that 'it seems the bottom of a big trough has been
reached and we are on the way up'.

That day the couple did some yoga in the 'warm sunshine,
followed by meditation lying in the sun'. He reports that he had
stopped the coffee enemas three days before, swapping them for
camomile enemas twice a day. They also fasted for the day—an
ongoing commitment not to eat on the first day of each month and
donate the value of that day's food to overseas aid.

> Borrowed from the Mormons it strikes me as an excellent idea, both
> for self regulation of diet, involving the benefits of giving the system
> a rest for a day, and a way of remembering the less fortunate of the
> world's population.

A couple of days later, Ian decided to ring the Commonwealth
Employment Service (Glenyss had been goading him for a while
to enquire about a relocation grant). He discovered that $350 cash,
plus one month's rent was available to them if they could justify a
need to relocate to take up a job interstate. Ian had already been
in touch with Ed Mintz, a veterinary surgeon he knew in Surfers
Paradise in Queensland, about a possible job. Mintz offered him
two days a week—and the relocation grant made it possible for
them to take it up. The couple headed north.

It is clear from his journal entries of the time that looking back on his early working days Ian felt that he had been successful as a vet because he had both an intuitive insight and would have a go at just about anything (he was also, by all accounts, a very accomplished surgeon and could relate very well with the animal's owners). In Queensland, working for Ed Mintz, a man he saw as 'thorough and super professional', Ian hoped to augment his intuitive skills with a little solid experience.

The couple had sold off as many possessions as they could and earned a little much-needed extra cash for the shift to Queensland. In Surfers Paradise they settled happily into a two-storey house in the waterside suburb of Biggera Waters. At the front of the home was a large double garage and it had a large kitchen and living room.

At first they slept on the floor in the living room until Ian built them a new pine bed. Woodwork had been an interest since early school days and he loved building furniture from 'sticks of wood'. The three bedrooms upstairs remained unused. The ground floor opened to a small lawn, where they did their morning yoga. At the back was a canal from which they would often pull fish for dinner—whiting, bream, mangrove jack, flathead and catfish. It was a pleasant place to be, although the job was not working out quite as Ian had hoped.

Mintz was 'a lovely bloke' says Ian today, but 'he was an absolute perfectionist. He would not let me do anything. So for three months I spent two days per week, between 8 am and 2 pm watching him work.' A further two days a week Ian was filling in at a local animal sanctuary desexing stray dogs and cats. The surgery was enjoyable and useful and Ian overcame the monotony in this repetitive work by becoming faster and faster at it. But overall, it was a frustrating return to the workforce—although there was plenty else to occupy Ian's mind.

Just before the couple moved north they had suspected Gail might indeed be pregnant. They had only moved to Surfers Paradise after Gail's GP had 'guaranteed us she wasn't pregnant,' says Ian. 'If she was pregnant we were going to stay in Victoria and if she wasn't we were going to move. He guaranteed she wasn't pregnant, so we moved.' Now in Queensland, the pregnancy was confirmed.

Having been told by his oncologist during the chemotherapy that the treatment he had was likely to leave him sterile, Ian has often wondered over the years if old Mrs Curl's spectacular healing methods had a major part to play in his capacity to become a father.

The pregnancy developed into an extraordinary and exciting time, steeped in possibility, and Ian was overflowing with love and the nervous anticipation of the birth of his first child.

It is a most exciting time. I have difficulty recording my elated emotions and concern for impending responsibilities. I am anxious to raise a child in the best manner.

On an inner level, however, the period in Queensland—and the months before and immediately after—represented a puzzling time for Ian. Physically there was also a serious setback: his chest was almost clear of cancer, his lung and pelvis tumours remained stable, but there was also a new pain in his spine.

Ian visited a local GP who specialised in back complaints and again he was sent for X-rays. 'When the GP read the x-ray report and looked at the pictures, he appeared very worried. He told me that based on what he could sense, he thought that I would be a paraplegic, paralysed from the waist down in a few weeks, perhaps months at the most.'

Ian's response was probably not what the GP expected. 'I laughed and said that after all I had been through, I was sure that this would be okay. I really did dismiss his prognosis out of hand. It was almost like it made me even more determined.'

Ian might have new pain in his spine but he also drew the conclusion that his healing, meditative focus must have been having more effect than he had imagined.

I cannot see a medical explanation for the facts, equating such a large reduction in one area [the chest] with growth elsewhere. It would give credence to the energy ideas that one area is cured, the other not. It may be that the mind has an even larger part to play than I thought—I certainly have been concentrating most of my energies on the chest bumps and their demise.

Ian believed that the reason why the chest was improving more rapidly than the pelvis was to do with the quality of the imagery that he was doing. He felt that he had greater success visualising his chest free of growth, because the lumps could be clearly seen, but not so much success with the pelvis because the growths were out of view and he lacked confidence visualising them.

Ian was at a loss which direction to now take—he had tried just about everything. He rang Ainslie Meares for advice, and Meares suggested two weeks of intensive meditation in Melbourne. Ian consulted another local doctor who suggested further chemotherapy, but Ian rejected it out of hand.

We are at a very critical time where I must show that the natural methods, the Divine Healing Power, is equal to the situation. It is unfortunate that my eclectic series of treatments, which have included chemotherapy, give the unconvinced a way out to explain my situation; my ongoing survival. For me too it is a test of my convictions. Chemotherapy holds no attractions but it remains difficult to see the best course to take.

Around this time, as well as uncertainty as to his next step, it suddenly struck Ian that up until his illness and operation he had never felt 'hard done by' before. 'I have always seen a purpose in everything and been content with my lot,' he wrote. Remarkably even through the early days after the amputation, depression was never a problem for the young vet, but now an element of self-pity had crept in for the first time.

Reading the diaries it is hard to ascertain how deep the self-wallowing was, although Ian does admit to spending idle time musing over how he could have spent the $100,000 he would have earned at the Bacchus Marsh practice by then, if the cancer had not suddenly appeared on the scene.

And then, in the next breath, Ian writes:

> ... how quick one is to lose sight of the benefits of one's situation and become caught by the aspirations of the general populace, losing sight of the higher ideals and one's true spirituality ... these present difficulties are hard to understand but they must be of our own making. Perhaps we have taken too much for granted. We will certainly appreciate home when we find it.

Now that the couple's first child was steadily growing inside Gail, and with Ian's job not turning out how he had planned, it was time to set down roots and settle somewhere suitable for the baby's arrival; and somewhere Ian could find a little more job satisfaction. After considering all their options and contemplating them deeply, the couple committed to moving to Adelaide, leasing a veterinary practice in the south of that city.

But first they had to honour a 'quiet promise' that Ian had made in India—to go back and thank Sai Baba if he recovered. The large growths on his chest were almost gone and Ian hoped to both honour the promise and, perhaps most importantly, restore his confidence in his ongoing healing into the bargain.

Ian's vitality and health were riding high at the time, but he also wrote that he still harboured a lingering 'fear of the spinal problem and the cancer as a whole'.

> My confidence is a little low probably because of the lack of harmony and prayer. Prayer leads to forgiveness and Grace, and they are what I feel I need at the moment. Is that the purpose of going to Sai Baba again—to seek the Grace of the Guru?

The only problem was, they were penniless. Undaunted, Ian and Gail booked two plane tickets to India anyway, filled with an unshakeable conviction that the funds to pay for them would manifest themselves. When it came time to pay for the tickets, the couple sent the airline what they thought was a 'dud cheque', says Ian. 'It was a great act of faith.'

Incredibly, their trust was rewarded. The tickets arrived and off they flew—completely taking for granted the fact that the funds had somehow miraculously appeared in their bank account to cover the cost.

It was only years later that they discovered what had happened. Ian had always held an interest in art and antiques and when there were funds available he would make purchases. As his illness had progressed—and they had moved from Kippen Ross, to Torquay and then to Queensland—it became necessary to gradually divest themselves of most of their possessions to pay their bills. Ian had reluctantly given a couple of things to his father to sell when the opportunity presented itself. The most valuable item was a much-loved original painting by noted artist Arthur Boyd.

The months passed and Ian completely forgot about the painting. Unbeknown to the couple, a few days before the plane tickets were to be paid for, the painting was sold. Ian's father had deposited the funds into his account without having a chance to mention it to his son before his departure. The amount covered the cost of the tickets almost exactly. Manifestation indeed.

In the couple of weeks before their departure Ian's journal is filled with insecurity and uncertainty. There was a great yearning for a spiritual breakthrough, mixed with confusion about the right path and a need for a stable place to call home.

> The things of the spirit have been so unclear for us lately, that to have a shallow foundation on the physical from which to work, makes striving so much harder.

And then a letter from friends in South Africa brought a 'great boost'. It expressed in words something Ian had not yet fully digested. The friends wrote that Ian's 'healing may be a light for others to follow'. The contents of that letter proved a powerful motivating force for Ian, reminding him of both his 'great responsibilities in this matter' and providing some portents of his future path.

We have been blessed to touch so many more. I cannot see how we can have had so much help in the past, and been led to so many who needed encouragement only to lose it now. The thought gives Gail great reassurance I know, and should help me in times to come . . . I feel sure my disease should be transmuted through service and cry out for the opportunity to give it. It has been frustrating these last few months not to be able to see direction or feel useful.

Norma too was corresponding regularly with the Gawlers with letters 'full of insight and understanding' and, sometimes, verse.

> Have faith little sparrow
> for the seed is here
> But the season is not quite ripe
> Yours is the gift of the golden pear
> if your Faith
> Stays big and bright

Norma's letters seemed to 'speak without words yet we need to get the letters to draw on her great help', wrote Ian. He realised the reason for feeling tense, irritable and disenchanted had been because of his sense of uselessness. Re-reading Ainslie Meares' book *Relief without Drugs* also brought Ian the understanding that he had allowed a great deal of physical tension to build up in his body over recent months. 'Since re-reading and practising his methods things have been much better. I feel the letting go. I do manage to release the physical tension, and more now, I enter into a different level of being. I am getting closer to the silence.'

Another point of uncertainty also revealed itself:

I continually affirm my allegiance to Christ in whom I have all Faith and direct my prayers. Here again is a source of conflict as I have difficulty resolving this allegiance with devotion to Sai Baba. I don't doubt the latter's powers or high development but I do have difficulty putting him on the same level as the man I know as Jesus the Christ. I want desperately to be able to do so and ask for a sign but nothing comes it seems. It appears my lot is to work things out for myself but I would dearly like to have more faith in Baba. Perhaps a second visit will resolve the matter. I fear being wrong as much as being right.

Despite this uncertainty, a few days before they left for India Ian had an important breakthrough.

It followed a frustrating visit to see Ainslie Meares where he had sought how to reach the 'deeper stillness' in meditation that Ian knew was there. Meares' response had been to simply to say that it was 'easy' and that all he had to do was 'let go'.

'I thought, you silly old bugger and I came away from that meeting really pissed off,' he says. 'I felt that he hadn't told me anything useful at all.'

Ian returned to Gail's sister's home, where they were staying, in a filthy mood. He shut himself away alone and lay down to meditate. 'I was cranky, so annoyed, so frustrated, that I just abandoned the whole idea of meditation entirely.' It was then that he had the 'profound experience' he so desperately sought.

> I seemed to relax very completely and become very still. I really do not know if I was breathing or not; certainly whatever there was, was very slow and shallow. Then I seemed to break through a hole in the centre of my field of awareness, to a calmer, stiller area and I heard myself cry out 'my soul, my soul, my soul'. It seemed to last but a brief moment and I was back in the normal state of deep relaxation.

After Ian came out of the experience, he was, as he remembers, 'manic for about an hour and a half', thrilled that he had broken through to another level in his meditation. The following night the couple visited old friend Tom Barrett and his wife Sue for dinner and 'I think I made an absolute fool of myself,' he says. 'I was completely out of character, talking flat out about all sorts of things; I was like the kid who had just broken into the lolly shop.'

He had broken through to a level he had thought he would never reach, and was bubbling with a sense of renewed, inexhaustible energy.

March 8, 1978. Sai Baba's arrival into the hall was greeted with an eruption of joyful clapping and singing.

Baba walked amongst the crowd for a little while and then took up his position in a gold-draped seat. Next to his seat was an enrobed and garlanded statue of Krishna. There were garlanded photos of the man everywhere and bowls of fruit offerings. The floor was decorated with flower petals arranged in delicate patterns. Baba talked for about an hour and a half, his words translated into English. Much of what he said Ian and Gail found too obscure to make much sense of, although a few things did cut through— including the importance of sticking to one path, the importance of following that path determinedly, and being of unshakeable faith.

The following days were spent in a routine of twice daily darshan and basking in Sai Baba's extraordinary presence. Baba spent time among his devotees and imparting wisdom from his chair. There was some casual recognition for Ian and Gail from Baba in the first couple of days, but Ian secretly hoped that 'an interview may be in the plan'.

Ian took it that all devotees and spiritual seekers had come to Baba with their own limitations and sought to be uplifted by his presence, but he could also see that finding the 'Divinity within oneself' was his ultimate goal.

'We must take advantage of the presence of the Avatar,' he wrote, going on to describe Baba as a 'Divine Manifestation—so it would seem very reasonable to address oneself to God through him. Surely this is worship.'

Ian was appreciative of any contact with the master, however small, and during one Thursday night's darshan Baba approached Ian and gave the second finger on his right hand a big squeeze.

I feel it will now have enhanced healing ability and feel further blessed and infused with His vibrations from close range.

Other days the couple received no recognition at all.

It was during this visit, however, that they were given a powerful demonstration of Baba's most astonishing gift: the ability to manifest objects, apparently out of nowhere.

At Ooty, the hill station he used as an ashram, Baba had decided to hand the buildings over to the local community as a kindergarten. Ian and Gail were fortunate enough to be present for the handover and to sit right up the very front at the official ceremony, with only rows of very young Indian children, dressed in their Sunday best, in front of them. Sai Baba and the children sang bhajans, the traditional sacred songs of India, and there was a 'very deep state of reverence in the air'.

Then Sai Baba asked the headmistress to step forward—at which stage the Indian mystic was between 4 and 6 feet away, says Ian. Baba put his arm out with his palm down and rotated it in the air. He then turned his palm up and there appeared, from nowhere, a statue of Shiva sitting on his palm that was 'about 3 inches high and about 3 inches across the base'! Ian was astonished.

He remembers carefully noting at the time that Sai Baba's sleeve was 'quite free of his arm' and his sleeve 'went only to about the elbow' as he held his arm out. For Ian there was simply no suggestion of a magician-like sleight of hand.

Sai Baba is known for having spontaneously manifested food, jewellery and objects, as if from mid-air, on a daily basis since he was a boy. Countless people have witnessed this phenomenon over the years. Many are positive they are true miracles, others are equally convinced it is nothing more than a magician's trick.

Anxious to find out the truth for himself, Icelandic social scientist Dr Erlendur Haraldsson (he was professor of psychology at the University of Iceland at the time, now retired) spent a period of ten years investigating reports of Sai Baba's mystical abilities during the 1970s and 1980s. Haraldsson spent a total of eleven months in India gathering material. His book *Modern Miracles* details his findings. In it he recounts countless eyewitness reports of Sai Baba apparently materialising from his hand everything from fruit out of season, to food so hot it is hard to hold, to gold chains, rings and statues.

Haraldsson met Sai Baba many times—and was allowed to observe his work countless times—but still continually asked the mystic to be tested under controlled scientific conditions. Sai Baba always declined, arguing that he could not use his powers for demonstrations. 'Divine power can only be used for the good and protection of devotees,' he had said.

On one visit Haraldsson had been talking with Sai Baba when the great man had mentioned something called a 'double rudraksha'. Haraldsson asked him, through an interpreter, what this 'double rudraksha' was but did not receive an answer. The conversation moved on, but Haraldsson wanted to know what this object was and would not let it go. He asked him repeatedly and insistently until Sai Baba, clearly impatient with the question, closed his fist, waved it around a few times, and then opened it again, saying, 'This is it.'

In his hand were two rudrakshas—or acorn-like objects—that had grown together. After Haraldsson and his companion had examined it, Sai Baba then indicated that he would like to make a present of it to them, took it back in his hands, blew on it and opened his hands again.

'The double rudraksha was now covered, on the top and bottom,' writes Haraldsson, 'by two tiny, oval-shaped, golden shields that were held together . . . by a short golden chain at each side.'

Haraldsson had the strong feeling the moment was spontaneous, but wondered if Baba could have planned the event. The academic later took the object to a London jeweller who confirmed that the gold shields were 22 carats. He also discovered that a double rudraksha was a 'rare anomaly in nature' and Indian experts he showed it to had never seen a finer specimen in all their days.

A number of Indian scientists have also observed Sai Baba over many years, including the director of the Indian Institute of Science and the former Vice-Chancellor of Bangalore University, both of whom were convinced of Sai Baba's genuineness. On Haraldsson's own trips to India to study Sai Baba, eight in total, the academic usually took a number of researchers. Twice he was accompanied by Dr Karlis Osis of the American Society of Psychical Research, once by Dr Michael Thalbourne of Washington University and once by Dr Joop Houtkooper of the University of Amsterdam.

They interviewed dozens of people who had known or worked with Sai Baba over the years and investigated reports of his miracles as well as 'critical rumours' hoping to get to the truth of the matter.

Without being able to demonstrate a scientific method, and depending essentially on the eyewitness accounts—and the testimony of their own eyes—they could not prove the veracity of Sai Baba's apparently miraculous abilities, but nor did they find any evidence it was a hoax. The book *Modern Miracles* is the result of their research.

After the handover ceremony at the kindergarten—and the utterly incredible materialisation of the statuette—the Gawlers decided to follow Sai Baba, much like many of his devotees would often do, to his next destination.

So sought after is the mystic, however (over one million devotees, including the then Prime Minister and President of India turned up to celebrate Sai Baba's seventieth birthday in 1996) that his whereabouts at any given time are kept relatively secret.

After the ceremony at the kindergarten, Sai Baba's motorcade came around to the front of the building and the great man drove off, with his most zealous devotees in hot pursuit. The Gawlers meanwhile were still at the kindergarten, content to take their time after being such close witness to the sweet kindergarten ceremony. And then the cars returned.

Sai Baba had got into his car, taken a couple of turns around the block, somehow shaken off most of the faithful, and then looped back to the kindergarten.

After an hour or so Baba and his entourage took off again and headed for Bangalore. This time the Gawlers followed along behind at a 'respectful distance' with their driver, Abdul, and a friend they were travelling with, a Canadian confined to a wheelchair.

Later, deep in a large state forest known for its wild animals including tigers, they came across Sai Baba's entourage parked at the base of a track winding up a nearby hill. The pregnant Gail and Ian were informed by devotees waiting in their cars that they were not to go up the hill. Ian, however, decided 'to give it a go' and persuaded Gail to head up the hill on foot to find Sai Baba, leaving Abdul and the Canadian at the bottom with the car.

It was the middle of the day, it was hot, and the hill became steeper as they walked slowly up the narrow road wending its way through the dense jungle of the state park. After about twenty minutes there was a sudden commotion in the undergrowth not far to the right off the track.

Immediately preceding this Ian had begun to wonder if they were doing the right thing. He says that silently he had asked for a 'sign' of what they should do—should they keep walking, should they go back? Now came a very clear and strong sign. 'It was obviously a big animal,' says Ian, 'and because I'd asked for a sign, I thought, cripes, if it is a tiger, then we have made a mistake.'

Whatever was crashing through the jungle was getting closer, and closer, then it broke through about 20 feet ahead of them. Out of the vegetation lumbered a big Brahmin cow—the sacred animal of India. It stopped in the middle of the road, stared directly at Ian and Gail 'as if to say, well, are you coming?' and turned and started walking up the hill, 'almost as if it was leading us upwards'.

The Gawlers followed the cow for another fifteen or twenty minutes, until she stopped, turned around and stared at them again, this time 'as if to say, you can go on ahead without me now,' says Ian. They walked on and once they had passed the animal, she turned and headed back down the hill.

A little bit further on the couple came to a fork in the road where they found five men, sitting. By now Ian, already well versed in metaphysics and the underlying meaning of a situation (and given their encounter with the sacred cow), took them to be a direct representation of the five senses—sight, hearing, smell, touch and taste—which, for any student of either Hinduism or Buddhism, are of key significance. On an ordinary level they might relate to the five senses, but they also relate to more transcendent truths on the wheel of life. As Ian was aware, the five senses give rise to feelings of desire or craving, which in turn gives rise to attachment, which in turn leads to the never ending cycle of birth and death.

In straightforward terms the Gawlers were wondering which of the two forks in the road to take and were clearly being instructed—on a symbolic level—to let their five senses, as represented by the five Indian men, guide them. 'We didn't actually say anything to these guys,' says Ian. 'They just pointed which way to go.'

By now the road was becoming steeper and the couple had been walking for about an hour. 'It must have been about two o'clock by then. We were hot. Gail was pregnant, and I was plugging away on my crutches,' says Ian. 'We were wondering what would happen next, when we turned the next corner and came across a policeman in the middle of the road.' The man called out to the Gawlers to turn around and go back. 'He was very emphatic but I just said to Gail to pretend he's not there and keep on walking. So we did.'

The closer they got, the more agitated the policeman became. He was shouting that the couple could not go any further and waving his stick imposingly above his head. The Gawlers just kept walking as if he was not there.

'As we got within 6 feet of him, it was just like somebody had pulled a pin. He collapsed. He couldn't handle it,' Ian says. The policeman's shoulders slumped, his stick by his side, he took a couple of stumbling steps to the side of the road and let them pass.

A further hundred metres or so, just before they reached the top of the hill where a colonial building with large verandas stood, the couple began to hear bhajans, devotional Hindu songs, filling the air. Moving closer, they saw that a circular road looped around in front of the building where there was also a large shady tree. The Gawlers decided to sit under the tree, enjoy the singing, and see what happened.

'We had barely sat down when the singing stopped,' Ian says, 'and Sai Baba's cars came from the back to the side of the building.' Sai Baba emerged from the building almost at the same moment. He strode towards the car and an open door, but then stopped and paused and walked around to the other side of the car where Ian and Gail were near.

'As he went to get into that side of the car he looked across at me, we made direct eye contact, and it felt like I had been hit between the eyes with a bolt of lightning,' says Ian. 'It felt like a blinding flash of light suddenly filled my third eye area', the spot between the eyebrows and just above the nose. 'It was physical. Tangible. It felt like I had been knocked backwards. I wasn't knocked off my feet or anything but it was very strong.'

Sai Baba drove past, very close to the couple and gave them a wave and a smile, and disappeared down the hill. All the other cars followed on, leaving Ian and Gail all alone.

Still recovering from the walk and their extraordinary encounter, they sat quite content to wait, expecting that Abdul would drive up to collect them.

And it was then that Ian had another of his breakthroughs; a sense that things were really falling into place.

In that moment it became obvious to him that a big reason for this particular trip to India was to question what to do with the rest of his life. And here, as the trip neared its end, they had become swept up in the metaphorical answer.

'On the spiritual path you have these opportunities to climb to a point where you can have a peak experience. This had literally happened for us by coming up the winding path to the top of the hill and having such a direct encounter with Sai Baba,' he explains. 'But what do you do from there? Do you just stay sitting on the mountain or do you do something with the experience, the insight? So we sat there for a bit and reflected. It seemed to me that if you do have that sort of experience, then the choice you have is to stay where you are, or you transcend and go off into space, or you go back down the hill and integrate—put the experience into your daily life.'

For Ian the metaphor was clear. It was as if he had been climbing a spiritual mountain for ages. Now he had reached the top and he had been introduced to a spiritual view. And there was nowhere else to go. Now he had to make his way back down into the marketplace and put his experience to good use.

Ian and Gail began walking back down the hill, still expecting to have Abdul reach them at any moment. But they walked on and on, until finally, after about 30 minutes they did hear the sound of a car approaching. They were amazed to discover that rather than Abdul, it was one of Sai Baba's cars that had come back to pick them up.

It turns out that their own driver had been pressured to take the Canadian to find a toilet. The diarrhoea he was suffering at the time had become worse in Ian and Gail's absence.

Meanwhile, well on the way to Bangalore, Sai Baba 'had somehow worked out that we were stuck and sent one of his cars back for us.' The car drove them via Bangalore to Whitefield ashram where Sai Baba was staying. There he had organised for his devotees to sing bhajans through the entire night.

'We stayed up all night singing and in the morning he came into the gathering,' says Ian. There was a group of 'three, four, maybe five hundred people' and he told them that anyone who had sung all night, as Ian and Gail had been, was 'absolved of all our previous karma'.

It was an extraordinary statement.

Sai Baba was effectively suggesting that in an eye-blink all the karma—all the harmful actions and their effects, amassed since beginningless time from countless previous lives—was summarily wiped clean!

The Gawlers flew on to the the city of Pune, in western India, for a few days to visit friends and hopefully meet Sai Baba once more at his ashram there. As it turned out, Sai Baba had left the site to spend time in Delhi. It was 12 March.

That evening in bed Ian spent a long time gradually relaxing his body, as Ainslie Meares had taught him—and which had become very much part of his daily routine.

He concentrated primarily on his foot, hoping to then move progressively up his body 'but it took a concentrated effort to induce much of a feeling of relaxation or letting go in it,' he says. Ian persevered and finally achieved 'reasonable relaxation', quickly followed by a 'great sensation of the energies associated with my pelvic bumps being whisked away.' Yet another important breakthrough.

> It was just as if a breath of wind had blown it all away leaving a clean hollow in its place. I feel sure, I am sure, the bumps will go quite rapidly now.

That night he slept well, woke at 6 am feeling cold and put on a shirt. He went back to sleep, only to awake at 8 am bathed in sweat.

Ian was still coughing intermittently and bringing up pieces of bone from his diseased lung. However by 18 March—the previous few days marked by back pain, heavy coughing and diarrhoea—Ian felt that a 'big block' has lifted and it has 'finally begun to flow. It has meant my back mobility has steadily returned with exercise . . . Gail's massages have helped balance things out greatly.'

By 23 March they were back in the presence of Baba.

> It felt like coming home to peace . . . Baba is a storehouse of all and acts for us to point the way along the path to our own self realisation and liberation. It is a great privilege to be in His presence.

Ian wrote at length and in great detail—possibly more than at any other time in his life, except perhaps in the Philippines—and his jottings from the time are questioning and introspective and relate to everything from the profound to the apparently mundane. At one moment he might be wondering aloud at the Indians' ability to be able to sit on hard surfaces for hours without concern, at another describing a lunch of vegetable soup, boiled beans, carrots and rice. You get the sense that every moment, however apparently small, was weighted with subtlety and meaning for Ian; every second crisp, vibrant and experienced in the present moment.

> It is incredible how just being around this centre of energies can have such an effect with so little happening on the overt, discernible side. All is subtle and in harmony.

On 24 March, Good Friday, Ian planned to offer the crucifix he carried on a chain around his neck to Baba to 'see if he chooses to do anything with it. Perhaps then I can reach an understanding of His relationship to the Christ.'

Quite explicitly Christ was the guiding light in Ian's life and, more than that, he also wrote on this, a pivotal day in the Christian calendar, that he hoped the 'message of the crucifixion and resurrection can be mirrored in my life that the lower self may die away completely and leave the radiant higher self a tribute to God'.

Later Ian held up his cross to Baba, who paused to look at it deeply then squeezed the forefinger of Ian's left hand 'near where the cross was resting'.

That day they enjoyed a lunch of brown bread, tomato and cheese, something he rarely ate. Ian wrote of how much they now enjoyed the most simple of foods.

> It is bad to enjoy exotic food. I think of how I used to seek it out and pay for it; now I am getting far more pleasure from simple fare. It will be good to return home and establish that routine also. I think the odd cassata or some such may keep my cravings quite satisfied as I turn fully to pure food. We have been shown so clearly the benefits of pure food in India. I feel it will resolve many of my difficulties. You just cannot improve on good, natural food. It can be made better, however, in the cooking process and there Gail is becoming an artisan too.

It was time to head home and, as Ian's journal entry recorded, they would be returning with hearts more full of joy, trust and belief than they could possibly have hoped. Ian had come to accept Baba as his 'spiritual guide and mentor,' he wrote. His faith, complex and sometimes confused at the outset of the trip, had found stability and focus.

> I still feel the Christ energy is the ultimate perfection for this planet and it is to its purity that we aspire, but I feel now Baba has me under personal guidance, that he is my Master who will ultimately lead me to that goal.

With their first child on the way and with Ian's health on the up, they were also headed home brimming with gratitude for their experiences and new understanding and with a seemingly boundless optimism for the future.

We both feel greatly contented and full to the brim with the joy of having been so close to Baba's influence once again. We received so much Grace it is hard not to feel unworthy. It makes us strong in our own Divinity to go back into the world and try again to live spiritually and help positively influence others. I feel we needed this extra strength to walk in the light of Spirituality and by so doing being a quiet, subtle example of the possibilities. All we do is becoming aligned with the inner I AM and we must be happier and more content as we approach true reality of expression. At times I pale at the problems we still have to resolve but yet there is a great confidence that the Divine Plan is in operation and if we obey the rules, follow the guidelines and remain within Baba's influence, all will be overcome. We have done so much in the last two years and changed so much surely for the better, that the prospect of maintaining that impetus over the ensuing years is very exciting. There are no limitations.

9

Old Noarlunga

Returning from Sai Baba for the second time with a 'confidence that service is our life and Adelaide is our home', Ian and Gail Gawler leased a veterinary practice in suburban Morphett Vale. Money was tight and Gail was six months pregnant. They stayed for about six weeks with Ian's cousin Glen at first, before moving into a new two-bedroom unit on the Onkaparinga river at Noarlunga, a small town just south of Adelaide, five minutes by road from the surgery.

Ian's health was mixed. He was feeling well and sleeping well. The growths on his chest were completely gone and there was little back pain and no pelvic problems. However, an incessant cough remained. As did the night sweats, arriving intermittently and unheralded.

On Monday and Tuesday 10 and 11 April he sweated profusely all day and night. He put himself on a mono diet—eating only grapes for ten days—hoping to clear out his system; the regular habit of coffee enemas also returned.

On the dietary front they had pulled back substantially from the zealotry of the Gerson days.

It is really good to be back on good food . . . I will eat as well as I can in the given circumstances. The big thing is not to make a thing of it. The meditation is going well. I seem at last to have caught the simplicity of it and instead of relaxing each section of my body I am doing it as a larger whole, using the mind more and feeling the whole body letting go, beyond relaxation into the calm of deep peace.

When Ian's leg was first amputated he meditated for half an hour, then for five hours when the secondaries were diagnosed. By this stage he had settled into 'about three hours per day' using a 'very simple and uncomplicated method of getting the body both physically relaxed and mind still'—very much along the lines Ainslie Meares had taught him. He had also used prayer and imagery, most notably at times when he was being treated. During the chemotherapy he had imagined 'the chemotherapy being effective, and it not affecting the rest of my body; just destroying the cancer cells.'

Meanwhile Gail's pregnancy was developing smoothly. The couple were keen to make sure their first child came into the world gently, at home, using the Leboyer birthing method.

Named after the French obstetrician Frederick Leboyer, the method ensures the birth happens in a quiet room rather than under the bright lights and clinical atmosphere of a hospital. Instead of the umbilical cord being cut immediately, under the Leboyer method the newborn is placed tenderly, still attached, onto the chest of its mother. Once the baby relaxes a little with the contact with its mother, it is then placed into a warm, body-temperature bath. This water supports the baby and enables it to relax even more. Voices remain hushed throughout.

Gail was adamant about having a gentle, non-conventional birth (remembering these were the days when newborns were still often held upside down and slapped on the behind to make them cry and draw their first breath). 'So adamant,' says Ian, 'that she did not even want to see a medico beforehand. She told me that me being a vet, she had full confidence in my being able to deliver our baby. I explained that while I was very keen to be there and of course had helped at the births of animals ranging from mice to horses,

I had never even seen a human baby being born and I felt I at least needed back-up.' So a compromise was reached in the form of Dr David Mitchell—the only doctor they could find who was delivering babies using the Leboyer method in Adelaide at the time.

Meanwhile, the couple were working very long hours getting the business established and Ian found he was getting unduly tired at the end of the day. Then his knee started to swell.

Ian had not had any formal medical tests done since the x-rays that had found new growths on the spine and predicted paraplegia. Now he contacted Adelaide oncologist Dr Alistair Robertson who, after examining him fully, ordered more x-rays. The results were very startling for a couple of reasons.

Robertson, looking at Ian's recent medical history, says today he would not have been surprised at all to discover that there was still evidence of cancer throughout his body. But remarkably, wonderfully, the extraordinary news was that Ian was in complete remission. 'So that was good,' says Ian, in typical understatement.

Robertson says the x-rays left him astounded. 'His chest x-rays showed an incredible improvement from the point of view of there being no evidence or minimal evidence of bone in his lung,' he says. Three or four years before, the x-rays had shown a mass of bone had grown inside his lung as the osteogenic sarcoma had taken hold. Now all the metastases 'with bone in them,' says Robertson— the secondary cancers that had grown on his hip, chest and inside his lung—'had more or less disappeared.'

As Robertson puts it, 'There did not appear to be a good reason for that, because although he did have some medical treatment, he didn't have very much. I was absolutely flabbergasted by what he had done, because osteogenic sarcoma is not a thing that people survive very long from—particularly when they have had metastases. From the point of view of oncology it would be very unusual for a person to respond in that sort of way and to go on improving.'

Robertson says he has only seen one other cancer recovery that even approaches such a miraculous turnaround in all his years of practice: a patient who had metastases from a primary cancer (and a patient in later years to whom he gave chemotherapy, he adds). 'She was a regular church-goer, prayed and had her whole family pray for her, changed her diet and did a whole lot of things. She is now cured from metastases in her liver from bowel cancer. And that is, again, more or less unheard of.'

What really struck Robertson on meeting Ian, though, was his 'serenity,' he says. 'It was very impressive and very unusual for the situations that I have seen him in.'

The most immediate 'situation' he is referring to being the fact that Robertson had to break the news that despite being clear of cancer, Ian was suffering with tuberculosis. And almost paradoxically, that was why his leg was swelling! Ian now had a condition which was labouring under the long and impressive title of hypertrophic osteoarthropathy. The TB in his chest was causing a reaction in his knee and this was producing the swelling.

Ian dug out his old chest x-rays from when he had first been diagnosed with secondary growth in his left lung. Sure enough, when Robertson examined them, although difficult to see, there was evidence of TB being present two years previously. This was around the time of his chemotherapy. It may well be that as the chemo dropped his immune defence, the TB flared. Having focused on the cancer growth in his chest, nobody, it seems, had seen beyond the tumour to see this other very serious infection. Suddenly the night sweats, the chronic cough, the loss of weight—all consistent with the symptoms of a tuberculosis infection—made more sense.

More than that—Gail suggests the presence of TB could possibly have been a key factor in Ian's getting well.

'That's something that has certainly passed through my mind since,' says Dr Robertson. 'There may be something in that. If an infection is a chronic infection [as it was in Ian's case] the build-up of immunity is very significant and I think that may have done something towards the cure of his cancer.'

The day after his diagnosis with TB, Ian went for an appointment with the Adelaide chest clinic. There, he and Gail confronted a 'rather forceful woman doctor who was keen to lock me up in one of their TB wards on the spot,' he says.

She explained that tuberculosis is an infectious disease, contagious to those in regular and close contact with the infected person. Then the really bad news. Babies, it seems, are very susceptible to TB. Having Ian in the same airspace as his newborn child was simply out of the question. Having Ian at the birth was out of the question. Having a home birth was out of the question.

Ian and Gail were devastated. 'This was a really cruel blow,' says Ian. 'I could barely believe it.'

The joy of being cancer-free gave way to a huge argument between Ian and the TB specialist who was determined that Ian should be admitted straight away into a specialist chest hospital. Ian was desperate to be at the birth and remembers suggesting perhaps he could attend in an aqualung. 'She thought it was a silly idea,' he laughs. 'I thought it had merit.'

Finally Ian said to her, 'If you put me in hospital, they will feed me crappy food and it'll give me cancer again and I'll die and my wife will sue you personally.' His serenity had momentarily vanished. In the back of his mind, Ian admits, he was thinking through how he would make good his escape.

It did not come to that. In the end the doctor agreed that Ian could go home on the proviso that as soon as his wife went into labour, he would have to check himself into the chest clinic and Gail would have the baby in a hospital.

Back home, the couple discussed their dilemma into the early hours. For Gail, it was particularly difficult. Fully expecting a natural home birth, she now had to readjust to being in a hospital, without Ian.

Finally exhausted, the two fell into bed at 1 am. At least now they could sleep and face the trials of their situation in the morning.

Or at least that is what they thought—instead, they had barely closed their leaden eyes when Gail's waters broke and she went into labour. Ian immediately got on the phone to Dr David Mitchell to call for his help. Having been so confident of a home birth, they had not even booked a hospital.

Mitchell, it turns out, kept a vineyard in his spare time and had been indulging with friends in the fermented bounty of his industry the previous evening. Now, in the early hours of the morning he struggled at first to understand what Ian was saying. Eventually he suggested that Ian take his wife straight to the local hospital at Blackwood. Mitchell rang ahead to organise it. Ian dropped Gail off in the early hours, they said their farewells and Ian drove off to present himself at the TB ward of another hospital.

Mitchell made his way to the maternity ward, and was 'revived with copious cups of coffee by the nursing staff,' says Gail. Two hours later, a healthy little girl was born. 'It was very straightforward,' says Gail. With the aid of a midwife, Mitchell delivered Rosemary using the Leboyer method.

Ian, meanwhile, was lying in a hospital bed alone, unable to be present at the birth of his own child. He would remain there for another week—in a 'very subdued' state, instructed he could not share the same airspace as his daughter until he had been given the all clear. 'The trusty medicos said that they thought it would take quite a long time, given my rather chequered medical career by then,' says Ian. He was told it could easily take a year, or four months at an 'absolute minimum'.

> Rosemary's birth in my forced absence has left me feeling like a shrivelled up dried up pea. It is as if the TB that has me in [one] hospital and she and Gail in another has shrivelled the last vestiges of my emotions. It is no doubt good that after two years of the infection I should find out about it the day before my child's birth, but its cruel ramifications strike hard.

Fortunately Ian was able to rent the flat next door to where the couple were living at Old Noarlunga and checked out of hospital after a week. His first sight of Rosemary was through glass (she is so 'small and petite', he recorded in his journal).

Soon all the outer windows of the flat were covered in marks where Ian had pressed his face against the window to look at his first born. Meanwhile he knuckled down and intensified doing the things he knew best to regain his health. He underwent conventional medical treatment for the disease, meditated three hours each day, paid particular attention to his diet again and recommenced the juices. He was given the all clear from TB in a fairly miraculous three weeks.

Back at work, things were soon up to their usual hectic pace. Gail, in typically accomplished fashion, had trained the nursing staff to keep the veterinary practice well run and shipshape in her absence and was often there with Rosemary in arms. 'I'd help in difficult surgery and things like that,' she says.

By October a vacant plot of land adjacent to the surgery, covered in rubble, was converted into a vegetable garden using Ester Dean's no-dig gardening method. Ian went to a series of lectures run by an authority on organic gardening, Peter Bennett. This complemented ideas gained at Findhorn and soon the garden beside the surgery was supplying a bountiful range of organic vegetables for the flat-dwelling couple. It was a significant moment and, as Ian wrote, one that marked a 'new phase in our lives in tangible form'. The garden also proved to be a major source of interest and discussion for people who brought their animals to the clinic.

As our embryonic family grows in the nourishment of mutual love so too will the garden flow, bear fruit and recycle the energies, building them stronger and finer in an ever- upward spiral.

Rosemary was thirteen weeks old at the time this was written and Ian also wrote that his wife was 'blossoming as a mother'. They were working towards becoming self-sufficient and so they planted butter-nut and bush pumpkins, cucumber, rockmelon, zucchini, beetroot, tomatoes, capsicum, lettuce, passionfruit vines and rhubarb.

Ian's weight had increased to 60 kilograms (nine and a half stone).

I am enjoying the secure feeling that extra padding brings. This last week I have begun to eat less as my weight seems to be peaking and levelling out. I feel less intrusion from pain than ever before and although the meditation times have not been long lately, all seems well.

Spring was in full bloom and Ian's journal was bursting with enthusiasm at the successes in their garden; he felt this sense of renewal was taking place 'within me as well'. His thoughts returned to the discussion he had had with Gail four years before, early in their relationship, when he made it clear he did not want the attachment and responsibility that a serious relationship would bring.

With their first child now born and the rigours and adventures of the road to health now behind them, how strange these words must have seemed to him then.

By 1978, looking back, Ian maintains that his reticence to get too involved or form a 'lasting bond' were based in a belief 'that I might have to leave society in the future and lead some form of isolated spiritual life. The image was not clear—just a sense of leaving what I was doing.' In light of the fact that he had always had trouble imagining himself beyond the age of 27 (he was, by then, 28) he now supposed that the cancer and amputation was the event he had foreseen.

What powerfully remained was the yearning for a spiritual life. Ian articulated a sense that his healing had left him with knowledge he could impart to others—although it remained to be seen how— but he was at least pleased to be giving 'service' at the veterinary practice to atone for 'the short-sighted motives of Bacchus Marsh'.

Having meditated lying down ever since the back problems had flared at Kippen Ross, now Ian returned to meditating sitting up. He would sit up in bed on top of a pillow, his back resting against the bedhead.

> I feel a greater tranquillity and depth . . . the nearness of the silence and all therein sends thrills of tremulous joy through my being.

Life with Gail and Rosemary was sweet.

> I am struck by what karmic links must had led Gail and me together and how we helped each other. She has put so much into my resurrection with massage, care, unceasing positivity and, in my turn,

Ian's paternal grandparents, Oswald
and Doris Gawler.

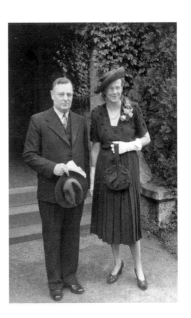

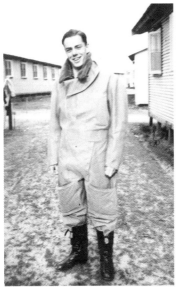

Ian's father Alan in new flying suit
and boots during navigator training
for the Royal Australian Air Force, Mt
Gambier, South Australia, 1941.

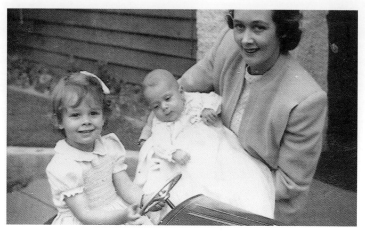

Baby Ian, 1950, with sister Susan, three years his senior, and their mother Billie.

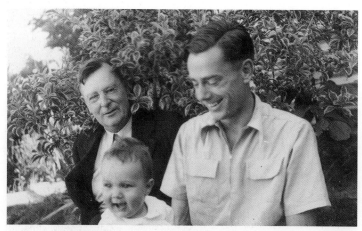

Christmas Day, 1951. Three generations of Gawlers—Ian with his grandfather, Oswald and father, Alan.

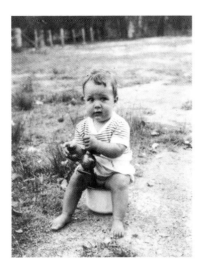

Potty training, 1951. The only time young Ian would ever sit still.

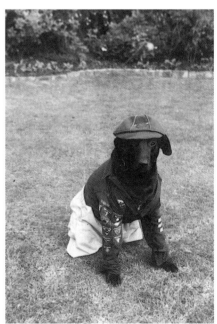

Ian's much loved and trusted companion, Bimbo.

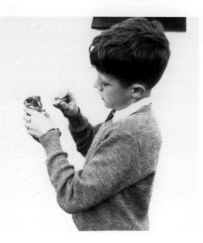

Feeding a baby possum. From an early age Ian had a love for animals and by 12 had determined to become a veterinarian.

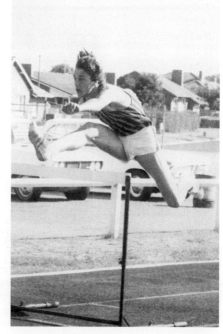

Hurdling, 1971. Ian went on to represent Victoria in the decathlon at the Australian national championships three times. The 110-metre hurdles is among the sport's ten events.

An X-ray of Ian's right leg on 30 December 1974 shows osteogenic sarcoma, a virulent form of bone cancer, spreading out from Ian's femur 'like a grenade in the early stages of exploding'. The X-ray was taken nine days before his leg was amputated at the hip.

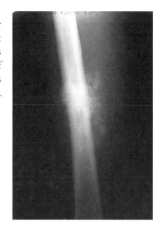

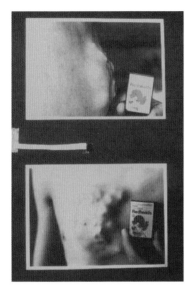

Later that year he developed secondaries in his pelvis, lung and chest. By late in 1976—when these pictures were taken—Ian's cancer had manifested as large bony bumps on his chest. Eighteen months later all signs of these bumps were gone.

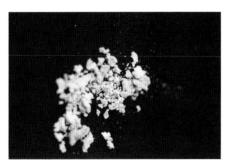

Bony spicules coughed up from Ian's chest over a period of several months as the bone cancer inside his left lung was breaking down. Most pieces were coughed up individually often amidst blood and sputum and each one was about the size of one or two grains of rice. (Photograph by Eamon Gallagher)

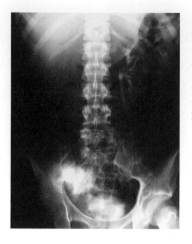

Pelvic X-ray 4 March 1976, taken at the time where the metastatic cancer is clearly visible as a large white mass. Early signs of cancer spreading into the fifth lumbar vertebra are also visible. The X-ray was taken at a time when Ian was experiencing his worst level of pain in his lower back.

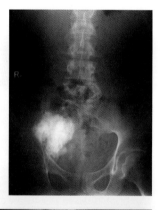

Pelvic X-ray 16 January 1978 showing how the cancerous lesion in the fifth lumbar vertebra had advanced in the intervening two years. This X-ray was taken at the time when one of Ian's doctors warned him that he was about to become a paraplegic, 18 months after a short course of chemotherapy and, remarkably, only five months before he was declared to be free of cancer.

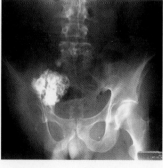

Pelvic X-ray taken 6 November 1980, showing how the pelvic mass had stabilised and how the fifth lumbar vertebra had shown an extraordinary regeneration.

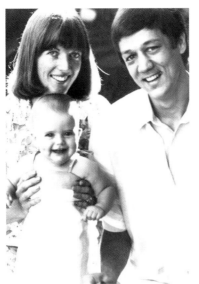

Ian and his first wife Gail with their first child, Rosemary, at six months in 1978.

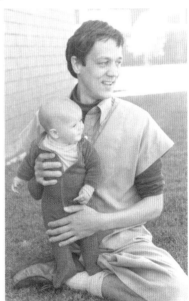

Ian and Rosemary, at nine months of age, 1979.

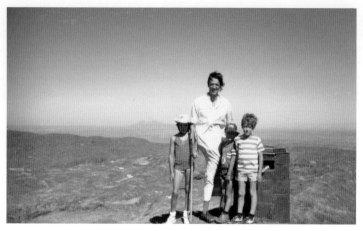

Ian atop Uluru (Ayers Rock) in 1988 with (from left) Rosemary, Peter and David. 'Now with greater knowledge of Aboriginal culture I regret having made the climb,' says Ian, 'but at the time it was a great experience.'

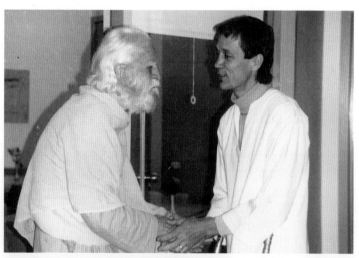

In the early 1980s Ian invited renowned Christian mystic and spiritual teacher Father Bede Griffiths to speak to one of his cancer self-help groups at The Gawler Foundation.

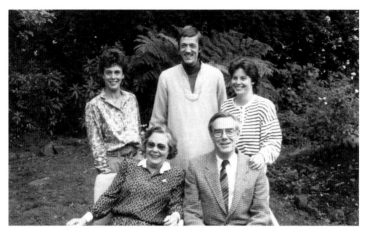

Ian's late father Alan and stepmother Glenyss Gawler. Behind them are his elder sister Susan (left) and younger sister Helen (at right).

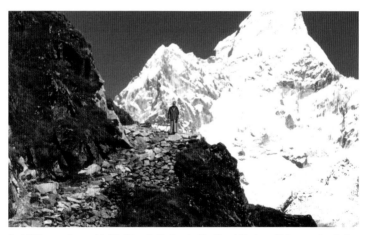

In 1999, together with his friends Dr Jamie Duff and Rejane Belanger, Ian led a meditation trek and retreat in the Himalayas, *Mindful in the Mountains*. The group walked for half the day and meditated the other half.

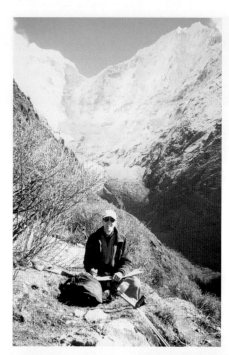

Sketching high in the Himalayas.

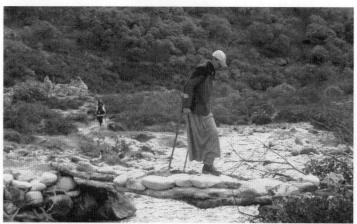

Crossing a stream at over 4000 metres.

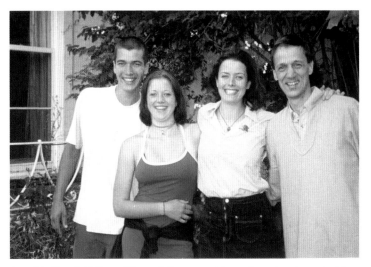

Ian with (from left) Peter, Alice and Rosemary (absent from the picture is eldest son David).

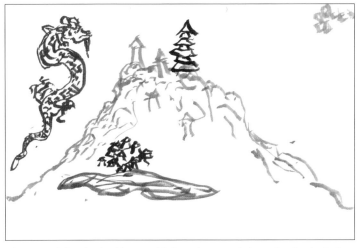

The original drawing by 11-year-old Quentin, created six weeks after he had surgery for a brain tumour, that inspired the title of this book.

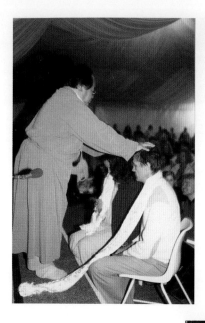

Ian's main spiritual teacher, Tibetan lama and author of *The Tibetan Book of Living and Dying,* Sogyal Rinpoche, blesses Ruth and Ian's union, 2000.

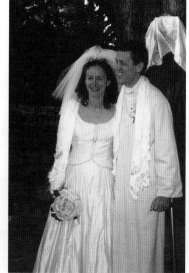

Ruth Gawler (nee Berlin) and Ian on their wedding day, 16 July 2000. The ceremony was performed under an oak tree in Melbourne's Royal Botanic Gardens.

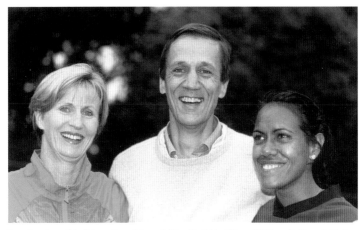

Ian Gawler with Olympic gold medallists Debbie Flintoff-King (left) and Cathy Freeman. (Photograph by Graeme Horner)

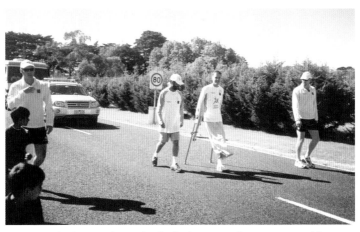

Ian carries the flame in the torch relay leading up to the Commonwealth Games in Melbourne, 2006.

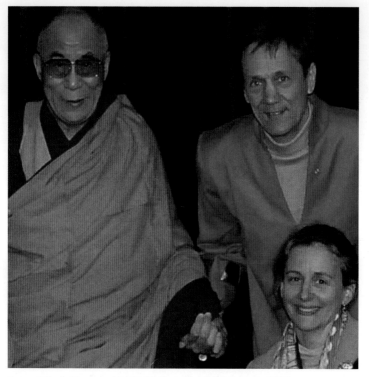

Ian and Ruth Gawler with His Holiness the Dalai Lama in 2007.

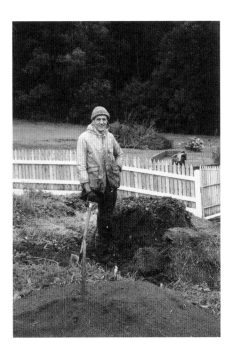

In his spare time Ian loves nothing better than working in his garden in country Victoria.

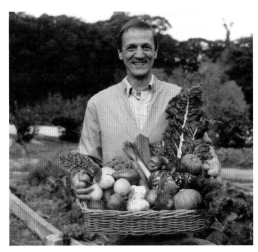

The fruits (and vegetables) of Ian's labours. (Photograph by Peter McConchie)

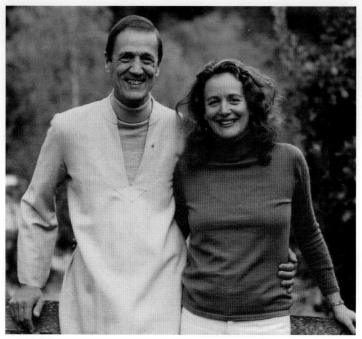

Ian and Ruth Gawler. (Photograph by Peter McConchie)

I have been able to reawaken her spiritually and lead her to many
new things which we can explore together.

On 21 October 1978 a report of Ian Gawler's illness and miraculous
recovery, penned by Ainslie Meares, appeared in the *The Medical
Journal of Australia*. The Gawlers' incredible journey was about to go
public.

In the report Meares charts Ian's recovery, mentioning the diet,
acupuncture, Filipino faith healers, chemotherapy and radiotherapy
and saying that his patient had 'developed a degree of calm about
him I have rarely observed in anyone, even in Oriental mystics with
whom I have had considerable experience'. Meares acknowledged
the 'extraordinary help and support from his girlfriend, who more
recently became his wife', but emphasised the intense and prolonged
meditation which had entered into Ian's 'whole experience of life'
and thereby reduced anxiety to an extraordinarily low level. This, he
suggested, in turn reduced the level of cortisol in Ian's system and
enhanced the activity of his immune system to fight his cancer.

The news of Ian's miraculous recovery—whatever the true
reason for it—would now gather a momentum of its own. Within
a week or two the mainstream press picked up on the report and
on 7 November stories about and photographs of Ian appeared on
page one of Adelaide's main newspaper *The Advertiser* and on page
three in Melbourne's *The Age*. Taking Meares' lead, both stories
emphasised meditation as the single greatest factor in Ian's cure.

The day after publication Ian wrote that the attention ...

... leaves me feeling more exposed and vulnerable and the
responsibilities weigh heavily ... an essential ingredient in my
healing has been the need to provide an example of what is possible
and now it becomes more important to keep fit and be seen to
manifest the ideals we propose.

Ian also wrote that he was pleased that Meares had recognised the
central role that Gail had played in his getting well 'even if we
choose to play it down to avoid excessive calls for help'.

Gail was busy enough with baby Rosemary and her responsibilities at the practice without having the pressure of this new clamour for help that the publicity would bring. Ian and Gail were equal partners in his return to health—without her support it is hard to imagine how he would have survived. It was by drawing on her extraordinary positivism, support, endless massaging, the tireless making of countless juices, dietary suggestions and undivided love that Ian made it through. It was Gail who convinced Ian's surgeon to allow him to travel to the Philippines and it was she who accompanied him on the pilgrimages to Sai Baba and Findhorn. Gail played a crucial role.

In any case, Ian was the actual individual who had recovered from the illness and made better copy for a journalist's story. Also, at the time, Gail was quite shy about publicity and actively preferred to stay out of the limelight. It was mutually agreed that it would be Ian who should and more easily could speak with the media, particularly given Gail's responsibilities as a new mother.

When the stories came out in *The Advertiser* and *The Age* Gail says she was all too aware that something 'potentially life changing' was beginning to unfold. The good side was that people from everywhere contacted the couple asking for help—often because they, or a friend or member of the family, had cancer.

Queries came in 'by the hundreds,' she says. 'So here we were, him just out of TB, the new veterinary clinic, the new baby, sitting up until the wee small hours answering letters by hand. So that really launched the work off but in a way that I wasn't personally happy with.'

Gail felt a 'huge, huge responsibility' that people were going to try and replicate their story, she says today, adding that she felt that people would try and meditate for five hours a day and neglect other approaches. Gail believed that Meares had overplayed meditation in Ian's cure. 'I know meditation can be very useful for a lot of things,' she says, 'but its implication in the curing of cancer I think has been really misconstrued.'

'Ainslie certainly associated the recovery with meditation,' explains Ian, 'and I'm sure that's true. I wouldn't have had the inner strength to go through all the things I did [without it]. And there is no doubt now, based on a huge body of research, that meditation does have very direct and wide-ranging health benefits. To me it is clearly a key, a major element in my own story and something that can help others to recover. But I do believe, like Gail, that it is only one part of a bigger picture. People often ask me what was the one thing that cured me. Was it the meditation, or the TB, or the diet, or the healers in the Philippines, or Gail's massage, or my own willpower—as my dad put it. I don't think that it was just one thing. I think that my recovery was the result of a combined approach; an integrated approach,' he says. 'And that's the approach I take to helping other people these days.'

In the early days, though, the Gawlers were still working out how best to articulate and disseminate the things that they had learnt in the previous couple of years. Meares' *Medical Journal* report, and the mainstream publicity it generated, not only emphasised the benefits of meditation in tackling cancer but it also stimulated large numbers of desperate people looking to take it on.

'We spent a lot of time in those early years [1979, 1980] following Ainslie's report speaking to people on the phone, and writing letters to them. It soon became obvious that we needed . . . [to convey] the same information in a more efficient and effective way,' says Ian.

'A book seems inevitable,' wrote Ian in his journal on 12 November 1978, as the media became more and more interested in his story. The following day Caroline Jones interviewed him for ABC Radio, together with a number of other radio interviews with commercial stations around the country.

Not long after, *Woman's Day* and *Women's Weekly* magazines ran large features and the volume of phone calls from cancer patients and their friends and families—mostly fielded by Gail—continued to grow. As for his health, Ian wore a number of nagging concerns: the pelvis was still sore and he was having acupuncture and homoeopathic remedies in an attempt to mobilise his upper back and neck.

In mid-November, back in Melbourne, Ian's much-loved grandmother Doris Gawler died. Doris developed a difficult cancer towards the end of her life, a cancer that was incurable by medical standards and she died quite quickly. It proved difficult for Ian to see Doris being confined to the conventional approach to her illness. He felt frustrated that his advice and experience were not sought and that he was too far away to be of any direct assistance; or even to be with her.

> I hope she was at ease with her difficult end stage and finally rose above the confusions and conflicts it produced ... She was a fine and loving person who gave me early security that persisted and grew so that I had a sense of roots and stability ... Her life was full and long. I loved her.

On the trip back to Melbourne for the funeral Ian also popped in to see Ainslie Meares.

Meares emphasised the need for Ian to avoid stress and also expressed his objection to Gail's 'lack of inclusion in the written articles,' wrote Ian.

> He was more pleased when told it was our choosing [to leave Gail out of the articles]. He was kind enough to say how he thought I could help many people and wanted to stress the need for continuous meditation and taking the inner calm into one's daily life.

The period marked a time that Ian and Gail Gawler were 'happier than ever before,' wrote Ian.

> We seem to flow together, to be better able to discuss things and add to each other. It is as if all the old conflicts have been burnt away leaving us without pretences, more open with each other and hence more content and loving. Rosemary seems to have catalysed this ... a channel for our mutual love.

Ian also expressed his wonderment at observing the blossoming of Gail as a mother, more remarkable for the fact that she had such a 'long ingrained hate for children and it is being transmuted now into heartfelt motherly love—beautiful to behold'.

As for his own development, Ian is very explicit in his diaries about this too.

> I have had premonitory mystical experiences—enough glimpses of quiet, enough awe of nature, enough to sense the Godliness in everything to stand convinced of the possibilities. It is just a matter of spending enough time and purifying the lower bodies to a point where they are not encumbrances and from there to sally forth. I have spent time lately meditating in front of Baba's photo ... I feel a great need to get a book going to put together all these ideas. The time is right and if it means leaving work I must have the courage to do it.

The Gawlers had a strong desire, primarily for Rosemary's sake, to move out of the flat and find some land where they could build a house and establish a new veterinary practice.

Both ideas would have to wait a little while longer, because they had another pressing need to return to the Philippines. Gail's father, Bob Kerr was suffering from end-stage emphysema, and he was hoping to reap some of the healing benefits his son-in-law had enjoyed. They left along with Rosemary and Gail's mother Olive.

The flight over was uneventful and the only hiccup upon arrival was another 'excited' immigration officer's determination to vaccinate all of them on the spot. Somehow they bluffed their way through as they had on that first visit.

In Baguio they visited a number of healers, including the venerable Mr Terte. However, he was not his usual self.

> Gone was the gentle giant who moved with modest strength and welcomed all with a self-assured, content and contained smile. Instead was a dishevelled man whose more than ample flesh sagged from weary bones.

Despite his obvious ill health Mr Terte operated on both Ian and Bob Kerr. Terte worked on Kerr's throat 'and seemed to relieve a lot of the tightness and congestion Bob felt there'. For Ian he removed three 'pieces of matter' from his chest. 'The matter was dark red and of a similar consistency to plasticine,' he wrote in his journal. 'I would not vouch for where it came from,' he added, although afterwards Ian admitted to feeling lighter and to breathing more easily.

The couples visited a number of healers over the coming days and then the Kerrs returned to Australia on their own. Bob Kerr had an anxious need to get home to familiar surroundings, remained quite ill and was severely stressed from the rigours of travel.

In the Philippines Ian and Gail stayed on and spent quite some time with Mr Terte, who by now seemed quite ill. Then suddenly Mr Terte was admitted into hospital with a serious infection in one of his legs. It soon became gangrenous and doctors wanted to amputate.

The first that Ian heard of it was early the next day when Mr Terte's daughter Arsenia approached him for 1000 pesos—then equivalent to around $175—for the operation. Mr Terte had been a healer for more than 40 years, and grateful patients had given him a lot of money over those years, but he had given it all away. He was penniless. The Gawlers gave them the money, although Ian felt Mr Terte would not survive the operation.

Later that morning Arsenia reapproached them. Mr Terte was so weak that he needed a blood transfusion before the surgery. 'We had to go into town with Arsenia, find someone on the street who was prepared to sell his blood, and had the right blood type, take them back to hospital, pay them and then organise a transfusion for Mr Terte,' says Ian. 'Not quite what we were used to back in Australia and more than a little surreal.'

Despite all this, by the following morning Terte had developed gangrene in the other leg. Surgery was abandoned and it soon became obvious that he was dying. And then came news that Gail's father had died back home in Australia. The Gawlers hurriedly arranged to return home the next day.

Before they left, late in the evening Ian managed to spend a last few hours with Mr Terte.

His daughter Arsenia's house was candlelit, the atmosphere sombre when Ian arrived. He was ushered into the small bedroom where Mr Terte lay back on a bed, surrounded by religious pictures and a few people Ian did not recognise. The others were ushered out.

'It was as if Mr Terte wanted to speak to me directly. He looked extraordinary. He was obviously dehydrated by now, his eyes drawn back deeply in his sockets. His mouth was sunken, his false teeth removed. It was clear that he was very close to death and that it was a real effort for him to speak. I had to climb onto his bed and get very close to hear what he had to say.'

Terte talked to Ian in quotes from the Bible. 'He said that healing took place under three things,' says Ian. 'It was faith, and prayer, and the Holy Spirit.'

Terte told him that faith represents the 'sort of thought that doesn't have any doubt about it. It's really very simple-minded and with a great deal of conviction behind it.' Prayer meanwhile 'involves an ability to have an interaction with a power greater than yourself, and to be able to ask for things to happen and to expect them to happen. And the Holy Spirit is that spirit in action, that energy in action,' says Ian. 'So this was a very profound, and at the same time, simple explanation of how that extraordinary healing takes place.'

Ian sat and meditated with Mr Terte for quite a while and hoped to be able to stay and be present to support him as he died. But reluctantly in the early hours of the morning he had to leave to prepare for an early flight out of Baguio. He was deeply affected by the 'coincidence' of being the one present for Mr Terte at the end of his life. 'Being given the benefit of his last words, having the essence of healing explained to me by him in circumstances which really were somewhat bizarre, all of this had deep impact and profound significance.'

Mr Terte died early the next morning just before they flew out. The Gawlers paid for his funeral.

Returning home to Adelaide it was finally time to put their plans for moving into practice and Ian's journal entry from 18 July 1979 is a point form list headed 'The Future? Where to be? What to do?'. 'Gayle's goals [Gail had changed the spelling of her name at this time]', wrote Ian, were: 'Self-sufficiency, vegies, fruit, goat, a sheep or two. No work unless helping with small practice. Healing with or without group. Spiritualizing: meditation in natural environment. Baby raising.'

Top of the list for Rosemary was 'room to romp harmoniously. A natural environment in which to grow spiritually. After two or three years, kindred spirits to grow with. Potential access to suitable education—Steiner school or similar'.

Ian, meanwhile, characterised himself as the income-earner with plans to write a book and make furniture. He rounded out his list with: 'Spiritualization: meditation, yoga, reading. Like to work without impinging on other activities. 2–3 days work.'

As for where they hoped to realise their dreams, these were listed to ideally unfold on '10 acres somewhere' with lots of big trees, good soil and flowing water. The land had to have private access, it needed to be 'undulating', surrounded by like-minded people and it had to be between 16 and 32 kilometres (or 10 or 20 miles as it was expressed) from the sea.

Their ideals were clear, but they were still open to alternatives. The real imperative was room to grow and for a place of their own with a garden. After looking extensively around the Adelaide Hills, they fell in love with a handsome stone cottage in Adelaide and decided to make an offer on it. The contracts were drawn up and Ian and Gail agreed on the maximum price they would pay.

'We decided that if this place was right for us, then the owner would agree to the amount we offered.' But the owner was fixed on a selling price just a little above the Gawlers' offer. The agent arranged for them to meet the owner, who asked Gail and Ian a little about themselves. They recounted a potted version of their extraordinary story of the last few years to the owner.

'And then she looked at us very wisely,' remembers Gail, 'and said: "You know, I could reduce the price on this house and sell it to you but it would be really wrong, because you two have much bigger work to do and you can't be here."' The agent, who had been carefully attempting to close the sale over the previous few weeks, just stared in open-mouthed disbelief. The sale was off.

Two weeks later Ian, Gail and Rosemary headed interstate to stay with friends who were developing a spiritual community at Mill-grove in the Yarra Valley, an hour's drive east of Melbourne in country Victoria. The Gawlers stopped in at a real estate agent at nearby Warburton. By now they were firm in their commitment to live in the country, or more specifically, find somewhere to match their list. They duly presented it to the Warburton agent, who took them immediately to a block of land near Yarra Junction. The block had everything they had dreamt about, including sweeping views of the surrounding ranges.

'It was just such a magnificent place we took the plunge,' says Ian. The land was owned by a dairy farmer, Len Rayner and his wife, and it had been on the market for five years. Rayner had subdivided his farm into a number of blocks—the one Ian and Gail plumped on was Lot 3, Rayner Court. However, Rayner really loved his land and was reluctant to actually let go. For years prospective purchasers had made offers that had been accepted by Rayner, and then at the last minute, just before the sale was to go through, the farmer would ask for more money. Numerous offers had fallen through. The Gawlers were warned of Rayner's quixotic approach and made their own offer: $54,000. It was accepted.

'The next day he rang back and he said it wasn't good enough, he wanted another $2000,' says Ian. Determined not to be put off, they agreed and the deal was settled.

It is so idyllic it is almost overwhelming. It still sends tremors of excitement through me thinking of it and its attendant possibilities.

Measuring 15 hectares (or 37 acres), 5 kilometres from Yarra Junction, the block was bounded at the back by the Little Yarra River. At the front the land was reasonably flat, rising to a small hill and then fell away quite steeply to the river. Most of the land was clear, with some mature gum trees and tree ferns at the back. From the hill, a perfect site for the house they planned to build, the views stretched down to the river and across to the mountains that ringed the property in the middle distance.

The site is thought to be an old Aboriginal meeting place, a sacred site and it is easy to believe.

In April 1980 they packed up their Adelaide flat, loaded up a trailer and headed for Victoria.

10

Rainbow Park

When Ian and Gail Gawler bought the property near Yarra Junction, an hour east of Melbourne, they knew it would be the permanent home they so desperately craved.

'It felt like the right place to be,' says Ian, 'the place I could live out the rest of my life and die happily when the time came.'

For now it was just a bare block of land. They had no house, no access track, no electricity, no sewerage and no mains water at their 15-hectare slice of the Victorian countryside. What they did have in plentiful supply, however, was natural beauty and an overwhelming sense of potential.

The Gawlers were living in temporary accommodation in Melbourne until the sale was finalised. Then, late on the day the contract was settled, Ian and Gail drove up to Yarra Junction and through the gate that led up to their new land. As a full moon rose over the mountains, they blissfully surveyed the small holding; their hearts brimming with a sense of possibility and good fortune.

Sitting near the meeting of the Yarra River and the Little Yarra River, 66 kilometres east of Melbourne on the Warburton Highway between Warburton and Lilydale, the township of Yarra Junction itself was not as picturesque as the rolling green, dairy and grape-growing countryside that surrounds it. That said, it had the authentic heart of a working country community, still relatively untouched by the Devonshire tea shops and boutique wineries that were opening up elsewhere in the valley. Besides, the Gawlers were moving into the area for the calm, natural splendour of the land.

By the time they did move onto their new property—by then dubbed Rainbow Park—Ian had lined up a contractor to put in an access road and to clear a space for a dwelling. Earlier Ian had employed one of Rayner's sons, Trevor, to put in a dirt access track and build a shed. The plan was that the growing family would live in the shed for six months while their house was being built.

As the plans for the house formed, Ian combined his long interest in architecture with the spiritual emphasis in his life and he plunged into the study of sacred architecture. The shed had a correctly proportioned pyramid placed above a skylight in its centre. The future house was designed around a hexagonal format with all the dimensions based upon the principles of sacred geometry.

However, the house was still only an idea when they first arrived. And the shed was unfinished. Gail's sister gave them a tiny, ancient caravan and delivered it to the land. The day they arrived, there had been some rain, the new road had no gravel on it and they were soon bogged. Len Rayner saw this predicament and came over with his tractor to pull them out. Delighted to be on their new land, but exhausted, they fell into the tiny caravan and slept.

In the morning, Rosemary, who, because of the size of the tiny caravan, had to sleep on the floor, was soaking wet. It had rained in the night and the caravan leaked. But she, like her parents had slept well and was just thrilled to be there.

When they arrived, Ian imagined that he would need to travel to Melbourne for work. Instead, much to his good fortune, it turned out that Yarra Junction was, he says, 'probably one of the few areas around Melbourne at that time that really needed a vet, but didn't have one'. Ian found a unit in the village for his practice and obtained council approval, 'So I very quickly had quite a good practice going.'

As for a permanent place to live, the couple had optimistic ideas of building their ambitious hexagonal house in double-quick time. Six months was the fantasy. Meanwhile their temporary home would be a shed, built for $4300, a little over 7 metres long and 3.5 metres wide. Rosemary was by then eighteen months old and Gail was pregnant again.

They settled into the shed, using the caravan as their kitchen. Then, when it became clear the house was going to take longer than they had first imagined, Ian built an additional small room to replace the caravan and to serve as a kitchen.

'Gail was pretty extraordinary with all that,' says Ian, 'because for a long time we didn't have a decent bathroom and we didn't have washing facilities, so we used to do all the washing at the surgery.'

The house was built in Ian and Gail's spare time. They employed the services of specialist tradespeople, but did a great deal themselves. Ian and his father did all the plumbing. The house's hexagonal-shaped structure was designed to admit as much natural light as possible. Built in local timber on a sandstone base, it had a big domed ceiling with a skylight over the central, main room, which also contained the kitchen. Bedrooms radiated off this central core. Ian and Gail's room had big picture windows overlooking the main mountain range. A wide veranda encircled the house, giving them somewhere cool to be in the heat of the summer and on rainy days it gave 'the kids somewhere to tear around without having to go outside'.

Building took much longer than anticipated and the shed remained home to the growing family for four years.

The Gawlers had chosen to live a simple, back-to-basics lifestyle, with a composting toilet and no power. They were loving it. Evenings were spent under the light of kerosene lamps and the fridge was powered by gas. Meanwhile the phone never stopped ringing with cancer patients and their carers, who had been inspired by the articles about Ian's recovery and were desperate to share some of Ian and Gail's experience and wisdom. Each phone call required sensitive and considered care—and it was Gail who continued to field many of the calls, at all hours of the day, with children to look after.

There was also a subsistence farm to maintain, countless seedlings to water and a fast-expanding vegetable patch to increase and maintain. Ian's health and wellbeing had returned to the point that 'the energy was bursting out of me', he says. 'I relished having a house to build, a vegie garden to establish and a new veterinary practice to develop.'

For Ian and Gail, being able to work flat out building a new family life and creating a place of their very own, was the manifestation of a long-held dream. At last the couple's extraordinary love and capacity for hard work had a means of expression.

In the early days water had to be obtained in a bucket from a dam that had been dug nearby. 'Gail often had a child on her back and another on her hip and a bucket in the other hand,' says Ian, 'and she would walk down to the dam in the mud to get a bucketful of water for the vegies. And then the phone would ring and it would be someone else with some incredibly challenging cancer problem . . . it wasn't unusual for her to get 30 calls a day . . . It was just amazing what she was able to do.'

Ian was, by then, busy running his now thriving practice, focusing mainly on small animals, and bringing in the family's income. Caring for horses had always been his first love, but now with only one leg and on crutches, he could no longer treat these large animals that required two free hands, brute strength, and a steady two-footed hold on terra firma. What he did find increasingly though—and had in the Adelaide practice latterly as well—was that people would make appointments to see him as a vet and when they got into the consulting room, with no animal in tow, they would sheepishly admit that it was actually human cancer, usually their own, that they wanted to talk about.

Typically people would ask him what was the 'one thing they could do' and Ian would tell them that in his view it was not so simple; that he believed in a multi-layered approach. And that would lead into a long conversation where he would advise them to consider their diet, 'what you do physically; you've got to look at what you do medically; you've got to use your mind, meditation— all these sorts of things'. And then they would ask Ian how to meditate 'and half an hour later you'd finish that conversation and somebody else would ring up asking how to meditate.'

It did not take long for Ian to realise that instead of having the same conversation with twenty people, if he 'shepherded them all in the same room,' he says with a characteristically laconic smile, 'I could have just the one conversation.'

In Adelaide, just after the first articles came out and the avalanche of phone calls began, Ian had written out a few key points over a couple of pages which he began to send to people. 'We were responding to people who were in a pretty desperate situation, and there were so many of them. That's when the idea of running groups formed,' says Ian.

So while from that moment on Ian and Gail were enthused about the idea of running support groups, it remained to be seen how the opportunity to do so would actually manifest. And then they had moved to Yarra Junction.

Having been inspired by Findhorn, 'once we bought the land we were really keen on the idea of establishing a sort of healing community,' says Ian. It was more of a loose idea than a concrete one. That said, in the early days just after they had taken possession of their new land, Gail turned to Ian and said, 'We're going to have that land next door one day. There's a healing centre on there. I can see it. I can feel it.'

Ultimately the goal was a holistic healing centre, but in the meantime Ian and Gail were keen to impart the lessons of Ian's recovery to anyone who was interested. Ian was clear in his mind that what he had done 'in terms of things like diet and meditation had a made a very significant difference to my recovery,' he says. 'And these were things that people could learn and anybody could get advantage from. At the very least the better people felt, the more peace of mind and the more sense of wellbeing they had, then the more likely they were to survive anyway.'

So it seemed that initially the most practical thing was to start a support group, to pilot that and see if it would be helpful or not. Any notions of an entire healing community was something to aim for later down the track.

The Gawlers sat down together and came up with a twelve-week program. It consisted of two weeks covering relaxation and meditation, two weeks on diet, two on positive thinking (including affirmations and imagery), one on healthy emotions, one on pain control, a week on death and dying, a week on the causes of cancer, a week on healing and a week on philosophy.

A serious bone of contention from day one between Ian and his wife, however, was that Ian planned to emphasise meditation and diet, yet minimise all the other more mysterious things that had facilitated his healing—the psychic surgeons, Sai Baba, Gail's constant massage.

For Ian, these factors, vital and powerful as they were, all constituted other people's intervention along his own healing journey—and while very useful for Ian personally, they could prove to be 'disempowering' for others, he says. Ian was more keen on taking an approach that emphasised the self-help and educational aspects. Outside help was talked about but was put into the context of his own story.

'We showed the film from the Philippines and we organised ... other healers to link up with our groups,' Ian explains. 'But I gave more emphasis to what people could do for themselves. This empowers people and helps them to develop a healthy, healing lifestyle—the essential ingredient for healing and ongoing good health.'

In a wider public context Ian did not talk much of the Philippines because the healing it offered was inherently 'complex in nature, contentious and difficult to access'. In the groups, however, faith healing along with the power of prayer and laying on of hands, were all discussed at length in the context of an overall picture.

'I talked of the self-help and manageable things like diet and meditation in public because these made good, immediate sense, were relatively cheap and accessible and gave people hope and a starting point,' he says.

Speaking today, Gail still feels that they did not give anywhere near the complete picture—especially given that people had typically sought them out hoping for the sort of miraculous salvation that Ian had found.

'Meditation is fantastic,' she says. 'I do it myself, I teach it, so I'm really into it but it has got to be out there in balance.' Also, as she points out, at a crucial point in Ian's own healing process—when he was suffering with serious back pain—meditation simply did not work for him.

It was when his pain was at its worst, back in 1976 that Ian parted company with Ainslie Meares and sought relief through acupuncture. While Ian only continued with a regular, sustained meditation practice throughout the crisis as best he could, it was not enough at the time to manage the pain. In fact, once Ian had recovered, he spent many months during the Adelaide period, developing his pain management skills.

'For me this led to a wonderful, personal breakthrough,' says Ian. 'During that period I cut one of my fingers with an electric saw. I was able to sew it up myself, using my veterinary skills and no anaes-thetic—and to do this completely pain-free. Then I had major dental work quite comfortably without anaesthetics. This was such a contrast to earlier days when I was so sensitive to pain, and a cause of great delight.'

With pain management skills now as a backup, meditation continued to be the very foundation for everything else Ian did.

It was utterly crucial. It gave him the stability and the inner peace to handle the rigours of his recovery, not to mention a better understanding of his place in a more profound picture. Meditation gave him an inner knowing, an openness and a confidence to pursue other avenues of healing—some of which were way beyond the edges of mainstream understanding or acceptance.

'The challenging thing is that quite a lot of what I did was quite esoteric and had quite a lot to do with energy medicine,' says Ian. There were three visits to the psychic surgeons of the Philippines (adding up to five months in total), there was his faith and involvement with Sai Baba, plus, 'Gail had done a great deal of massage for me. There is no doubt she has quite a healing gift in her own right,' he says. But when they began the groups 'we really downplayed a lot of that,' he adds. 'I made the judgement that it was enough to be getting nutrition and meditation out into the public arena, when there was so much opposition to the notion that either of those two things could help people with cancer. To then link up [cancer treatment] with magnetic healing or some of the more paranormal things that we had done, I felt was just going to negate the whole thing.'

Unfortunately though, this also meant that Gail's tireless and extraordinarily loving contribution to Ian's getting well was not underlined as much as it possibly could have been. 'She often felt that when I talked in public about what had really helped me to get well that I gave too much emphasis to the nutrition and the meditation and not enough to all the help that she had given me,' he says, 'and all the different people who had given me different healing gifts in that more esoteric sense. And there certainly was an error of omission in that sense.'

At the time though, it seemed a minor omission, and probably was. Driving Ian was a big and noble vision for the couple's work; that it could be a catalyst to beginning to bridge the gap between what was possible via mainstream medicine and what was 'possible through the patient's own resources'. It was about trying to empower the people with cancer to be able to seek out the very best of care from an array of places—as he had—conventional, complementary and, if they were up for it, esoteric.

'The words weren't formed then,' he says, 'but it was very much about fostering integrated medicine and looking at the patient as an integrated whole of body, emotions, mind and spirit and working in an integrated, multidisciplinary system where you take the best of all the different forms of healing that are available.'

His heartfelt, secret motivation meanwhile was to help foster in others his own realisation and recognition that 'suffering offered such a wonderful opportunity for transformation in people's lives,' he says. 'That it was a real gift to be able to help people move beyond the real suffering and despair that they often feel when they get diagnosed with a major illness.'

It was a radical and spiritual take on healing, wellness and the place and value of serious illness in ordinary life. It was also the springboard for the twelve-week program. All they needed was somewhere to hold the sessions.

So it was that in September 1981, the Gawlers rented a room in a building in Riversdale Road, Hawthorn—a suburb of Melbourne—with a group called the Findhorn Festival Group for their budding cancer support groups. This group was established by people who had been to, or were interested in, Findhorn and its principles. They welcomed renting space to Ian and Gail for their new venture.

However, late in the week before the first session was to be held, it occurred to Ian that they had not thought to do any advertising or marketing at all—and as yet no-one had booked in for the program. Ian rang the medical reporter at *The Age* newspaper on the Thursday.

'I told him what I was doing, and asked him if he would be interested in doing a story,' he says. On Friday, Ian was interviewed and his picture was taken in Melbourne's Treasury Gardens as he meditated under an elm tree. Come Saturday, a large feature story appeared on the front page of the paper, accompanied by the photograph.

Ian and Gail had decided to have a public meeting the following Tuesday so that people could register their interest, and discuss what they planned for the groups. The first twelve-week support group was planned to begin the following day. After the newspaper article, the phone 'rang hot' and 50 people turned up to the first meeting. Thirty of those signed on for the first group.

Ian worked from extensive notes he had devised before the first meeting and then 'from week to week it was a matter of working out what we were going to say'.

They might have been flying by the seat of their pants, but they were drawing from the hard-won lessons of Ian's increasingly well-known recovery.

'In retrospect, it was actually a blessing that we were completely new to all this,' says Ian. 'I had never been in a group myself, never had any training to run a group. So while I had read a lot on psychology and esoterics, the group thing was completely new. I had to put myself in the shoes of someone else with cancer and think, if that was me, what would I need to know, what would I need to learn?'

To begin with, the format was half an hour of meditation, followed by an hour of discussion. Within two weeks it became obvious that more time was needed and the sessions were extended to two hours a week, a format that remained for years.

The first groups ran on Wednesday afternoons. Within a couple of weeks the demand was such that they started an additional group on Wednesday mornings.

When they first set up the sessions there was a lot of discussion between Ian and Gail about whether they should charge an attendance fee or seek payment by donation—whatever the individual was able, or felt happy, to give. 'We were both quite keen on doing it by donation,' says Ian, adding that then he spoke with Ainslie Meares about the issue and Meares was unequivocal in his advice: if the groups were run by donation people simply would not value them.

'And we were broke anyway,' says Ian, 'so we thought we would charge a modest amount and that would be the way to do it.' They called it the Melbourne Cancer Support Group, charged $70 per person for the twelve week program and initially conducted it as a private business.

'I found there was so much I could talk about from a health and educational point of view,' he says, adding that he understood that other cancer support groups around at the time tended to focus more on free-wheeling discussion. This meant that people often just talked about their problems.

'We didn't do a lot of that, and I think that was probably one of the reasons why our groups worked so well, actually. Each of our sessions had a particular theme such as nutrition or meditation. In those early days I figured that everyone knew about all the problems associated with cancer and did not need to dwell unduly on them. What people needed, and what we aimed to provide, were workable solutions to their problems.'

As time went on, they also recognised that it was the couples—the cancer patients accompanied by a partner—who seemed to be doing better than the people participating as individuals. Also, in those early days, most of the participants had been through all the medical options and had been told that there was nothing more that could be done. Suddenly the Gawlers were instilling people with a new element of hope. It proved a radically new, exciting and positive atmosphere—but they had a lot to learn about presentation.

As a fair example of his naivety in conducting groups, for the very first group session Ian lined up his participants in rows in front of him and fundamentally gave a lecture. He intended to ask them if they would like to sit in a circle after the first couple of weeks 'when they were a little more comfortable with the whole thing, but I actually found the thought of being in a circle a bit intimidating myself,' he says. And then halfway through the second week someone in the groups suggested that they sit in a circle instead—which they did.

'It took me years before I felt really comfy having open discussions with the groups,' Ian says. 'It was much easier to just tell people what to do—which is what I did in those early days. As the years went on, I learnt from the participants, and from other study, and gradually developed a much better capacity to facilitate the groups and their dynamics.'

In the early years the groups concentrated mostly on what the solutions were and spent little time going into people's emotional life or giving them a chance to express their feelings very much. 'While emotions did come out quite a deal, we did not block them and I think we dealt with them well when it did, we certainly did not encourage it. We really were focusing on what is popularly know as positive thinking,' says Ian.

Later groups were given many more avenues for being emotionally expressive and validating their feelings and fears within the group setting. But in those early years any ongoing support took the form of the Gawlers giving participants their home number. 'A lot of people rang and Gail spent a lot of time with them on the phone,' says Ian.

The Gawlers were enthusiastically creating an innovative, compassionate, instructive and inclusive cancer support group, from the ground up and with remarkable success, but the finetuning took years.

For the first couple of years, for instance, the groups would typically run for two hours and then when they had finished everyone would have a cup of tea. Or more correctly what would happen would be that people who were gregarious and talkative would hang around and have a cup of tea, but the more reserved and introspective—the ones who probably needed to stay and talk—would disappear and miss out on the benefit of talking with others.

'And then dear old Jim [Maliaros] came in one day and said: "Why don't we meet for an hour, then have a cup of tea and then come back to the session?"' Ian thought it a fine idea and the groups have been doing it ever since. 'This small change took seven years to work out and it meant that everyone, quite naturally, had the opportunity to talk with the others in their group. People talked more, people interacted more. It made a huge difference to the quality of the program.

'I think in the early days what compensated for our lack of skill was the real dedication to wanting to help people,' adds Ian. And it worked—and for people from all walks of life.

Jim Maliaros had been diagnosed with cancer of the prostate, with secondaries in other parts of his body, and his doctors had told him that there were not any effective treatments they could offer him—in fact there was very little they could do for him at all. 'As Jim recounted it, he got the message: go home and die,' says Ian.

Jim had emigrated to Australia from Greece as a teenager, to come and live with an uncle and build a new life for himself. He had married, had three sons and by the time of his diagnosis owned his own supermarket—which he managed with his wife.

Jim took his diagnosis particularly badly. He was 'devastated', says Ian. 'He stopped work immediately and he went home—and as he described it to me—he closed all the blinds in the house so that he could cry in private. He'd only pull himself together when either his wife or any of his sons came home from work, uni or school.'

Then one day, Jim had gone down to his local newsagent to get the paper and he saw Ian's book *You Can Conquer Cancer*, just out, next to the papers. 'It struck a chord with him,' says Ian. He bought the book, read it and then discussed it with his wife. He described being 'really puzzled'. On the one hand, he had been told by his doctors that there was nothing much that could be done for him and yet here was a book that was saying 'you could change your diet, and exercise, and meditate, and help your immune system, and through that perhaps you could recover'.

Ian's groups were running not far from where the Maliaros family lived and Jim's wife registered him for the program. In those days payment was upfront and, at least in the first few weeks, Jim has said the only thing keeping him going was the fact that he did not want to waste the money his wife had already paid.

At first Jim found it difficult to believe that things as simple as a change in lifestyle, diet and meditation could possibly be of benefit. However, his family encouraged him and even his sons supported their father by going on the same diet. Meanwhile he started meditating.

'Jim had some pain,' says Ian, 'and he found this started to diminish fairly quickly. Also he couldn't help noticing that his state of mind was getting better; so he kept coming.'

Jim had been told that he would be lucky if he lasted until Christmas. 'By the end of November when he finished the course he was looking pretty good and it didn't look like he was going to drop dead by Christmas,' says Ian, adding that he suggested to Jim that he go back to his doctors to see how he was doing.

Jim was not so sure. He told Ian that the doctors already had said that 'they can't do anything for me, and the last time I went to see them, they gave me such bad news in such a bad way that it took months to get over it. So if things have got worse, there is nothing they can do, but if they are worse then at least what I'm doing is making me feel good. If things have got better I don't want to change either. I'm really enjoying eating this way now and I'm getting a lot out of the meditation.' It was as if for Jim, the cancer had become a minor issue, and living well was a new and exciting focus.

At the end of November Jim enrolled in the next twelve-week program, completed it, and then did the following one. All the while Ian continued to suggest he have his health checked out by his doctors.

Finally, eighteen months after commencing the groups, he did. 'First off he had a bone scan which showed that his bones were all clear,' says Ian, adding that he then went and had everything else 'scanned and poked and prodded'. He was all clear. 'I remember him ringing up one Tuesday night, we were at home and I think he would have been about 40 miles away,' says Ian, 'but I reckon I could have heard him without the telephone, he was so excited.'

And then early the following year Jim was talking to one of his son's friends, who, like his son, was studying medicine. Jim was telling him the details of his illness and recovery. Apparently the young medical student could not make sense of it. He really attacked him over it and said that Jim had wasted his time and that the only reason he had got better was that he was just one of the lucky people who had experienced a spontaneous remission. Jim went ballistic and yelled and screamed at his son's friend that there was nothing spontaneous about his recovery and that he should broaden his horizons.

'I guess from a medical point of view he had had a spontaneous remission,' says Ian, 'but then as Jim put it there was nothing "spontaneous" about it.'

Jim had followed to the letter what Ian suggested he do, and for him it worked. More importantly, though, Jim said that when he had been diagnosed he was given no hope. 'Now I feel like I'm living,' he had told the young medical student, 'and even if I die tomorrow I'm going to die feeling happy and fulfilled. I think I'll live for a lot longer and you and the doctors have got no right to try and take that hope away from me.'

The young medical student was echoing conventional medicine's tendency—perhaps unknowingly, certainly unthinkingly—of 'pointing the bone' at cancer patients. 'It can be devastating,' adds Ian.

Instead Ian was advocating a positive outlook, with an emphasis on meditation. His approach offered no guarantee of a cure, but clearly opened up possibilities and focused upon a 'committment to what works'. Ian Gawler's emphasis is on empowering a patient to take charge of their own healing and build enough confidence to take responsibility for their own choices—conventional and complementary.

'But do you go beyond one doctor's advice?' writes Ian in one of his recent newsletters. 'Do you seek second opinions, speak to friends, read books, and get on the internet? And if you do all that, how do you decide? What is right and what is wrong?'

And that's one of the important ways meditation can help. Meditation calms emotions and thoughts and often leads to our 'inner voice of intuition speaking to us confidently and clearly'.

Ian suggests that our two greatest assets in the decision-making process are our intellect and our intuition. 'But Western science with its basis in logic has almost overrun intuition as a valid means of decision making'. Meditation can help restore this balance. As well, meditation has a now well proven capacity to relieve stress—a serious hindrance to getting well and being well.

That said, teaching meditation can have its own challenges, as it did for Ian.

The form of meditation Ian was teaching early on in the programs was very much in line with the one he had been taught by Ainslie Meares. He began by helping people to physically relax first, and then to watch their thoughts come and go 'without trying to *do* anything', says Ian.

'People who were coming to us were putting a big value on meditating,' he adds, 'particularly people who felt they were at the end of the run with conventional medicine.'

They were also convinced that if they were going to get better, then this was one of the important things that was going to help them, so they placed a huge amount of emphasis on doing it right. 'And they could get quite anxious. And so if they were not careful, they would turn what was meant to be a stress-relieving situation into a highly stressful one.'

The method Ian taught early on was effective for those who were willing to persevere—and did not put too much pressure on themselves to perform—but for others it could lead to more frustration and stress.

Also, Ian was finding that people were coming from sessions with Ainslie Meares reporting the same problem. 'He was very dogmatic in how he taught meditation,' says Ian. 'If people got it, it worked really well, but if they did not, they felt like failures.'

Ian realised that he needed to learn more ways of introducing meditation. He sought out and studied with Zen masters, Christian mystics and Tibetan Buddhist teachers. This led to a much more comprehensive method which made meditation more accessible. Ian somehow found time to squeeze the study into his already busy life.

Early in the 1980s, twice a week, Ian would drive to Melbourne to run the groups and spend the rest of the week working in his veterinary practice at Yarra Junction—and then head home to work flat out on their steadily developing home and garden. On top of that there were children number two, three and four—all arriving in quick succession, all home births in the shed—to nurture.

Dr Peter Lucas, based an hour away in Melbourne, was on call for any unexpected eventuality for the birth of the couple's second child, due August 1980. If it proved to be straightforward, then Ian was to act as midwife. As it transpired, when Gail went into labour it soon became clear they needed help.

'While I'd helped lots of animals of all shapes and sizes give birth, I had quite a lot of trouble working out what was going on with Gail.' She had been bearing down for a long time. Ian rang Dr Lucas and asked that he head for Rainbow Park just as soon as he was able.

Dr Lucas arrived and broke Gail's waters and the baby came out like 'a cork out of a bottle of champagne . . . he came out in one hit, it wasn't a gradual process. In fact we missed catching him as he was flung out.'

David was born posterior and Rosemary, observing the event with saucer eyes, 'did get a bit of a fright' says Ian.

The birth of Ian and Gail's third child was idyllic. It was a Saturday afternoon, March 1982, and a beautiful day. 'Peter was born at twelve noon,' says Ian, 'and it was very easy and relaxed.

'They were very happy times, but there was a lot to do getting a vet practice going, building a house, trying to get a vegie garden going and having kids regularly,' he says.

Child number four, meanwhile, Alice Mary, came in a rush after Gail went into labour in the middle of a cancer group in Melbourne in 1983.

The couple hastily finished the meditation session, jumped in the car, Ian drove home at high speed, Gail barely had time to lie down on the bed and Alice was born. Most people might make with extreme haste for the safety of a hospital when a new child is on the way, but the Gawlers—passionate advocates of home birth as they were—were desperate to get back to the familiar surrounds of their shed, with their other children around them.

Rosemary, then five years old, had been present at the births of her brothers, although it's doubtful how much she would have remembered of them, but she was very keen to watch what was going on. Ian recalls that she was very much part of the birth and really enjoyed it.

Peter, born the year before, was asleep and David, then going on three, also watched with interest. Rosemary, David and Peter then showed this 'wonderful sense of loving,' says Ian. 'Real, genuine, completely unconditional love that they showed for the new sister. And it really was beautiful. It was very touching.'

That year Ian enlisted another vet, Terry Iken, as a partner to work in the burgeoning vet practice. 'It was such a relief to have somebody else in the practice,' says Ian, adding that he soon suggested that Terry buy him out and take over the entire practice—leaving him to concentrate on the cancer work. Terry jumped at the chance and the Gawlers began making their living from the groups. 'We weren't charging much, but so many people were coming and we were living very simply, so we made ends meet,' he says.

As for firm business or financial plans—they just did not have any. 'We believed in manifestation. We just had this constant view that if you are doing good work and if you go forward with confidence that it will work out,' he says. 'In fact in our view it was actually counterproductive to make a business plan in the conventional sense because that reflected a lack of trust in a higher principle. We had an absolute conviction that if we were doing the right thing then it would work okay.'

Much like for those at Findhorn, faith was the Gawlers' core philosophy.

By the end of 1983, Ian and Gail Gawler had four groups meeting each week, with over 100 people in all—and Ian running most of them. As the children got older, Gail became more directly involved with the groups but in the early days she concentrated on handling the never-ending avalanche of telephone inquiries.

Ian meanwhile continued to make all of the media appearances, ostensibly because Gail was 'very shy', he says. Accordingly, as time went on, the media's focus would remain predominantly on Ian, despite the fact that the couple worked—especially as the children grew up and became less dependent on their mother—very much as a partnership.

'Later when she got a bit freer and more involved in the work, she decided that she wanted to be seen for what she was doing,' says Ian, 'but by then the media was not interested. I don't think she ever understood how all this transpired.'

So in the mid-1980s, it was quite common that the couple would do interviews together, but that Gail's input would end up on the cutting room floor or edited out of the newspaper story. 'She thought it was some sort of conspiracy,' he says. 'She took it personally rather than understanding that by that stage I'd already become an established media figure. It was difficult for her.'

And then in 1983 came a frightful family emergency, just as a journalist from a women's magazine was due to interview the couple for yet another profile on their work.

The couple had been busy tidying up and had put a fair bit of rubbish in their Tarago van to take to the tip. Gail meanwhile had gone inside to meditate. There were a couple of other things to load into the van and Ian got behind the wheel to move it forward.

Peter was a few metres behind the van and Ian had asked him to stay where he was while he edged the van forward to load in the last bits of rubbish. Ian moved forward, little more than a car length, and felt a sickening bump.

Twenty-five years after the event Ian's eyes still register the terrible shock of the moment and glisten to the memory. Sickened to his stomach, he got out of the car and was thinking, what am I going to find? Peter, eighteen months old at the time, was in that childhood phase where he loved waving goodbye to people. He must have run forward and had somehow got himself in the way of the van. He was knocked over and the left front wheel ran directly over his head.

'I jumped out of the car, ran around to the passenger's side and there he was, lying on his back with a big tyre mark over the side of his head,' says Ian. The tyre had split the skin and Peter was yelling at the top of his lungs 'so I knew he was alive'. Ian bent down and took Peter's head in his hands and he could feel 'all the bones crunch. It was soft and moving around.' Drawing upon his veterinary experience, Ian felt sure that his skull had been crushed, yet he was alive! He remembers noticing that the skull was not obviously distorted, but at the same time having the clear feeling of 'bone against bone'.

What happened next is one of the more powerful moments of his life. Ian quietly and inwardly affirmed 100 per cent that his infant son was going to be okay.

'I knew that was what I had to do. I put all the doubt out of my mind. I reckon it's the most confident I have been of anything in my life,' he says.

'It was a sheer act of will.'

By this stage Gail had come out of the house having sensed that something was awry. She was confronted with the harrowing scene. 'There was blood everywhere,' she says.

They quickly put the seriously injured Peter and a very concerned Rosemary and David into the car and rushed to the hospital at nearby Warburton, where he was immediately examined and his head x-rayed.

Miraculously there were no fractures. It was decided Peter should still be rushed to the children's hospital in Melbourne for more comprehensive investigations.

There were no signs of internal damage. 'He didn't have . . . an intra-cranial haemorrhage or anything like that,' says Ian. 'It was an absolute miracle.'

In the early hours of the next morning, Peter was anaesthetised and the wound on his scalp repaired.

Years later, when Peter was about seven, he walked past his parents' bed at home. There was a book by spiritual teacher Ram Dass lying on it, which Gail had been reading. The book described the experience of dying and the moment of death. In it was an illustration Dass had drawn of the visual experience of that moment of death that people sometimes described to him—and it had been left open at that page.

'I saw Peter walk past the bed,' says Ian. 'He saw the book lying open at this particular picture and his eyes lit up. He had this amazed look on his face. He turned to me and said, spontaneously, "That's what I saw when you ran over my head."'

Not that it was Peter's only near-death experience in his early childhood.

It was Boxing Day, 1987, and Ian had taken the children in the car on the very short ride to the water pumping station that was down the hill from the house, right beside the main dam. Ian asked David, who was about seven at the time, to hop out and turn the tap on so that the water could make its way to the house.

'He fiddled around for a while and came back and said that he couldn't do it,' says Ian, who then got out of the car himself to turn on the tap. This completed, he turned back to get in the car only to look up and see the car slowly gathering momentum—and heading for the dam!

It hit the dam, which was well over 4 metres deep, at a 'reasonable clip and skimmed across the top of the water like a stone', he remembers—with three of the children still inside. Rosemary had managed to get out. Ian leapt from beside the pump and dived out into the dam as the car started to sink.

The two boys were in the back and Ian managed to pull them out as the water level in the car rose rapidly. Alice was in the front seat and had hold of a doll that she had been given for Christmas. 'She didn't want it to get wet and so she didn't want to get out of the car,' says Ian, adding that by now the water had filled up in the car to the top of the dashboard. 'The car was going down really fast, so I just reached into the front seat and pulled her out between the seats. I just got her out as the car went under,' he says.

As the car disappeared, Ian was left in the middle of the dam treading water clutching three young children who could not swim.

Juggling them forward, making sure each kept their head above the water for a moment or two, Ian struggled back to the edge of the dam. There they all sat for some time, soaked, shocked and lucky to be alive. Meanwhile Gail, who had again been meditating at the time, sensed something was wrong, came out of the house and was appalled to see her family sodden and dazed walking back up towards the house.

Gail was less than amused. For Ian it was merely an unfortunate accident, but for Gail it was more proof that her husband was what she calls an 'edge rider'—someone who enjoyed risk-taking and tempting fate. It is a criticism she levels at him for a lot of his behaviour.

'I think people who have nearly died can come back and they can be really "hot" for the edge. He was always right on that edge himself,' Gail says, adding that she felt this became a serious issue at times when their children had also found themselves swept up in Ian's way of being.

Despite the family tensions, exacerbated by how full their personal and professional lives were at the time, the 1980s had proven to be rich and exciting times.

At first the work had been run as a family business. As it became clear that the groups were being helpful and the work expanded Ian formed the view that creating a charity made perfect sense. His motivation was, as he explains, based on the fact that they did not 'want some entrepreneur coming in and making heaps of dough out of what was intended as a humanitarian ideal'. That said, a charity needed to be managed by a voluntary committee and there was the real possibility that such a committee might have ideas that were in opposition to the young couple's own. For this reason Gail strongly preferred the idea of maintaining their work as a family business. This was a source of heated debate between the two, but Ian insisted on the charitable structure.

In December of 1983 the Gawlers established a non-profit, non-denominational, registered charity initially called the Cancer Care and Contact Association, to support the work of the Melbourne Cancer Support Group. They also applied for, and received, tax-deductability status.

The first committee included Maurice Watts, an engineer by profession, as president. John Kelly, a merchant banker, became the first treasurer; while Kate Mottram, a personal friend and an administrator by profession, was the secretary. The rest of the committee consisted of Ross Macaw, a Queen's Counsel and husband of Ian's sister Susan; Nancy Cole, who was a nurse; and book editor Susan Gabor.

At the same time the Gawlers appointed Mike Sowerby to do individual counselling on a one-to-one basis. Although not formally trained in counselling, Sowerby had been studying third-year veterinary science in 1979 when he had been diagnosed with cancer in one of his kidneys.

Sowerby had decided to ignore the diagnosis at first and continued with his studies. By the end of that year he had become quite ill with secondaries and was given between six and eighteen months to live. Then he had contacted the Gawlers, while they were living in Adelaide, and had become interested in the couple's ideas about diet and meditation. He had also been to see a Philippine-based faith healing couple, Helen and David Elizade, who were visiting Australia.

After eighteen months on the Gerson diet and three hours per day of meditation, 'I felt I was genuinely healing for the long term,' he says in the book *Surviving Cancer*, edited by fellow cancer survivor Paul Kraus.

'I was using the lymphatic lump under my arm as the indicator of my healing progress. It would get bigger, smaller, harder and softer. This was like a litmus test of my progress or lack of it . . . It took some years before I was free of the gross physical symptoms i.e. lumps.'

At the time Sowerby was in his early twenties and then spent the following years devoting his time to organic gardening and farming. He then met his soon-to-be wife Sue, who Ian and Gail had met at Findhorn and introduced to Mike.

With Sowerby on board, the popularity of the Gawlers' work continued to snowball. It was clear that the program was meeting a need and was effective. Also it was clear that the running of residential groups was an inevitable next step. To this end plans for a residential building were drawn up, but with an estimated cost of $2 million it was far from clear how the funds were going to be found to build it.

Fundraising was a constant activity. In 1984 a major raffle was held, as were a garden party and two benefit shows at the Athenaeum theatre in Lilydale. Kirsten Coates, whose fiancé had recently died of cancer, also completed a sponsored ride on her pushbike from Darwin to Melbourne in aid of the Gawlers' work. A sum of $30,000 was raised that year.

Late 1984 also saw the release of Ian Gawler's book *You Can Conquer Cancer*. Originally conceived as a workbook for the twelve-week program, it proved a runaway success. It went into a second edition within months.

Around the same time Ian also began to organise seminars, including one by Elisabeth Kübler-Ross, the American bestselling author of the classic *On Death and Dying*.

Also in 1984 Ian organised Cancer Perspectives, a landmark two-day conference at Melbourne University, featuring thirteen different people outlining their approach to cancer. It was attended by 350 people.

'The whole idea was to present an integrated view and to give specialists who had different points of view a chance to speak,' says Ian. The Gawlers were keen to foster cross-pollination and interaction between medical disciplines—mainstream and complementary, as well as the natural therapists. The aim was to engender a little mutual understanding and the real sense that each could not only learn from the others, but that they were all reaching toward a common goal.

Speakers included a professor of surgery who taught meditation, a psychic surgeon, an iridologist, an oncologist, a naturopath, a radiotherapist, a psychologist and a GP who pioneered the therapeutic use of vitamins and minerals.

As a sign of the medical climate at those times, two leading surgeons from the University of Melbourne, Professor Gabriel Kune and Associate Professor Avni Sali, both received letters from their dean advising them that it would be preferable if they did not speak amongst such diverse company.

'To their credit,' says Ian, 'they did and the conference became a landmark event in giving voice to a more expansive, more integrated approach to the management of cancer.'

Avni Sali's commitment was such that he later joined The Foundation's board and has served continuously since. He has been a powerful advocate of integrative medicine and is currently President of the Australasian Integrative Medical Association.

Within a matter of a couple of years, the group had grown from its humble beginnings in a house shared with the Findhorn Festival Group in Riversdale Road, to a respected and progressive organisation, underpinned by a bestselling book, that could attract international speakers of the calibre of Elisabeth Kübler-Ross.

Ian and Gail's places of business, on the other hand, remained small, suburban and low-key for years. After Riversdale Road they moved into a succession of different venues in suburban Hawthorn and Canterbury. The name of the group was changed to The Australian Cancer Patients Foundation which better reflected the focus on helping to manage, treat and prevent cancer. Its office in Melbourne became known as The Melbourne Living Centre.

Office work and administrative meetings were held in a small shop, next to the ambulance station in Canterbury Road, East Camberwell for a time, while the groups were held in a private home around the corner in Surrey Hills. Then they moved to their own house in Burwood and the groups met in a church hall down the road. Next they moved to an old two-storey Federation bungalow on Mont Albert Road, Mont Albert, where finally the administration and the groups could be contained in the one building.

One evening Ian remembers holding a particularly memorable meditation session. The session had begun as usual, Ian guiding them progressively into a relaxed and peaceful meditation. Soon the group had settled into a deep and profound stillness. Opening his eyes seemingly 'a few minutes later' Ian was surprised to discover an almost empty room, one lady knitting in the corner, another reading a book. An hour and a half had in fact passed by—and not wanting to disturb their teacher's deep meditation most of the class had gradually, and quietly, disappeared.

The Foundation was next welcomed into a section of an old nunnery in Mahoney's Road, Burwood, which was big enough to spread out even more so that as well as being able to accommodate the groups and administration, they could add a bookshop and counselling rooms.

The first residential seven-day cancer program began in December 1985, at Mannix College at Melbourne's Monash University. Again, this trial proved successful and regular residential programs began early in 1986 at Jumbunna Lodge a few kilometres from Yarra Junction.

Jumbunna Lodge was always intended as a temporary venue because, early in 1985, the big dream of having a permanent residential healing centre on the land next door to the Gawlers' own property—as Gail had envisaged from those very first days—became a tantalising possibility.

It turns out that around the time the Gawlers purchased Rainbow Park, the 15-hectare property next door had been bought by a builder. He had erected a large shed on the property for his purposes, but he had then got into building tractors. This venture had failed and now he was looking to sell it all.

Suddenly the Gawlers' big dream was looking like a realisable prospect. All they had to do was convince their committee.

The committee thought it was 'a great idea but said that there were no funds for this; we don't have any money,' Ian recalls. The Gawlers might have based their work on a profound trust that things would spontaneously manifest when there was genuine need, but the committee—now headed by Ian's own father Alan—did not share their attitude. 'We said: we've got faith,' says Ian, 'what more do we need?'

The committee remained unconvinced.

'We were quite adamant that this was the right place,' says Ian, 'There was no doubt in our minds that we had to buy it and we worried that if we didn't, somebody else would jump in.'

At this particular point in its development, 1985, The Foundation consisted of Ian and Gail Gawler, with Mike Sowerby employed as counsellor, and a receptionist. Ian, Gail and Mike decided they would offer the committee an ultimatum. The committee would have to agree to the purchase or the three therapists would resign.

'We thought we were making them an offer they could not refuse. But to their credit, they were quite unfazed,' says Ian. 'They said okay, go ahead and resign.'

Needless to say it was not the reply they had anticipated. The trio took a day or two to regroup and work out their next course of action (in truth, they had never actually intended to resign and their bluff had been well called).

They resolved to call an extraordinary meeting of members and did so on 29 April 1985.

The meeting convened with 80 or so members turning up. 'It was very amicable,' remembers Ian, 'and the committee spoke really well, but it was a pretty weird meeting.' The committee's line was that given there were no funds to finance the purchase, it would simply be irresponsible to go ahead. 'We didn't even know at that point where a deposit was going to come from,' says Ian, adding that he then stood up and agreed with the committee that the lack of funds was a 'reasonable concern' but that if you 'have faith then you just go forward and expect it to work out—and we are totally confident—it will.'

The committee's reply was that they did not believe in faith this way, and could not operate like that. The Gawlers' concerns about having a committee running their organisation had been realised. Worst of all, though, this stumbling block was the very basic tenet of their reason-to-be.

Ian told the meeting that 'everything we do has faith running through it as a major principle' and the proposition was put to the vote.

Before the meeting Dorothy Edgelow remembers Ian asking her if she would mind signing up her family as additional members.

Meanwhile back at the meeting, the ten or twelve additional members of the Edgelow family were yet to turn up, but just as the voting began 'my troops all walked in,' says Dorothy.

The committee was outvoted, almost unanimously. They resigned on the spot. A new committee was voted in and Dorothy Edgelow was appointed fundraising manager.

Her first act was to organise a bush fair at the nearby property she shared with husband Ken. It rained all day and $7000 towards the sale was raised—not enough for a deposit on the land, so the Edgelows' donated $10 000 of their own money towards it. This was added to by $10 000 from Sandra and David Bardas of women's clothing chain Sportsgirl and an additional $10 000 from Bill and Julie McHarg of Colliers International. Bill accepted the role of Foundation president.

The land was in The Foundation's hands and the dream of a residential centre could at last be realised.

11

Turning Suffering into Happiness

In 1987, computer programmer Ray Perich had been diagnosed with cancer and was lying in the Royal Brisbane Hospital depressed and desperate. And then a friend dropped in one day and gave him a book. 'There was a photo on the front cover of a scrawny bloke with one leg wearing a sort of a frock,' remembers Ray.

It was *You Can Conquer Cancer.*

Told by his doctors that the cancer in his bile duct had likely already spread to the liver, pancreas and bowel and that he had two years to live at best, Ray says that Ian's book was, 'the first thing that gave me any hope that it was actually possible for me to survive.'

Ray had learnt to meditate years before. It had seen him through a tough time, but he had not stuck with it. Now in desperate straits again and inspired by Ian's book he immediately re-started a regular meditation practice, learnt to relax, listened to music and 'lived largely on fresh juices that my mother and sister made and brought in at visiting time'. He also used to regularly daydream, imagining himself in the bush. 'I could hear the birds, hear the wind in the trees, I could smell the forest. I did this for hours a day,' he says.

Unbeknown to Ray he was practising a powerful imagery technique. 'Apparently when you're doing something you love, you release endorphins into your bloodstream,' he says. Imagining you are doing something can have the same effect as actually doing it. The endorphins 'are your body's natural painkillers and anti-depressants', Ray later learnt, 'but they also boost your immune system, your first line of defence against cancer'.

Ray left hospital after a month, weak and skinny, but alive. He was looked after initially by his mother and sister, while his doctor was Dr Ruth Cilento, someone not only famous for her work with cancer patients but who had started her own cancer support group in 1983. Dr Cilento put him on a diet very similar to the one that the Gawlers recommended. And then Ray attended one of the Gawlers' ten-day residential programs at Jumbunna Lodge. He found it 'inspiring and helpful'. Ray's full story of survival is told in *Surviving Cancer*.

Charged around $500 each for full board, the residential sessions at Jumbunna led participants through the same subject matter as in the twelve-week course, with around three hours meditation per day. The people who 'lived in seemed to gain more than the people who came on the day basis,' says Ian. 'They had the opportunity to have some time out—a break from their home or their work or whatever it was.'

The residential program offered a structured ten days sharing the knowledge that Ian and Gail had learnt and developed on diet and nutrition, meditation, relaxation and a positive state of mind, as well as how to overcome obstacles to peace of mind and find meaning and purpose in life. There was plenty of time for participants to share their experiences and to ask questions in a group situation—plus get the support of people facing similar challenges.

Participants were accommodated in a dormitory setting, divided into men and women, and although many participants initially had reservations about sharing with others, the contacts made and the profound communication that living and eating together facilitated became a central tenet in the group's success.

The thorough, intensive nature of the residential program offered people a more profound chance at healing; an environment for people 'to go into their own nature and their own intentions a lot more deeply', says Ian.

At the time of Ray's diagnosis in 1987, the program was well established at Jumbunna Lodge. Meanwhile, fundraising continued in earnest to make the Gawlers' vision of a permanent retreat centre next to Rainbow Park a reality—now that the land was secured.

As the momentum of the fundraising increased it became increasingly clear that the name of the organisation was a problem. 'We were continually being confused with the Australian Cancer Council, the Cancer Council and other organisations. I was put under a lot of pressure to accept a change to "The Gawler Foundation" which from all our advice at the time suggested would be easier for people to identify with.'

Just as, at the time, the 'Pritikin' diet was well established, the Gawler name was becoming well known as representing a particular way of approaching cancer management.

'However, we also were moving more and more into disease prevention and wellness programs; as well as conferences and trainings for health professionals. While I was deeply concerned about the personalising of the name, and my own ego issues, I reluctantly agreed and we became The Gawler Foundation.'

Maija Kepars, a public servant living in Canberra attended two residential programs run by The Gawler Foundation in the early 1990s and found for the first time in her life that she was 'in a group that was totally accepting of the other person.' Maija had been diagnosed with breast cancer in 1991 at age 59, and had opted for a radical mastectomy of the left breast. She had also had some lymph glands removed from under her arm—where the cancer had spread—and had undergone radiotherapy treatment. 'My prognosis wasn't very good,' she says.

Doctors had suggested she probably had two years to live. Not knowing where else to turn, when a friend had recommended The Gawler Foundation she had signed on, unsure of what to expect. 'Meeting others and making friends at the groups was the most moving part for me,' she says. 'We really didn't know very much about each other to begin with and the only basis was that we all had this illness. There was so much love.'

Maija remembers sitting in her first group on the first morning and 'I couldn't move and I couldn't say very much. I was shit-scared and after that I just cried for a day and a half, just didn't do anything, just cried,' she says. 'Every time I opened my mouth I cried and cried and cried. I think I was getting rid of my tension, firstly because I hadn't really been able to discuss my illness with anybody and secondly, it was this incredibly good feeling from the other people who would hold my hand and give me hugs. It was just so overwhelming . . . people could open up and talk about their fears. Suddenly there were no constraints. It was the biggest discovery. It was like chocolate to be able to talk about myself and be listened to. And it seemed to work for everyone like that because otherwise they wouldn't open up . . . there's really something about group therapy if it's wisely done.'

Meal times proved a time for a little raucous laughter. 'I have never seen a group that laughed more and cracked more jokes than during meal times,' says Maija. 'It was like being in some vaudeville show and that's quite understandable because if you can't cope in any other way, you start laughing about it.'

But coping was precisely what was learnt in ten days, not to mention skills developed to work out the elements of their existing lifestyle that might have made them ill in the first place. Returning home from the program she meditated 'every day at three o'clock for an hour and a half,' she says. 'Meditation doesn't come to me very easily because I'm super active. The easiest was the diet. I didn't have any coffee or tea or sugar or meat for something like five years.'

Importantly, too, Maija changed a lot of her 'attitudes' and her way of relating to the world and others. She went from someone who worked tirelessly for everyone around her, to someone who learnt to slow down a little, to say no more often, and take some time out for herself.

'That was the biggest switch,' she says. 'I think sometimes these big illnesses do us a lot of good, you know. They say that a life that hasn't been analysed—an unanalysed life is not a life worth living and to a certain extent I think that is true.'

Ray, too, learnt to reinvent himself, 'changing the way I operated in and related to the world,' he says. 'I used to have the typical cancer personality,' he says, 'the nice person, always doing things for others, low self-esteem, unable to say no, wanting people to like me, living my life according to other people's expectations.'

Ray learnt to say no and learnt to put himself first, becoming 'not so much selfish as self-compassionate ... if someone asked me to do something I would think about it first instead of immediately saying yes ... I am no longer the compliant person I once was. Which means that now some people love me and some do not; and that is okay.'

In *You Can Conquer Cancer* Ian talks about the 'nice' person cancer profile.

> Trying to please other people is a fine ideal. It is the motivation behind it, however, that creates problems for cancer patients. For them, this begins as a conscious means of coping, a defence mechanism, not a pure motivation. It is taken up as a premeditated defence mechanism and means they become reliant on factors outside of themselves, outside of their control, for their fundamental happiness and sense of worth.

Cancer patients are also frequently 'emotionally tight', he adds today. 'They prefer to keep their emotions to themselves and they have difficulty in expressing them even if they want to. It has taken me years to feel comfortable telling people how I feel about them, particularly if I want to express my feelings of love.'

If there's one fundamental thing that Ian has learnt of his own healing, it is that his existing nature and his inner patterns were a key causal factor in his own illness. For Ian though, his emotional reserve and the habitual 'silence' that Gail talks about were only the more obvious patterns contributing to his lack of balance and contentment—his dis-ease. Inside Ian, though, it was the far more subtle blockages—finally shifted with the help of Sai Baba—that remained the deeply challenging ones to transform on the path to getting, and being, well.

For others, like Ray Perich, learning to recognise your habitual patterns and working to transform them can prove a faster process. It is a deeply personal, introspective transformation that can ultimately only be affected by the individual—with a little meditative insight, a healthy lifestyle, not to mention the counsel of therapists such as Ian and others in a similar boat, as support. Perhaps this is where having someone like Ian involved is so useful. For him the process was long, involved and complex. He really had to study it in great detail to work it out for himself.

They say you teach what you need to learn.

Maija, now 75, says she is getting 'healthier and healthier. I'm feeling better now than I did ten years ago and I think that is partly because I have changed a lot of my attitudes.'

Only a few months after Ray Perich had consciously changed his way of being and relating to others, 'a strange thing happened,' he says. 'I realised one day that I actually felt good about myself and that despite having cancer and a death sentence hanging over me, I couldn't think of anyone I would swap places with. In that moment I knew I would make it.'

That same year Ray Perich came in contact with the work of Ian Gawler, 1987, Ian received official recognition for the work he was doing when he was awarded the Order of Australia Medal in the Australia Day honours list. He remembers receiving the letter of notification in the post. 'I can honestly say that I have never been so surprised by anything in my life,' he says.

At the awards ceremony he chatted to professional cyclist and Tour de France hero, Phil Anderson, back home from his base in France to pick up an award. Gawler remembers being 'blown away' to discover that Anderson had heard of, and admired, his work, just as athlete Debbie Flintoff-King approached the pair to say that she understood that Ian knew a bit about meditation and was an athlete and wondered if he could help her.

She told him she had two issues. One was that she had trouble sleeping before big events and, two, she thought she was a bit down on her self-confidence.

At the time Debbie was number two in the world in her chosen event, the 400-metre hurdles. She had already been to a couple of sports psychologists trying to find the extra edge she knew she needed to be number one. The Seoul Olympics were little more than a year away.

As it turned out, the sports psychologists had suggested Debbie use imagery as a technique to improve her times. They had suggested that if she could visualise the perfect race in her head, then she was more likely to be able to do it in reality. 'They told her that she should imagine that she was in her own body running a race,' says Ian. The only catch was that Debbie had trouble imagining herself in her own body.

'When I talked to her this became apparent very quickly. She could imagine seeing herself running like on a video but could not imagine herself in her body as if she was actually doing it,' says Ian.

It also soon became clear, both from talking to her and watching videos of her races, that Debbie ran a perfect first 200 metres and finished very well, but she would 'fade out on the bend' in the middle of the race. 'It was like she was very present and mindful in the first 200 metres,' he says, 'then she went mindless around the bend and then she would take off again up the straight.'

Ian taught Flintoff-King how to meditate in a series of weekly sessions over a couple of months. He gave her meditation tapes that he had recorded to listen to on a regular basis. Debbie also took up yoga. 'He taught me how to relax and what to do when I was getting nervous,' she says. Ian also suggested she meditate for at least twenty minutes regularly each day as 'an accumulation rather than when I needed it, so it was something that could relax me more. He also helped me a lot with the visualisation because I found it very difficult to imagine in my mind an actual hurdle race. So we spent a lot of time working on running the race in my mind and where there might have been mistakes or whatever, and then fixing them in my mind so that they worked well in the race as well.'

The sessions really helped her feel peaceful at the beginning of each race, she says, knowing that she knew exactly what she had to do. 'A few times I had had problems at hurdle seven where I "changed down" with my legs. I was running a certain pattern with my legs whereby I would use the left side of my body for the first six hurdles and on the seventh hurdle I changed to my right side,' she says. 'I had trouble seeing that smoothly, so he helped me.'

Before the race she would run through it in her mind, so that when the starter's gun went off she knew 'exactly what I had to do. It just happened. And it made all the difference, because I only needed that little bit extra having been number two in the world for the two or three years before that.'

And then came the Olympic final of the women's 400-metre hurdles in Seoul, 1988. Flintoff-King had always been second to East German Sabine Busch, but by the time of the Olympics a new contender had emerged, the Soviet Union's Tatyana Ledovskaya. The Australian beat the Soviet by 0.01 seconds in the semi final.

Commentators suspected Ledovskaya was keeping something in reserve for the final. And indeed in the final two days later, with only 50 metres to go and with the Russian clearly ahead, it looked like they would be right.

Watching it on television during a retreat by the beach in Lorne, Victoria, Ian remembers the excitement of the race. 'Actually for me, although I was a decathlete, my most competitive single event had been the hurdles. So here I was, watching vicariously as someone I had come to know so well was striving for an Olympic gold medal.'

Debbie and Ledovskaya crossed the line locked together. The relief on Ledovskaya's face was palpable. She thought that she had won. The announcers declared Ledovskaya the winner immediately following the race—and then the photo finish was called for.

'Debbie was there on the outside of Ledovskaya and she was still determined to win.' She threw herself at the line and lunged forward as Ledovskaya leant back in relief. The photo revealed that Debbie Flintoff-King had pipped Ledovskaya by 0.01 seconds at the finish line for the second time. 'That last little bit to get me over the line was my meditation and yoga for sure,' she says.

Debbie Flintoff-King was the Olympic champion. She had needed her coach and husband, Phil King, not mention her own dedication and hard work to take her to the very pinnacle of her chosen sport but she had Ian Gawler to thank for the vital competitive edge that had taken her over the line.

Now in her late forties and retired from athletics, Debbie still meditates regularly and says she suggested meditation and yoga to another of Australia's world-beating runners over 400 m, Cathy Freeman, winner of the 400 metre Olympic gold medal at Sydney in 2000. 'Cathy ended up at the same yoga class as me,' she says. Ian has since also worked with Jana Rawlinson (nee Pittman), a World and Commonwealth champion in the 400-metre hurdles, on visualisation and meditation techniques.

On one of the walls at The Gawler Foundation today is a picture of Ian Gawler with Debbie Flintoff-King and Cathy Freeman at a Melbourne function. It is patently a thrill for Ian, the ex-athlete, to have had such a key role in Flintoff-King's success and he also clearly loves to meet with others who have triumphed against the odds.

On a pinboard in his office there are pictures, among others, of Ian with Tim Macartney-Snape, who, with Greg Mortimer, was the first Australian to conquer Mount Everest and was later the first to climb it from sea level to summit; as well as war hero Weary Dunlop. Macartney-Snape and Dunlop were keynote speakers at one of The Gawler Foundation's annual conferences in the 1980s. Dunlop, an old friend, also spoke as special guest at the launch of Ian's first book, *You Can Conquer Cancer*, in 1984.

Up on the wall there is a photo of Ian with US singer/songwriter Joan Baez. There is a picture of Ian with His Holiness the Dalai Lama; with his main meditation teacher Tibetan lama Sogyal Rinpoche, author of *The Tibetan Book of Living and Dying*; there is one with swimmer Shane Gould; another with Judith Durham of 1960s pop band The Seekers; there's one with TV personality Rove McManus and his late wife Belinda Emmett, a past patient at The Foundation; and there is a picture of Ian with US doctor and social activist—the man who injected humour into health care—Patch Adams.

Patch Adams founded the Gesundheit! Institute in West Virginia in 1972 as a 'creative response to the health-care crisis in America: spiralling costs; dispirited caregivers; and alienated patients', he says. The doctor's life and work—which includes heading a team of doctors dressed as clowns to connect with and lift the spirits of their patients—was dramatised in the 1988 film *Patch Adams* starring Robin Williams.

Patch was brought out to Australia to speak in the early 1990s at the Mind, Immunity & Health Conference—an annual event founded by Ian—and was invited to drop in to The Gawler Foundation to speak.

'The only day he could come was when we had a residential program with a group of cancer patients and the topic of the day was death and dying,' says Ian.

After greeting Patch on arrival, Ian emphasised to him before he went in that the group was talking about death and dying and that maybe he should begin in a 'somewhat serious manner'.

Patch opened the door to be met by a cancer support group who were all wearing Groucho Marx glasses, noses and moustaches. They were blowing whistles and throwing streamers. 'They really got him off guard. It was fantastic,' laughs Ian. 'He did a double take, took about five seconds to get in the mood, and then he went right off.'

Patch—a tall, gregarious raconteur with long red hair pulled back in a ponytail—was in his element cracking jokes and sharing anecdotes all about death and dying. The group loved it, except one particular woman.

She was, it turns out, facing up to the challenge of a particularly difficult, and usually terminal, cancer. She did not think that death and dying was a laughing matter. 'She didn't think Patch was funny,' remembers Ian, 'and the more that people around her were laughing, the more serious and the more grumpy she became.'

Patch was beginning to wind up his session and had started talking about how he thought that people take dying far too seriously. Dying could actually be fun, he said, adding that 'if he was in hospital and he thought he was dying what he'd want to do would be to get out of bed and sing about it'. Whereupon he started shuffling around the room and doing a chicken dance and singing 'Oh boy, I'm dying. Oh boy, I'm dying.' The room was in hysterics—except for this one solitary woman.

'It was too much for her and she exploded,' says Ian. 'She addressed Patch quite belligerently. It's all very well for you people, she said. It's all very well for people like Ian and Gail, who were young when they got sick, what about people like me?'

Patch stopped in his tracks, wheeled around and looked at her, his face in mock seriousness. 'Oh you poor woman,' he said. 'Just think, if only you had got cancer twenty years ago you would have your own healing centre by now.' And then he bounded across the room towards her, leapt up in the air, landed on her lap, wrapped his arms around her, cuddled her and started talking quietly to her. 'He's actually a very skilled therapist,' says Ian. 'It was almost as if he blew her mind and then began to talk of what was really possible for her.' Ultimately the outcome was that she 'completely shifted' through that encounter.

The woman lived locally, had already been to a twelve-week cancer program, but she 'wasn't doing well. She had been in a really dark state of mind,' says Ian, 'I had suggested she come to the residential program to see if something more intense would help to swing things around. Then she had this amazing encounter with Patch and she came away from the program with a completely positive attitude. She went on to have a complete recovery.'

By the time of Patch Adams' visit the residential programs had moved into the purpose-built healing centre the Gawlers had envisaged on the next-door property all those years before. The first live-in groups were held on The Gawler Foundation's land in 1991, but it had been a long and hard road to get there.

Indeed, it had been seven years previously that the extraordinary meeting of the members had been called and they had bought the property with a view to building the residential centre.

When the Gawlers first started running groups the intention had always been to run residential programs and the original plan had been to build something substantial from scratch. The dream was a circular building on top of the hill—so that everybody had a view from their rooms. They wanted something that worked like the 'rim of a wheel' with bedrooms on the outside and a lecture theatre and administration in the centre.

By 1986 it became clear that raising the sort of money needed to build such a place was a hurdle too high even for the extraordinary Ian and Gail. Besides the land already had a huge warehouse, 48 metres long and 24 metres wide, further down the hill. The cost to convert the warehouse into the core of the new healing centre would be substantially less.

Major raffles were held to raise money, as were luncheons and art shows. There were seminars and car raffles. In 1985 a bush dance was held in the warehouse, attended by 600 people.

All through its history The Gawler Foundation has had to work exceptionally hard at raising funds through any means it could. It has been a particular frustration that the organisation draws very little of the millions donated every year for cancer research.

'I feel that we are doing direct, constructive work, and getting very little support relatively speaking, compared to when you look at the millions of dollars that get put into cancer research . . . looking for bigger and better drugs,' Ian was quoted as saying in 1987—and little has changed today.

That said, the organisation has attracted the support of a loyal army of volunteers and some very generous benefactors over the years. As well as the income it receives from its programs, The Foundation relies on the largesse of its many friends. It has fund-raised about 25 per cent of its income for many years in an effort to keep its fees to a workable minimum.

Furniture has been donated over the years, hundreds of volunteers have offered thousands of hours to the organisation since its inception and while to date there has been no government funding, cash donations flow in from everybody from benevolent corporations to past patients grateful for the help they have received. Without such people The Foundation simply would not exist.

'The fact of the matter is that over the years The Foundation got into some quite difficult financial situations,' says Ian, 'and what would happen then is that people who were supportive would end up bailing us out. We were always on the edge financially because if we had the money we would use it for something.'

Just to complicate matters, Ian felt the need to take the year of 1990 off. This idea had formed back in 1985 when Ian considered that his work would benefit by a dispassionate review. 'I felt that if I took time away from the place, I could reconsider what we were doing and how we were doing it and make adjustments as needed. However, as 1990 approached, I was feeling increasingly tired and the elective year off that had been planned, loomed as much more of a necessity.'

At the time he said he was tired of saying 'I'll do it later' to the children and wanted to spend more time devoted to them. By 1989 it also became clear that Gail too felt she needed time away from the rigours, stresses and trials of the organisation and resolved to join her husband in a twelve-month sabbatical.

It did not quite pan out as they had hoped. As Ian puts it, the organisation very nearly 'imploded' without the couple's guiding hand. Eight months into the year off, it became clear that disagreements and infighting at the Melbourne centre in suburban Burwood were threatening to undermine the entire organisation.

Ian and Gail called a general meeting of the membership and put it to them that they could either continue having The Foundation split into two locations, at the Yarra Valley and at Burwood, or they could concentrate all their efforts at the Yarra Valley with the residential groups.

'It was pretty much an overwhelming decision that we should concentrate on the groups,' says Dorothy. And so it was that the Burwood centre was given funds to effectively split from The Foundation and be run by its own management.

The crisis was something of a watershed for the organisation and for its existing philosophy. 'From that we started to become more conscious of setting up a tighter business structure,' says Ian.

From 1991, with The Foundation back on a more stable financial footing, the Yarra Valley Living Centre was gradually completed in stages. Ian wrote a letter for participants and friends of The Foundation to help begin the building, a total of $30,000 came in in response. It was enough to convert one-third of the warehouse into office space and build a large meeting room where the groups could meet. Participants on the ten-day residential program were brought in daily from Jumbunna Lodge for the program and then returned to the lodge to sleep.

In 1992, a major loan of $650,000 was negotiated. Office space and new accommodation blocks were then added and opened in 1992 and 1993. The residential programs could now be held fully on site.

From 1993 The Foundation rolled on relatively smoothly. Outwardly it was a period of relative calm and it was certainly a period of consolidation.

It was also the year, on Gail's fortieth birthday, when she changed her name to Grace. She had previously changed the spelling of her name to Gayle, but now opted for a completely new moniker. 'I'd always hated my name with a vengeance,' she explains.

You Can Conquer Cancer and a second book, published in 1987, *Peace of Mind* continued to sell in volume all around the world and have since been translated into a number of different languages including German, Spanish, Thai, Hebrew, Hungarian and Italian.

Ian was increasingly invited to address conferences and workshops around the globe and his extraordinary abilities as a communicator were helping mind–body medicine to gain ever more mainstream acceptance. Mind–body medicine takes an approach that also considers emotional, mental, social, behavioural and spiritual factors and their effect on health and wellbeing.

In 1991 he addressed the annual conference of the Royal Australian College of General Practitioners. In 1993 he was invited to speak at the International Mind–Body Conference in Israel. Two years later he spoke at major health conferences in Britain (The Question of Hope, in Bristol) and Holland (The Hospital as Temple).

In the years since, the list of major mainstream health conferences in both Australia and overseas he has addressed is an imposing one.

It was in 1984 that the Gawlers had initiated The Foundation's own annual conference, starting with Cancer Perspectives. And then in 1993 and 1994, while attending a conference in the United States—the National Conference for the Clinical Application of Behavioural Medicine—Ian developed another big idea on the conference front.

'At the second of these conferences that I attended, Bernie Siegel [a surgeon, pioneer in the empowerment of cancer patients, and author of the bestseller *Love, Medicine & Miracles*] made a great speech,' says Ian. 'He got up and said this is one of the best conferences in the world with one of the worst titles.' Also at the conference was Dr Candice Pert, a legendary pharmacologist famous for her groundbreaking research in the immunology field and the treatment of HIV/AIDS. There were Miroslav and Joan Borysenko, authors of *The Power of the Mind to Heal*; as well as Dr Emmett Miller, medico and bestselling author in the mind–body field.

Ian was thrilled to be among peers at a time when he felt isolated in Australia. 'There was this real sense of fellowship and support,' he says. He returned to Australia from the 1994 conference and resolved to establish a similar conference in the antipodes—and, as is typical of Ian's modus operandi, decided it should be organised immediately.

A friend put him in touch with Brigitte Zeller, a Swiss national living in Australia and an experienced organiser. The two of them decided to set a date in March 1995, only three months away.

They booked a hotel and conference centre on the Victorian coast at Lorne for the long weekend in March 1995. 'I was very keen on body surfing, so I thought I might be able to get into the surf as well,' reveals Ian. He rang and personally convinced Emmett Miller and the Borysenkos—plus a couple of other international speakers—to make the journey halfway around the world at short notice for 'a fraction of the money they were charging in the States'. Then Ian lined up sixteen Australian experts to speak. 'It was frantic, we really worked flat out and Brigitte was just extraordinary,' says Ian. 'She is very Swiss, very organised, she looked after the detail and that's what had made it work.'

Australia's first specific multidisciplinary conference for practitioners of mind–body medicine, the Mind, Immunity & Health conference, was a resounding success.

Ian's motivation for the conference was to build a sense of community around mind–body medicine. 'One of the reasons I was keen to do it was that many people interested in mind–body medicine in Australia at the time were working in isolation,' says Ian. 'They were either working as sole practitioners, or if they were working in a hospital or a practice they were the only ones interested in that field. Quite often their colleagues were either just putting up with it, or sometimes they were even antagonistic. They didn't have a sense of support. And that was the thing that was significant about the conferences—not only were they a training ground but they gave people collegiate support.'

Over two hundred people turned up for that first long weekend, half of them GPs, as well as nurses and psychologists. It became an annual event. 'I received a lot of letters from the medicos after the first one saying it was an eye-opening event for them,' says Ian. 'They said it was really exciting but they were really struggling with how they could integrate the things they had learnt into their practice. After the second one it was lovely because I got a whole lot of other letters saying it was starting to make sense now, they could see how to use it,' he says.

Dr Marc Cohen says that these conferences were a 'huge boon to the whole complementary health sector and to the research units and the practitioners in Australia.' Cohen is Professor of Complementary Medicine at Melbourne's RMIT University and past president of the Australasian Integrative Medicine Association (AIMA).

'The conferences were really important for my own professional growth and my professional career, and then when Ian announced after five years that he wasn't going to run them anymore, a whole lot of people were devastated.'

Ian was finding that the work to keep the conference program running ('even though I really loved it') was too much to handle alongside the mountain of other things he was doing. Then Brigitte

Zeller had decided to return to Switzerland. Ian felt Brigitte was virtually irreplaceable.

'She was so good. We worked so well together and became good friends,' he says. 'I reckoned that the chance of finding another person who could do it so well, and in a way that was also enjoyable, were impossibly slim.'

So Ian stood down and Marc Cohen decided to take it on. Now under the auspices of AIMA, it is known as the Holistic Health Conference and it is still going strong.

'Looking back at the things I've done, those conferences are one of the things I feel happiest about,' says Ian, 'because they had a part to play in AIMA getting started and because of all the good they've done to establish integrative medicine in the medical community.'

During the 1990s the Yarra Valley Living Centre blossomed. Countless trees were planted on the property by volunteers. Renowned herbalist Dorothy Hall set up an imposing herb garden in concert with Gail, now known as Grace, and an organic vegetable garden provided much of the fresh produce. Dorothy Edgelow, as the catering manager, was lovingly churning meals out of The Foundation's kitchen for the residents.

Outwardly hugely successful and offering priceless help to cancer patients, inwardly The Foundation was not without its management problems, staff intrigue and difficulties. By the end of 1995 The Foundation was standing on shaky ground financially once more. At the time the organisation was looking for a new general manager—a position which was filled by Siegfried Gutbrod, a former senior executive with a large multinational company.

Gutbrod had become disenchanted with the corporate world and was looking for a more altruistic challenge. Originally he was interested in simply joining the board at The Foundation, but Ian suggested he apply for the position of general manager that had recently fallen vacant.

Gutbrod brought a stabilising influence to the organisation, not to mention instilling a more orderly administrative routine. By all accounts, up until then management and human resources skills had not been The Gawler Foundation's strong suit. Grace often took a tough approach to staff management and Ian, although rock-solid in his vision, had a less hands-on and more conciliatory approach. When there were problems it led to insecurity and confusion. Indeed 'there were a lot of bitter feelings in The Foundation when I came, as well as fear', says Gutbrod.

However, Gutbrod was well in tune with the Gawlers' spiritual ideals. In fact this was precisely what attracted him to the job. Gutbrod had been involved in the Rudolf Steiner movement for years and was familiar with the idea of manifestation and sought to combine this with effective management and accounting.

'I think I introduced a combination of good accounting but also working with the laws of manifestation—trusting that things would manifest,' he says. 'We had wonderful experiences of that where we as a group could just hold the trust and the money would miraculously appear out of nowhere.

'The attractive side for me, coming from the corporate world, was that we could very consciously work with these spiritual concepts alongside established business practices.'

Ever since they had established their organisation the Gawlers had to work flat out not only maintaining the extraordinary level of care they offered to clients, but also spending a lot of time propping up an unorthodox business structure that had a very small margin of error. The laws of manifestation might have worked for them for years, but the approach meant they were always sailing close to the edge of financial crisis or oblivion.

That said, the edge has always been where Ian has lived most of his adult life—and the place he has felt most comfortable.

The lifestyle also did not come without its effects on the home front.

'Mum and Dad were both busy people,' says son Peter. 'We spent a bit of time with babysitters.' The family rarely had the chance to take holidays together. So in 1993, when Rosemary was fifteen, they decided it might be one of the last chances to take a holiday with all four children together. Ian arranged to fly from Israel, where he had been invited to speak at the International Mind–Body Conference, to the United States where he met up with Grace, who had been visiting the US for work. They then flew to Hawaii together to meet up with the children, who had been put on the plane from Australia by friends.

The family took a couple of days driving around and then settled down on the island of Maui to enjoy some time relaxing at the beach. Grace was happy to read a book and Ian and the kids were eager to get into the water. Known locally as Big Beach, the waves at the beach were not so big—'three or four foot' as Ian remembers them and the Gawlers, minus Grace, were soon enjoying the water.

Grace can remember lying on the beach with a book and thinking all the troubles and stress of Australia were 'behind me now. This will be a great time for me to relax.' And then within two minutes David was by her side saying, 'Quick, quick, Daddy's hurt himself.' Assuming it was a joke, Grace waved him away and got back to reading her book. Peter soon rushed up with the same message. He too was summarily dismissed. But then, by the time Rosemary had come up saying the same thing, she began to worry.

'I looked up and peered over my sunglasses and there was Ian as white as a sheet, sitting at the edge of the surf holding his arm.'

Ian, a confident and accomplished body surfer, had gone out and caught a couple of waves breaking close to shore. Ian was not used to these 'shore breakers' (they were of a type not usually found in Australia) but here in Hawaii he was enjoying the sensation of taking them for a brief ride, sometimes being dumped harmlessly as they broke near the shore. 'I thought, oh yeah this is fun, and went out again. The next minute I'm on top of a three- or four-foot wave and I look down and all there is is sand,' he says.

Ian crashed, his hands out in front of him, onto the unforgiving sand. The top of his arm, the humerus, broke into five pieces.

Grace was furious. 'I thought it was a really foolish risk he took, not looking at the beach and just going straight in,' she says. Ian, in his defence, thought he had been caught out by a chain of circumstances and it was nothing more than an unfortunate accident.

Whatever it was, it meant that Ian had to spend the rest of the holiday—and indeed the next two months back in Australia—in a wheelchair, unable to get about on his crutches. The family holiday, meant as a much-needed stress-leaving break from their incredibly busy lives, had become, at least for Grace, yet another stress-inducing schemozzle.

It was yet another significant factor in a marriage that was slowly but inexorably moving towards breaking point.

12

Falling Apart

Apart from the precious few who were privy to the intimate details of their turbulent domestic life, Ian and Grace's separation shocked everyone in the couple's orbit to the marrow.

Outwardly they were two enormously strong-willed individuals who had their differences and disagreements, much as any couple, but their marriage was unshakeable, forged and strengthened in the bonfire of Ian's illness and miraculous recovery. Or so it appeared.

The Gawlers were a couple that had been through everything, conquering seemingly insuperable odds, together. Grace had supported her man through inconceivably harrowing trials. She had been utterly devoted to him, had been his nurse, masseuse, lover, cook, healer, mother to his children and the co-conjuror of their great dream and adventure, The Gawler Foundation.

Ian, in return, had been a loving, caring and attentive husband and father and, in the course of his extraordinary journey to good health, had inspired and supported Grace in her own career aspirations and spiritual progress.

For many years Ian and Grace had spent much of their time together. Initially the couple travelled together, but later Grace could not manage travelling with all the children. Then, as the tensions between Grace and Ian built in the later years of their marriage, for Ian it became 'almost like a relief' to travel to get away from the conflict at home and have a break. At home in Australia meanwhile, everywhere he went, people would approach him. They would even interrupt family outings with their stories of difficulty. Ian would patiently give them time, but lack of anonymity and repeated intrusions only added to the stress for Grace. Meanwhile for Ian, work became a refuge.

From the very beginning Ian had devoted much of his time to his work. Ever since the early days when he worked prodigious hours in the practice before his illness at Bacchus Marsh, Ian Gawler has had extraordinary capacity for applying himself to the job at hand. Working on Foundation matters until one in the morning, or even three, became typical. Weekends were often filled with work around the property or on outings. On Sundays Ian typically took the children and their horses to compete in regular events, all over Victoria.

Grace too had a superhuman energy and facility for labour.

'One of the things Grace was keen to let people know was that she could wear six hats at the one time,' says Dorothy Edgelow. 'And she was justified in saying that, because she could. She used to manage the front office at times and held seminars. She was all over the place doing everything.' Dorothy was a firm friend of the family and was The Foundation's catering manager for many years—taking nothing but the deep satisfaction she felt working for The Foundation as payment. She is also the author of *A Recipe for Life: The Gawler Foundation Cookbook* (volumes 1 and 2) and would often help out looking after the kids, when things became simply too hectic.

'In the many years I was there—and I suppose I was only there when they were very busy—I never saw them sitting down at the table together.'

In the early days, living in the shed at Rainbow Park, Ian worked long hours in his practice down the road in the nearby township. Twice, and then four times per week, he would travel the two-hour return trip to Melbourne to lead the cancer care program. Grace meanwhile shared part-time nursing duties at the veterinary practice and had co-directorial duties in the cancer care program.

Meanwhile the work the couple managed to fit in on the farm, particularly Ian, was also prodigious. He somehow, for instance, found time to plant over 2000 trees. Ian has a passion for trees—and with open paddocks to begin with—he located and planted many rare and exotic trees, as well as many natives.

All the while Ian was building their home, often with his own hands, and together the couple somehow found the time to nurture their four young children. As Rosemary says, 'I am incredibly thankful to my parents for the time that they put into us kids. Regardless of what they had to do and how busy they were they always put us at the top of the list.

'Particularly when we were small, mum and dad tried to involve us in everything. I think that was more out of necessity than anything else. They worked so hard. If they didn't involve us we would have been farmed out and never seen or heard of again,' she says. 'I can remember going to programs at Jumbunna Lodge on music night and we would sing along with all the patients.'

Rosemary also remembers the countless times over the years when either Grace or Ian would drive them, with their horses in tow, to horse riding events on the weekends. 'There was a hell of a lot of preparation time too,' she says. At the event Rosemary remembers that her parents 'would sit in the car and work frantically. Then they would watch us do our event and then they would go back to the car and work frantically for the rest of the afternoon. They were always there, yet there were a lot of parents who would simply drop their kids off and disappear.'

Gradually as The Foundation expanded, the pressures on both of them multiplied exponentially. There were programs to lead, employees to manage, clients to counsel, fundraising to manage and supervise, conferences to organise.

These were stimulating, exciting and challenging times, but time was the real issue and there were many competing demands on both of them. Tensions surfaced and festered.

It would be easy, but simplistic, to draw the conclusion that the workload was a major cause of Ian and Grace's problems. In fact as Ian says, 'in my view the *relationship* was the problem with the relationship. Grace did a lot, we both did a lot and certainly all of that real pressure contributed to our problems, but it was a symptom as much as it was a cause.'

More specifically, one of the huge contributing strains on the marriage was the fact that Grace had been gradually building a list of grievances she harboured toward Ian. Grace gathered a long list of events for which she found it impossible to forgive her husband. These included the family car ending up in the dam with her children in it, not to mention her husband breaking his arm in the surf in Hawaii on their family holiday. Top of the list though, was the accident with Peter.

It is clear that Grace does not blame her husband for what was an appalling, unforeseen accident when Peter was run over, but she could never forgive him for going away to lead a seminar in Queensland the following weekend. 'That one was a severe dent in our friendship, relationship, companionship,' says Grace.

At the time of the accident, August 1983, Ian was committed to go to Brisbane to present the 'first talk of significance that I did in terms of the cancer work'. He was due to speak for two days at the Relaxation Centre in Brisbane. Two hundred people had registered for the weekend. The accident happened earlier in the week. Faced with the dilemma of cancelling the workshops, or leaving Grace alone with the children, Ian chose to leave.

For this Ian is contrite. 'I think that it is probably fair that she had a grievance about that. However, we did discuss it at the time, Grace agreed to me going and, on my part, I knew how strong she was and thought that she could manage. In the event, she found it really difficult and was angry with me. I guess the tragedy is that she never got over it and that in itself became very difficult,' he says. 'That situation with Peter was . . . very difficult . . . for me . . . and, if I had my time again, particularly knowing the consequence of how it affected her, I would have made a different choice.'

'We couldn't change what had happened, Peter was fully recovered, and I was sorry that I had done it. I feel like it had been a simple error of judgement in our busy lives. But the difficulty that came out of it was that she wasn't able to forgive me for what happened . . . no discussion in ensuing years would help her understand I was sorry I did it. I was really sad it had caused her as much grief as it did,' says Ian, 'but we couldn't change it and the only choice was to forgive. You move on or you hang on to it. And that became one of a number of things that, for Grace, were unforgivable in our lives together.'

Grace did not see the dam and the Hawaii incidents as unfortunate mishaps, or as the inevitable adventures of a full and rich family life, as Ian did, she saw them all as evidence of her husband's wilful recklessness and neglect and laid the blame for them squarely on his shoulders.

Meanwhile there was no let up in their working life—and tensions inevitably surfaced, some which were to remain unresolved.

There were their ongoing differences of opinion and styles: Grace's preference for a business model, Ian's for a charity one. Grace still thought the program focused too much on diet and meditation to the detriment of some of the more esoteric factors in Ian's recovery. He continued to attract most, if not all, the publicity— and consequently, as Grace saw it—the credit for the work of The Foundation. And then when Ian was awarded the Order of Australia in the 1987 Australia Day honours list, Grace was overlooked.

'I said to Ian, I don't think this is really fair,' she says. 'I'm sort of half of The Foundation, I'm co-director, and co-founder and I've been part of this the whole way along. I said it's not about ego, it's just about rightness. And he said, "Oh I'm receiving it for both of us." It's been very helpful for him to have received that but it wasn't helpful for me.'

'It was actually the programs that were the main problem,' maintains Dorothy Edgelow. In her view, 'Grace had developed a different way of dealing with the physical and emotional problems, particularly with women.'

Grace was of the view that women could be more frank and share a better sense of camaraderie in a single-sex group. She convinced Ian of the efficacy of her way, he readily acknowledged the value of Grace working more directly with women, and supported her in this. However, her direction subsequently began to diverge ever more from her husband's.

Perhaps if the couple had managed to establish a more stable home life, the divergences and disagreements at work might have been more easily absorbed or resolved. The couple had shared so much, so closely in the early days, but there were, as Ian admits, 'flaws in the relationship'. At times work and family life blurred into one difficult or incommunicative reality.

There was also a great deal that they did agree on. For instance, the Gawlers generally found it very easy to work together when they jointly led groups. They had always made a great team. However, when they did see things differently it would lead to bitter disagreement, with neither side willing to back down.

'Differences of opinion were very hard to resolve because we were both quite strong-minded people,' admits Ian, adding that, 'I was the one that was there every day and had a sense of what needed to be done and Grace would only come in intermittently.' Ian's decisions often prevailed.

Ian Gawler has a quiet authority; whereas Grace had an entirely more imposing, domineering personality. 'She would walk into that kitchen and the doors would fly open, and you stood back wondering what she wanted this time,' says Gail Lazenbury, then a member of the kitchen staff, now catering manager at The Foundation. 'You didn't say no.'

'On his own Ian would not have been able to get to the level he has,' notes Dorothy. 'He had the vision but he couldn't have done it without Grace. She was the one who sorted it all out and put it into perspective. He had the ideas and she would get all the nuts and bolts into place . . . she was the below-the-surface driving force.'

Grace had worked so hard to save his life and now she was a full-time, overworked 'protectress' (as one person who is close to the Gawlers put it), who had very little support of her own. She had children to nurture—a lot of the time without Ian around— and she had missed this kind of care herself.

Ian and Grace are both driven and accomplished individuals, but their will manifests in different ways. Patients during the 1980s and 1990s might have been forgiven for thinking that Grace was the one who ultimately ran the place with a firm hand. In truth, it was Ian who had a tighter grip on the tiller, and he did so with a quiet but immoveable efficiency.

'When you work with him you can't change anything,' says Rudi Uriot his personal assistant for seven years (2000–2007). 'He is very much in command. He will listen to you and say yea or nay. He has this subtle way of just pursuing what he wants.'

Ian 'likes to be in control,' adds Dorothy, 'and Grace didn't like to be controlled. She wanted to build and work on her own theories and work on her own passions.'

More than that, though, serious differences of opinion on how to handle staff would occasionally surface—not the least because the couple had two very different approaches to management. Ian approaches staff management—like everything he does—with forgiveness. Grace, on the other hand, as she herself admits, was more 'principled in saying no—one strike and you are out'.

Ian is acutely aware of the impact and life consequences of an employee losing their job. He always looks for a peaceful solution. Ian sees the good in people, regardless of the circumstances. Grace had a very clear-cut idea of who was in the right and who was in the wrong.

Mix this divergence of management styles with the knowledge that The Foundation had what was effectively a two-headed leadership, then it is little wonder that when any staff crisis did emerge—as they do in any organisation—that there would be some serious problems in its resolution.

It is also little wonder, given the co-directors were also married, that these issues would lead to considerable tension between the two of them on the home front.

On this score, a number of incidents stand out.

The first involved a therapist, Sarah, (name changed) trialled to work on a new program. As Ian frankly admits, while working with Sarah it became very clear to him that there was an attraction between the two of them, although he tried to give her no indication of this fact, nor did he act on his instincts. Nevertheless, as he puts it, he 'spent about a day thinking about it—and I was thinking about it quite seriously because it [his relationship with Grace] hadn't been all that easy. Also, monogamy has always come very easily to me. I had never been tempted to have an affair, never been interested. And—this is true—in a spiritual sense I always thought that this was one of those temptations I needed to confront; to be tested by. So here I was, with an attractive woman, feeling tempted. Fairly quickly, I thought no, I don't want to do that, it's crazy.' More than that, though, Ian then remembers feeling chuffed that his faithfulness had been tested (albeit only by a fantasy in his own mind) and that he had managed to come out the other side with his integrity intact. He resolved to tell Grace about it when he got a chance, but before he could she had picked up on the attraction in her own intuitive way. 'By the time I told her,' says Ian, 'the shit hit the fan.' Sarah's employment was discontinued at the end of the program.

'I actually did speak to her [Sarah] about it many years later, but at the time she couldn't work out what had happened,' says Ian. 'On the surface everything seemed wonderful and then she was told at the end of the program that we did not want her to work with us again. She was flabbergasted.' Neither Grace nor Ian explained the true reason to her at the time.

This was not an isolated incident. A number of people lost their jobs over the years at The Foundation, for apparently innocuous reasons. Others that should possibly have been let go, were not. Grace was a formidable boss who was not afraid to resolutely act in what she saw as The Foundation's best interests; while a number of people have described Ian as shy of direct confrontation or conflict, particularly in the working environment.

One of the most contentious issues in The Foundation's history meanwhile centred around a new therapist named Gary (name changed). This issue also had serious implications for the Gawlers' personal and working relationship. It concerned a serial problem that developed around matters of professional conduct.

To protect the vulnerable, forming a sexual relationship with a client is regarded as professional misconduct. Gary had come on retreat at The Foundation before he was likely to start work and then formed a relationship with one of the female participants he met at the retreat.

It was not really appropriate, as Ian puts it, but it was not strictly unethical given that Gary was not yet employed and was not acting as a therapist on the retreat. 'I talked to him about it being a bit edgy and not really ideal and told him not to let it happen again.' In hindsight Ian now realises the conversation was not as strong or as clear as it might have been, adding that he is 'much better at being clear and direct now. It took me 25 years to learn it. I found that it was very hard in the early days to be really directive with staff. I have always preferred to work with people who worked out the right way to function and who could self-regulate themselves.'

Unfortunately, however, Gary was clearly not somebody with the ability to self-regulate. After about eighteen months the first relationship had ended and then he formed a new relationship with a recovered patient. 'Again it was not a straightforward situation. He had very little to do with her while she was on the program, but he was there as a therapist while she was on the program,' says Ian. Quite some months later the woman volunteered her services to help The Foundation and it was at this stage that a relationship formed.

Ian counselled Gary again, told him how difficult a situation he had created and made it clear that what had happened was unacceptable. However, he resisted firing Gary, telling him that it could clearly not happen again. Grace was appalled. 'The energy of it was huge,' she says. 'The implications . . . were huge and our committee at the time didn't want to do anything about it because they weren't really people who were in the professions.' As far as Grace was concerned, the situation was unethical and Gary should be fired. 'It was like if one person did it, it almost gave permission for others [in The Foundation to do the same] and I got to the point where I thought: I can't deal with the energy of this,' says Grace. 'Here I am working in a women's health practice and what's happening here?'

Meanwhile the situation only got worse. The second relationship eventually broke down and then Gary announced that he had formed a relationship with another past patient he had met on the programs and they were to be married.

'This time it was clear-cut, although it was particularly traumatic,' says Ian. 'I was really concerned for his new wife, but he had to go. I fired him, he took it very badly and there were some ugly confrontations before he left. It was a very difficult thing for me to have to do, even though it was necessary.'

Although Gary was fired, Grace thought the damage had already been done. 'I think she was of the view that he should have been fired on day one, when he became involved in the first relationship,' says Ian. 'Obviously I took a different view.'

'Ian's never been good at that kind of thing all his life,' says Grace. '[In the veterinary practice] I was the one who went after the bad debtors. He doesn't like confrontation.'

'If I have ever approached depression in my life,' adds Grace, 'it was at that time. It was so, so big.' Grace had opposed her husband publicly in committee meetings over the Gary saga, as she felt she must, and she said it 'was like putting the nail in the coffin' of her relationship with him. 'And I can understand it from his point of view,' she says, 'because this was all built up and he felt humiliated that his wife had gone against him quite publicly in The Foundation.' Ian does not remember feeling humiliated.

Running parallel to this was the fact that the new general manager, Siegfried Gutbrod, did not often agree with Grace's way of approaching things either. 'He didn't like me doing my women's health groups in the way that I'd been doing them,' she says. Siegfried, for his part, says he 'cannot remember any particular issue I had with the way Grace was running her groups.'

Siegfried and Ian developed an efficient management structure and they gradually became firm friends. 'I think that we complemented each other,' says Siegfried. 'I reported partly to Ian and partly to the board. We were very friendly with each other but I called a spade a spade and that worked very well.'

Events had conspired to Grace feeling 'disempowered,' she says. 'And I thought either I'm going to grow a cancer in myself if I stay or I have to go.'

Grace left The Foundation to create her own business in 1996 first from a bedroom in the Gawlers' family home (son David magnanimously offered his own bedroom to the cause and took over the shed as his pad) and then Ian helped her buy a small house nearby for her work, which was to focus on women's health.

All the while though, Grace and Ian's relationship at home deteriorated further. Debts were mounting. Blazing rows were common. Or, as Ian puts it, for years all that needed to happen was the mention of a name or situation that angered his wife and Grace would fly into a rage that could last hours.

Son Peter remembers there being 'three or four years' late in the marriage when there would be 'a lot of arguments and that sort of thing'. 'I don't really know or want to comment on what they were about but there was a lot of arguing going on between him and Mum,' he says.

Siegfried remembers seeing Ian come in to work looking physically and emotionally drained. 'Many a time I'd see him coming in at eight o'clock into The Foundation and he was devastated. He talked for half an hour or an hour just to debrief or whatever,' he says. 'There had been enormous fights in the morning and he had to be ready to face groups.'

'At the end of our relationship,' says Ian, 'there was the breakdown of the ability to have a useful conversation about minor things, let alone major things.'

Grace's expressions of unhappiness and anger meanwhile had become such regular occurrences—over a period of years—according to Ian, that he started purposely triggering them in the hope that Grace would recognise the absurdity of the situation. 'I'd only have to say "Peter's accident" or the name of one of the people that she had taken exception to and she'd fly straight off into a tirade. It would last for hours. I would try to engage her rationally but it was unrelenting. She would not stop if I asked and pursued me if I tried to walk away. In the end I realised that the only way I could stop it was to swear at her, because when I swore at her she would take offence and retreat into the victim role,' he says, 'It was incredibly frustrating and sad. I tried all sorts of things. I used to say, "Look, would it help if you got a stick and just beat me for a while?"'

From Grace's point of view, Ian was retreating into silence, as he did so often in the early days. It only compounded her anger. 'Quiet people and silent people tend to get together with gregarious people. In the beginning it really works, but after that it really doesn't . . . and that was certainly the case with us. We worked well as a team but as soon as things got bigger, that's when we really got into problems,' she says.

From his point of view, Ian just felt he was being habitually harangued.

It was an untenable, potentially explosive situation and something had to give. On a number of occasions it descended into low-level physical violence on both sides. 'It was really a mess,' says Ian. 'That was the atmosphere it was getting to.'

Grace moved into a separate bedroom. Ian says, 'The kids were in that atmosphere. It was terrible. It was terrible for all of us.'

Pages and pages of Ian's journal from the time are devoted to the depth of Grace's rage and his despair regarding what to do about it.

17/7/97. Another week of constant unrelenting conflict. It is hard to imagine having your worst argument 2–3 x daily. After every moment that Grace has me alone (even relatively—how impossible all this must be for the children) she is launching into me . . .

10/8/97 . . . I have put all my efforts into staying with Grace, absorbing the rage and hoping it will transform into loving kindness. It is so hard to have to function in an unfriendly atmosphere, to feel unwelcome in your own house.

27/8/97 . . . I have put up with her style (rage, blame, denial of involvement) for so long I have nothing left. I am being driven out of my own home . . .

24/9/97 . . . I seem to have no choice but to leave. I still struggle with the dilemma. There is the spiritual tie which is so strong and the commitment and yet how can this endure the crazy psychic and emotional abuse Grace keeps hurling at me . . . it seems to me I have suffered enough now. I do not deserve this ongoing abuse . . .

The end of the relationship finally came when 'Grace said repeatedly that she didn't believe in forgiveness,' says Ian, 'she told me that she didn't want to forgive (and was happy to take the resentment to her grave) . . . she said: "Well, I'm happy to keep doing this, I can do this until I drop dead,"' he says. 'I know what she is like; she could have.'

At the very core of Ian's beliefs and ideals is a basic tenet of forgiveness; more than that, it was a core philosophy of The Foundation and something Ian has suggested to his clients as being a fundamental prerequisite for the long road to getting and being well. Grace's clear conviction was that he had done things that were unforgivable. It was enough, says Ian, to break the sacred vow—for life—he had made in marrying Grace. The marriage was over. It was November 1997.

Siegfried Gutbrod received a phone call one Friday morning that month from Ian asking him if he could come and stay. 'Two hours later he was there with his horse float,' he says. Inside were a few of his belongings. 'She was away for the day and he moved out and that was it.'

Grace had been running a breast cancer retreat in nearby Healesville that ended that day and when she returned home he had gone, with, as she maintains, no warning. She says she was aware that her husband had been keen to have a serious discussion, but it had not eventuated because they had both been too busy. 'So this was a very big shock,' says Grace, adding that she had arrived home on a 'really high note' from a retreat shared with a 'fantastic group of ladies' only to find Ian gone and her kids 'in a mess'.

'Dad finally saw fit that they couldn't resolve the issues and thought it would be better off for everyone if he left,' says their son Peter. 'Which I think was a good idea looking back on it now. Things were not very pleasant for any of the kids at home and I'm sure they couldn't have been pleasant for Mum or Dad either.'

Ian says that he had made the decision to leave on the Friday—after first telling Grace he planned to move out on the following weekend, because he knew the only peaceful way of doing this was to do it without her being home.

Ian's journal records this a week before he left.

> 23/11/97. Grace came in later and asked when I was leaving. I said at the weekend. She said good, that suits her fine. I said we need to discuss how it all happens, but that has not happened. What a relief leaving will be ...

Ian had also given forewarning of his intentions to the three older children Rosemary, then nineteen, David, seventeen, and Peter, fifteen. Peter remembers helping his father load up the trailer with Rosemary's boyfriend Tim.

With Alice, only fourteen at the time, however, he found himself in the heartbreaking situation of only being able to tell her at the last minute. Ian did not think his youngest daughter was old enough to cope with any indications he was about to leave. 'I had urged Grace a number of times to meet with me and the children so that we could talk about my leaving. She had refused. I don't think she really thought that I would do it. So with Alice I had this really difficult situation.' Ian told her he was leaving that day as he took her to school. 'I didn't want to just leave her, I didn't want to not tell her. I don't know if that was a mistake, but it certainly felt terrible for me and it affected Alice badly too,' he says, adding that he felt he had no other choice.

Grace, it seems, never thought that her husband would *actually* take the radical step of leaving the family even though he made it abundantly clear he was about to, was very distressed and took it very badly emotionally—and, as things quickly transpired, physically.

In fact Ian's leaving quite possibly hastened a recurrence of a uterine prolapse. Grace had suffered her first prolapse several years before, possibly as a result of all the heavy lifting around the farm, as well as having had four babies—one a difficult birth—and possibly as a result of a genetic weakness. 'My mother had never spoken to me about it,' she explains, 'but apparently it's in the women of our family.'

At the time of the first prolapse, surgery was recommended but Grace refused. 'She really felt that such surgery would be an invasion of her body, she talked of it being like surgical rape,' says Ian.

Grace managed the condition non-surgically and recovered, but it recurred several times over the years. Now, three days after Ian left her, it recurred much worse than ever.

This time surgery was unavoidable. Grace rang Ian, told him how scared she was of the surgery and asked him to accompany her. 'I was really taken aback by all this,' says Ian, 'but I really understood Grace's fear and predicament, and said that I would do it, but that was all I would do. She was on her own again after the surgery.'

Ian spent all of the next week in Grace's hospital room, including sleeping each night in a chair at the end of the bed. Then they went their separate ways again.

Ian was staying with Siegfried. He took the spare room at Siegfried's place and slept on a mattress on the floor.

The stay was planned to be only 'a few days' at first, says Siegfried but it stretched out to six months. 'He went through agony,' he says, 'and I suppose his way of coping was to throw himself completely into work.'

Ian had moved in at the end of November and by February began a Masters of Counselling course at La Trobe University. 'He worked day and night. When I went to bed at ten o'clock he would sit up and do his uni work,' remembers Siegfried. 'So I think that was his way of coping apart from talking a lot and meditating a lot.'

In the period immediately after the separation it was particularly difficult, not only because Grace and the children were living right next door to The Foundation, but mainly because Grace was consumed with rage at the fact and the manner of her husband's leaving.

'I had no objection to what happened,' says Grace, 'because I think it would have happened anyway. It was the way it happened. I would have waited until the children were older. We would have lived our separate lives, like so many couples do. We would have gone our separate ways but we would have done it in such a way that the other person didn't have to fall over with an illness.'

Grace refused to talk to Ian after her hospital stay. Ian also says Grace made it a question of 'loyalty to her' if their children saw or spoke to him. He continued to pay the bills and finance the family.

'I went to the house only once or twice in that short period [after he had moved out] and each time there was a scene,' he says. If he tried to call, and Grace answered the phone, she would hang up in his ear. Ian subsequently became isolated from his own children for quite a while. The children were told that he had abandoned them all.

In the longer term Ian moved into a small house in East Melbourne alone, drove to work during the week and would see his children as often as was possible on weekends.

Ian would drive the hour from East Melbourne to the Yarra Valley and then 'he'd take us out for dinner or a movie' in the city, says Peter. 'He'd drive us home at midnight . . . and then drive himself home, so he made a fair effort to be there for anything we needed.'

Incredibly during the time of Ian and Grace's separation The Gawler Foundation functioned as normal and gossip was kept to a minimum.

'It was quite controlled and how they kept it controlled was an amazing feat,' says Gail Lazenbury, 'especially in a small place like the valley. The whole thing could have exploded or the whole place could have imploded quite easily.'

Gail Lazenbury remembers Ian calling staff meetings to inform them of what was going on, both immediately after the separation and during the conflict between them that continued on for years. He would 'explain the situation as it was because he wanted to stop us going out to the neighbours and saying: "You'll never guess what . . . she did this . . . and he did this"'.

'The hardest thing, as far as the staff were concerned was not while it was happening, it was when it was all over and the residents were saying "Where's Grace?"'

As a close family friend, Dorothy Edgelow found the separation particularly difficult and felt badly for them. 'I was in the middle and I sympathised with them both and I did a lot of time supporting Grace and Ian,' she says.

As for the Gawler children they 'have been severely affected,' says Dorothy, who spent a great deal of time with all of them before and after the split. 'In their growing-up years they were all very much alone anyway. They certainly had many, many hours to look after themselves and work with themselves. They are very, very strong. All of them. I think younger kids would have fallen in a heap with what was going on.'

The strains on Ian and Grace were enormous and both suffered immeasurably. Grace was ill and distressed and angry and coping as a single mother on 15 hectares. She says people in the local community jumped to their own conclusions about the split. At Yarra Junction, 'when I was able to get down there' she discovered that people 'would no longer speak to me,' she says. 'I said to the local feed store man: "You're really cool with me, I've got to ask what's going on." And he said: "We don't think much of people who leave men with only one leg …" It was hard. I lost a community and friends and I was getting more and more isolated.' The debts were mounting and people were not being paid.

Ian meanwhile was living in his rented East Melbourne house alone and suffered terribly from being separated from his children. He saw a counsellor regularly, contemplated and meditated for hour upon hour and expressed his grief in a daily art journal. As an escape, when he found the time, he took to visiting his good friend Dr Jamie Duff and wife Rejane Belanger at their home in the countryside near Coffs Harbour, New South Wales.

Jamie and Rejane share a mud-brick home they built themselves at Bundagen, a sustainable community nestled in the Bongil Bongil Coastal National Park.

Owned as a cooperative, Bundagen was established 25 years ago and is now home to around 180 people. The community's homes are connected by footpaths—instead of roads—and cars have to be parked on the edge of the 320-hectare hamlet. All of Bundagen's energy needs are met by solar power and its water needs fall from the sky. The three guiding principles of the community, which is different to a commune, are environmental responsibility, social harmony (it has a 10 pm noise curfew) and economic independence.

'He found this place a real hideaway,' says Jamie, who was clearly able to give Ian emotional solace at a time of desperate need. 'They're like brothers,' according to a mutual friend. 'We share the same sense of humour,' adds Jamie, as well as the same birthday, 25 February, although Jamie is two years older.

Jamie Duff is a general practitioner and mountaineer, originally from the north of England. He has been part of numerous Himalayan expeditions and was the doctor on the south-west face ascent of Everest in 1975, led by Chris Bonington. He was also expedition doctor on Australia's north-face ascent of the same mountain in 1984, accompanying Tim Macartney-Snape, Lincoln Hall and Greg Mortimer. Although his doctoring duties for both expeditions precluded making the final push to the summit ('I've never had any desire to climb right to the top of Everest', he adds), Jamie has climbed the south-west face of Changabang, soloed the north-east ridge of Khumbutse and made the first ever crossing of the North Col of Everest. He is also co-author of the standard first aid reference book mountaineers take with them to the peaks, *Pocket First Aid and Wilderness Medicine* and he is the co-developer of the Portable Altitude Chamber, a lightweight and relatively affordable way to treat altitude sickness.

Ian and Jamie share an interest in meditation and Tibetan Buddhism and it was on one of his recuperative trips to Bundagen that Ian expressed a wish to see Everest. The two of them came up with the idea of leading a meditation retreat to the Himalayas.

In 1999 a group of seventeen people, led by Jamie Duff and his wife Rejane, with Ian as its meditation teacher, met at Kathmandu in Nepal and flew on to Lukla, a small village at 2900 metres above sea level and the starting point for the trek towards Everest.

The trip was three weeks in all and the trek part of an adventure that was fundamentally made up of walking for half the day, and learning about and practising meditation for the other half.

The group would set out early in the morning in silence. Jamie has discovered over the years that if you trek while in a meditative frame of mind, mindful of every step and everything that is around you, keeping silent, then the 'walking is much easier and much more enjoyable'.

Ian Gawler had special lightweight titanium crutches made for the trip and would 'just pole his way down the trail every day,' says Jamie. 'It was incredible. Here's a guy who has had his leg amputated and he's on crutches and he never fell over once and the terrain was bloody difficult. Fit young people find it difficult.'

Fashion designer Sally Browne was also on the trip and says that Ian had a 'marvellous way of just going on. He'd just swing his foot through and he was a faster climber than a lot of people.'

A video taken by one of Ian's fellow travellers shows footage of Ian making his way up precipitous and rocky paths with remarkable dexterity. At the age of 49, and with only one leg, Ian cracked on every day with the commitment and agility of an athlete half his age.

The pressure on his arms and armpits must have been relentless. In fact, as Jamie explains, the work required in walking with crutches is equivalent to having to carry an additional third of your body weight around. 'Ian was like an all-terrain vehicle,' he says. 'Never got carried, never got supported. Incredible. The villagers would just stop and watch him go by. I don't think they had ever seen anyone on crutches.'

Sally Browne remembers Ian would power on as fast or faster than anybody else on the trek. In the afternoons he would also then lead the meditation sessions. After the rigours of the morning's trek, sometimes negotiating narrow and rocky paths next to sheer cliffs, or wobbly bridges strung across rivers on chains, it was 'amazing to see him so focused and yet still able to give to people,' says Jamie, 'and be there with a meditative focus and hold the group, and never get grumpy, and never get tired, and never lose his sense of humour. That's a really impressive feat.'

That said, Ian did sometimes look strained on the trip and he did lose 2.5 kilos in weight. Physically the trip took its toll.

Mentally and emotionally, though, Ian could not have been in better shape. It was already eighteen months since his separation from Grace and he had met someone new.

13

Ruth

It was late in 1998 and Dr Ruth Berlin was not having the best of mornings. Her younger son, Misha, had woken up with a sore throat and was crying that he did not want to go to school. She had a full list of booked patients at her general practice and she did not want to cancel them. Now she had to organise and take Misha, seven, to be cared for by a friend. Life had been pretty tough for a while. 'I was in a really hard place, feeling like I had wrecked my family, while on the surface I was putting on a brave face for the world,' she says.

And then, just as she was pulling out of her driveway in Old Eastside, a suburb in Alice Springs, a long box arrived by courier. Opening the box, she screamed in delight. Inside was a red waratah in full bloom 'very alive and fresh and beautiful'. Ruth admits to talking aloud to herself about the gift for the rest of the day. 'I remember being in the car and having the flower in the box next to me on the passenger seat, aware that now I was going to be somehow protected and cared for.'

Then, as the day went on, with one patient and then another to see in the poky office of a rundown building, the deeper intentions of the man who had sent it began to seep into her consciousness.

It was from Ian Gawler.

A bit later that evening, while cooking dinner and preparing the kids for bed, Ruth remembers thinking, 'He's sending me flowers. He's getting confused. I did not want anything romantic. I had decided that life had become as complicated as I could manage, and that "relationship" was something I was no good at.'

At the time Ruth Berlin was working in general practice in Alice Springs, living each day at a time, in the isolated desert town which she called home. She was far from her parents and brother and sister. The 'Aboriginal Industries'—as they were referred to, tongue-in-cheek, by the people who worked in the region's health, education and administration—commonly attracted energetic, rebellious souls. She had been living there since 1990, originally moving to the Alice to work in an Aboriginal outpatient facility that serviced many traditional people. They came barefooted, smelling of smoke from their fires and talking in languages that had never been written. The dialects of the Aboriginal people filled the waiting room and corridors of the fresh, new buildings. It felt a bit like Kenya, where she had worked before her children were born. She felt useful, and some of her patients' pain resonated with her own pain.

In 1993 she gave birth to a stillborn son with Down's syndrome and separated from her partner, John Wakerman. John was the father of her two healthy sons, Saul and Misha, aged six and two and a half at the time. She had only recently recovered from a severe, chronic back problem and major depression. Originally offered long-term medications and surgery by her colleagues she had instead turned to yoga and psychotherapy for a solution. After a long and difficult rehabilitation her body was painfree and the depression had lifted. She wanted to help her patients with the techniques that had helped her and started to incorporate psychological therapy into her mainstream medical practice.

'I was a bit over-zealous with some of this to start with, because I wanted others to experience the profound healing which I had experienced. So I would see some of my patients any time of the day or night when they called me for help on my mobile.' Her daily life was repeatedly interrupted with calls from patients and out-of-hours consultations. It was another reason why life had become so tough for her.

And then a colleague slid a brochure under her nose.

'This is the kind of thing you may be interested in, Berlin,' he said with a smile. It was a flyer for the Mind, Immunity & Health Conference to be held in Lorne, Victoria in March 1996. It could not have come at a better time and arrived with the added bonus that the Northern Territory Government would foot the bill for the airfare and accommodation to assist in her ongoing professional development and training.

There was also the added attraction that after the conference had concluded, there would be a great opportunity to visit her brother David, who was principal cellist in the Melbourne Symphony Orchestra. The two of them had a close relationship and shared many understandings of life. She missed spending time with him.

The conference itself proved a revelation. There were overseas experts in immunology and mind–body medicine, as well as a Tibetan master, Traleg Rinpoche, and Rabbi Laibl Wolf. There was yoga and there was meditation and for her there was an atmosphere of lightness and effervescence, she says. During the conference she attended a casual breakfast with six others; one of whom happened to be Ian Gawler, the conference's convenor.

Ruth remembers him to be gentle and kind and appropriately inquiring. Beyond that, there was nothing exceptional about their first meeting, she recalls.

The following year, in March 1997, Ruth returned to the conference and was surprised to discover that Ian had remembered her and said hello. Later on they found themselves together in a post-conference workshop run by a Jungian analyst from New York who was expert in analysing people's drawings. As part of the workshop, participants were broken off into groups of three to each draw their own families and to reflect on each other's drawings. Ian and Ruth shared the same group. Ian drew six figures on a page—representing himself, Grace and their four children—and Ruth remembers being really struck by the fact that they looked like they had nothing to do with each other. Each person was drawn separately and doing individual things.

The small group had a discussion around the drawing. It was clear to Ruth that the Gawler family was hardly connecting at all. 'I remember thinking it strange because there was a general impression of the Gawler family being very united, but I was not being particularly preoccupied with it,' she says. That November Grace and Ian separated.

At the Mind, Immunity and Health conference the following year, in March 1998, Ruth's perception of Ian was that he looked 'fragile and thin. I saw somebody who was clearly suffering,' she says. 'It was almost like all the energy had drained out. He was depleted and had lost some weight. He looked sallow to me, and I remember thinking that this wonderful innovator and teacher needed help. Repeatedly I was thinking—somebody do something!'

Ian came and sat next to Ruth during the supper on the first evening of the conference. She was surprised by how familiar and friendly he seemed towards her. He talked to her like they had been old friends. Later the following day he asked her to join him for the Speakers' Dinner. Ruth declined the invitation, telling him that she was not a speaker and it would have been odd for her to be there. She was feeling quite confused about what was happening because she felt a natural ease and confidence when they exchanged their views, but she had never imagined herself to be a part of his world.

With him, she felt like there was a mutual recognition. A mutual acknowledgement of courage in the face of adversity, a deep respect for the truth and a natural affinity. There was also a profound understanding that she had glimpsed when she had looked in his eyes.

Some of her confusion also came from her own situation. She was living with her boyfriend David in Alice Springs at the time. For a few years she and David had attempted to forge a deeper relationship as they repeatedly separated and came together again— at least six times, she recalls. 'It was very sad, what we put each other through.'

After the conference, Ian would ring her from time to time,

usually in the evenings and wanted to talk at length. It felt like a privilege to Ruth that he sought her counsel and support.

For Ian's part, Ruth represented someone who was prepared to talk about things that 'other people might prefer to keep to themselves,' he reveals. 'She had an emotional honesty, an openness that was really delightful.'

Ian Gawler had come from a polite Protestant background, where feelings were not routinely shared and private thoughts were left unsaid. Ruth Berlin, on the other hand, had a Jewish upbringing in a house full of music, emotional self-expression and intellectual discourse about human rights, science and the arts. 'Everyone talked at once and listened occasionally!'

Ruth was born in Capetown, South Africa on 19 January 1958. When Ruth was two, her family moved to Holland—briefly—then emigrated for four years to Israel, followed by another five years in Britain before emigrating to Australia in 1970. There she went to Sydney Girls High School, was dux of the school in her leaving year and graduated from Medicine at Sydney University in 1981. She worked in Kenya for a couple of years, as well as briefly in Malaysia. It was then that she moved to Alice Springs in 1990 with her partner John Wakerman. Sons Saul (born 1986) and Misha (1991) come from her fifteen-year relationship with John, a fellow graduate from her years in medicine. The couple never married and separated in December 1993.

Ruth is an attractive, very intelligent, disarmingly candid and vital woman with a penetrating gaze and a genuine interest in the welfare of others. She is given to frank, warm and open exchanges—unlike the more guarded nature of Ian and his forebears whom she regards as 'English' and 'Victorian' in their communication with each other. She asks direct questions and gets direct replies, ostensibly because of her own candour and love of interesting dialogue.

After that conference in 1998, Ian began to ring Ruth more regularly and she soon became aware of what difficulties he was facing. 'I was really ready to be a safe sounding board for him,' she says. They talked about his feelings around the separation from his children and the problems he was having with access to them. They would talk in the evening, sometimes for an hour at a time, and their conversations were a precious time for Ruth too. She often found herself alone at home and although she was getting better at managing solitude, it was a gradual process. Periodically she would lose herself in a crisis of existential despair and feelings of abandonment—particularly when her children were away from her for weeks at a time, on holidays with their father. Her friends were no comfort to her in these times. Often she would go out into the desert and look up into the sky in the blazing heat, and question everything she had done. She would wallow in feelings of loss for hours, often using a long walk through the nature reserve to Alice Springs' Old Telegraph Station, as a way of working it out of her system.

One day Ruth was walking through the country in the late afternoon. The sky was turning a mauve-pink as the sun set on the horizon where the MacDonnell Ranges stretched from east to west. Above her head, iridescent and boundless, was a deep blue sky. The sandy red path meandered through the witchetty bushes, Eremophila and corkwood trees as it went north along the banks of the dry Todd River bed. There was deep comfort in its arid resilience and it spoke to her directly of the capacity to endure in the face of the hardness of life. She loved the palpable stillness that the evenings often held. But that afternoon any comfort was eclipsed by the feelings of grief that welled in her heart. She had run out of hope in her relationship; she was away from her children too often; she was a single doctor in a small country town; and her friends thought she had lost the plot after giving birth to a stillborn child. 'I had reached the lowest point of my life,' she says.

Halfway into the walk, in the middle of nowhere, Ruth's feelings of utter desperation had mounted to the point that she remembers looking up towards the sky and addressing God in the most heartfelt, despairing and direct way; with tears streaming down her face, she moaned out aloud: 'I can't do this by myself anymore. I can't do it. I need your help.'

Until that point she described herself as someone without any spiritual beliefs. Up until this moment, 'I didn't have any prior sense of connection with God,' she says. 'In fact my relationship with God had remained something of a cold war. It was like: I don't think what you are doing in this world is very nice.'

Ruth had been practising yoga regularly since school days and read books of a spiritual and esoteric nature, but she admits that she had not connected these with anything in her own inner life. Yet, now, in this moment of deep crisis she was calling out loud to a God she had not acknowledged or recognised or believed in. 'It was the most extraordinary feeling that came through my body. I felt so weak but instantly there was this deep sense of relief,' she says. 'It was like the war I had been fighting was over.' It was a classic surrender.

The fundamental change she underwent was indeed, as Ruth explains, a recognition of God's presence. But this acknowledgement came with a blinding sense that she did not have to do it alone. 'I had been brought up to believe that, whatever happened, I had to do it myself. That was the image I had of myself. There was a lot of strength in that, but a lot of pain.' Something fundamental in her inner life had shifted.

And then a month later, on another particularly difficult day, the fresh waratah bloom arrived.

The waratah is a native Australian shrub that grows to about 3 metres in height and it is the official floral emblem of the state from which it originates, New South Wales. The plant comes from the Proteaceae family and the flowers—which blossom in spring—are red, bulbous, other-worldly and magnificent.

The waratah is a very significant flower for Ian Gawler because he connects it directly with his mother. Along with daphne, it was her favourite flower. This connection was deepened by a remarkable Aboriginal experience.

Ian had organised a conference on survivors in 1992. His old mentor Sir Edward 'Weary' Dunlop had been one of the keynote speakers along with the Aboriginal elder and leader Burnum Burnum.

While Weary had spoken of his experience surviving the Japanese prisoner-of-war camps and returning home alive, Burnum Burnum spoke on how indigenous people had survived for 40000 years or more before white rule in Australia.

The next day, Burnum Burnum conducted an interactive workshop. He told a story of a young Aboriginal couple who fell in love but for whom such a relationship was taboo under their tribal law. He enlisted Ian's oldest daughter Rosemary to act as the young girl and chose other children and parents for the other roles. In the story, the young couple run away, are pursued by their tribe, have a series of adventures, get caught and the young man is speared and killed. The young girl, heartbroken, collapses and dies. As Burnum Burnum told this part of the story, he had Rosemary lie on the floor and curl up in a ball. Then he covered her with his huge traditional possum cloak before producing a real live waratah—which no-one had caught sight of until that moment. For Ian the workshop had been an electric experience.

Burnum Burnum explained that he was telling the traditional Dreamtime story of how the waratah came into being. It grew out of the blood of the broken heart of the young lover. For Ian, Rosemary, his first born, reminded him of his mother and here was such a dramatic link. This link was further reinforced by the fact that there was a waratah on an antique chair given to him by his grandmother, carved by her uncle.

The actual bloom Ian sent came from a bush he had planted at The Gawler Foundation's garden when it was first established. Ian had snipped off the most exquisite flower on the plant and sent it to Ruth.

Ruth was deeply moved by the gesture, taking it as a gift from the universe, a perfectly timed expression of life and beauty in the middle of a hard life. And then the more personal implications of its arrival slowly dawned on her.

'The waratah has a significance for him beyond any flower,' she says. Ian, it transpires, had told Ruth the Burnum Burnum story at the previous conference and had offered to send her a flower when they were in bloom. That said, the flower had taken on a deep symbolic meaning by the time it arrived.

'So I rang him up and said: Ian what do you mean by sending me a flower?' says Ruth.

Ian's reply was long and meandering, more about the planting of the bush in The Foundation's garden, as Ruth remembers, until she asked again.

'No, what does it mean?'

'I'm being friendly.'

'Bullshit, I said—at this point I could not contain myself—men send women flowers because they are interested in some kind of sexual or romantic involvement.'

There was silence at the end of the phone.

'And then he said something like: well that's a possibility.'

For the first time, it really hit home to Ruth that Ian was seriously interested in her. 'For him what he meant when he sent that waratah was that it wasn't just a romantic interest but for him it was like he was sending his heart and he was saying: this is marriage, long term, everything,' she says today. At the time she had not yet fully grasped all this. 'He was clearly the most mature and the most assured man I had ever met,' says Ruth. 'And then I heard this voice in my head that said, if you turn this down you won't get another offer like this.'

Crucially too, her experience in the desert a month before had left her open to the possibility of really opening up her heart to someone else—in a way that she never really had before.

'From then on my responses to him were different,' says Ruth, adding that the phone calls increased and she begun receiving more presents in the post, including music and roses. It was very much an old-fashion courtship. They arranged to meet in January 1999 in Sydney, while Ruth was in the city on her annual visit to her father and stepmother.

From Circular Quay on a bright warm day, they took a water taxi to Doyles restaurant for lunch overlooking the harbour at Watsons Bay and Ian ordered a glass of champagne and then a bottle of wine. Neither made a habit of drinking much usually, in fact Ian had only recently began to drink again a few months earlier, after abstaining since his illness 24 years earlier. Ruth ended up feeling quite drunk and insisted they go for a walk.

Watsons Bay is a picturesque suburb at the southern head of the entrance to Sydney Harbour. Established in the 1780s, it started life as a fishing village, but is now a well-heeled locale with multi-million dollar homes—although it still retains some of the charms and heritage of its humble, weatherboard-built beginnings.

From Doyles, Ian and Ruth took a walk after lunch towards the lighthouse that protects ships from the cliffs and rocks at South Head, but only made it as far a small sheltered and sandy cove, Lady Jane Beach. Lady Jane Beach is a nudist beach.

When they got to the far end of the beach, Ruth suggested they go for a swim and proceeded to strip down to her knickers. They did not have bathers or towels with them. 'I wanted to test his courage,' she says, adding that it dawned on her that Ian was a 'quite well-known person'—and a man with an old-school upbringing. For him to take off his kaftan and jump into the water in his underpants would be quite a challenge.

Ian remembers understanding the import of Ruth's request quite clearly. While internally he laughed at her capacity to challenge him so directly, it was a moment that clearly required a decision. He stripped off and entered the water; now unable to suppress the laughter. Ruth was amused to see he favoured old-fashioned y-fronts.

The swim was a direct challenge to a man she was all too aware was eight years older than her. 'Older men can seem to be a bit kind of fatherly and I didn't need a father, I have a good one,' she says, 'and I didn't want to be with someone who was boring in that non-spontaneous way.' He passed her 'test' with flying colours.

The following day they took the Manly ferry together and Ian talked candidly about being on the vessel with his mother as a young boy and it being a very cherished memory. Habitually cautious in the face of emotional intimacy, Ian had begun to really open up with Ruth. She took his hand, as they sat side by side, coming back to Circular Quay.

They spent most of the day together and Ruth confessed to Ian everything she could about her complex past. 'I put all the laundry out,' she says. 'I didn't want another relationship that wasn't open.'

She was not entirely sure how it would be received because up until then she had assumed by Ian's demeanour that he was quite a conservative man—with ascetic tendencies. She had supposed that Ian had some difficulty in being 'emotionally open' and had found this to be very limiting in past relationships. 'I thought that people who are "spiritual" could be quite uptight,' she adds. 'I think there was a bit of me that was worried he was going to be a bit Spartan.' The lavish lunch, the champagne, the wine, and the swim eased her apprehensions. It became clear that rather than being conservative or uptight, the apparent emotional reserve was more a function of respect for others, and, his inclination to be very careful with matters of any delicacy.

Indeed in return for Ruth's confessional, Ian also revealed to Ruth that he was in a lot of financial debt as a result of the separation. A new relationship was clearly not going to be without its own problems.

Until then she had 'no idea what an acrimonious divorce situation he was in,' she says. In the phone calls he would allude to his and Grace's difficulties, but had not outlined the specifics. Now she was beginning to understand that his was in 'a league beyond' most separations she had known. 'He seemed to be under constant attack.'

Although very intimate in terms of communication, at this stage, Ruth reveals with her characteristic candour, the couple's new relationship did not yet have a sexual dimension. And even when that began to develop it had a very defined boundary—set by Ian.

In late May 1999 Ian had flown to Alice Springs to speak at the annual mini-conference that Ruth's medical practice held at a cattle station south of Alice called Ooramina. The conference had been established as a regular event; a team building exercise for the doctors and a chance for their families to get to know each other. Ruth saw it as a way for her and Ian to be together, as well as a chance for him to share a little of his wisdom with her colleagues and engender 'a more positive approach to illness,' she says. 'I hoped that some of his ideas on mind–body medicine could permeate their narrow thinking.'

The night of the conference, Ruth and Ian slept under the stars, their swags next to each other. Ian read her inspirational and spiritual works by Sufi poets Rumi and Hafiz. 'This was very clever because poetry was something I had written all my life,' says Ruth. 'I was very attuned to it. I used to read poets as a pastime. My mother used to write excellent poetry.'

Preferring John Donne, T.S. Eliot, W.H. Auden—classic poets in the English language—Rumi and Hafiz were not poets that she had ever come across. 'In fact it was more interesting than some of the poetry that I had read—there was like a renaissance for me in it. And he was reading me this—and his swag was right next to mine—and there was the sense that he was definitely wanting something physical to happen.'

Ruth's relationship with David had ended soon after her return from Sydney and Ian had already been separated for eighteen months by now. Nevertheless, Ian was very clear that he did not want to consummate their relationship until his divorce was complete. 'He had quite a clarity on that,' says Ruth. 'He said that on a spiritual level he had taken a vow and there had been a marriage.' Only after the divorce was through in July 1999 did he feel free to be sexual 'naturally', says Ruth, adding that what he meant by this was that, until then, intercourse was out of the question.

'I was quite surprised because there was obviously this great yearning in him,' she says. 'I was a bit relieved on some level but I was also struggling with whether he was making excuses or was he really clear. I'd had a complicated sexual history and I was hoping that was going to be finished with that.'

Ruth's concerns proved to be unfounded and once the divorce was finalised in July their relationship developed and deepened naturally. But there were still real geographic limitations. They had to settle for only seeing each other every two months for the rest of 1999, taking turns to travel between Melbourne and Alice Springs. They talked on the phone every day for an hour—'which was pricey and, to me, a bit bonkers,' says Ruth. 'But Ian insisted.'

Ian was delighting in Ruth's capacity to be emotionally open with him and the feeling she gave him of being emotionally safe.

He marvelled at being able to speak with her on any subject and to not feel threatened or attacked. Besides, the long conversations meant that they were getting to know each other really well.

'My sense of this,' says Ian, 'is that often when mature people first meet, sex happens quickly and becomes quite a focus for the relationship. Because Ruth and I waited and because we were so far apart, we talked on the phone a lot and the relationship developed as a deep friendship. Out of the friendship, and after the divorce, then the sexuality developed in a very loving and natural way.'

By October of 1999, the long-distance relationship was feeling really unsatisfactory for both of them. Something had to give. Someone had to give. They began talking about the possibility of Ruth moving to Melbourne—and then on 23 November, which was Sai Baba's birthday, Ruth was walking in the desert again when her mobile rang.

What followed was another lengthy conversation about the relationship. Ian had realised well before what a commitment it would be for Ruth to move and he was planning to ask her to marry him when they were together again the following January. But suddenly there seemed an urgency in it for him.

Ian asked Ruth to marry him.

While Ruth had never been married before, she says that she actually thought that if Ian and her were going to be together then she wanted them to be married, adding, however, that it proved very difficult for her to say yes.

First, there were her children—settled at school and needing to be near their father in Alice Springs—and there was still a lingering sense of denial that Ruth was carrying about how much she really did need support and a good adult relationship. 'So when Ian rang up and asked me to marry him I said: "I don't want to play games. I don't want to play games. I don't want to play games."'

Ian asked her again and Ruth said yes.

A month later Ian flew up to Alice to give her an engagement ring in the same place she had taken the call a month before.

Then, in June 2000 Ian drove up to Alice Springs to help Ruth pack and sell her house and furniture. Although Ian was carrying a heavy debt from his past life and divorce, they decided to spend the proceeds of the sale of her house on their wedding and honeymoon.

'I didn't want to spend it clearing his debts,' she explains. 'It was a bit crazy, but there was an aspect of our relationship where we wanted to start with nothing together, so that whatever we had together, we made together. It was like a clean slate.'

They were married on a clear winter's day in July 2000, in the Melbourne Botanic Gardens under the boughs of a huge and magnificent oak tree, its branches bare but pregnant with the potential of the coming spring.

14

The Dragon's Blessing

It was mid-March and the day promised to be unseasonably hot. Not long after nine in the morning, day five of a ten-day residential program, and it was already nudging 30 degrees outside. Inside the Yarra Valley Living Centre's main meeting room the air was altogether cooler and utterly, profoundly, quiet. The broad green leaves of the oak tree on the lawn beyond the window were still, as if set in a perfect and understanding solidarity.

Sitting in a horseshoe shape, in purple high-backed chairs, were 21 women and nine men. The youngest in their twenties, the oldest over 70, from all around the country and from disparate walks of life. Had they not shared a common bond, perhaps their paths might never have crossed. Apart from those who had come to support their partners, they had all been diagnosed with cancer. Some knew that their doctors were of the opinion that quite possibly they had little time left to live; others had been given a more open-ended prognosis.

The apprehensive silence that had enveloped the room was easy to understand. The focus of discussions earlier in the week had included nutrition, meditation and mind training. This day's subject was death and dying.

At the front of the room, having just sat down in a blue armchair was Ian Gawler, his left leg curled up underneath him and his crutches on the carpet beside him. He was yet to speak. Now he looked up and surveyed the room with friendly, compassionate and knowing eyes. He was calm, unhurried and intimately understood the group's palpable unease.

He told the room that when he was fronting his first group in 1981, on the week that had been slated to discuss death and dying, the 30-strong group had suddenly dwindled to six. 'The next week, everyone was back and everyone seemed to have very good reasons why they couldn't make it the previous week.'

Death is not something most people want to look squarely in the eye. It is something we commonly ignore as if it simply does not exist or only happens to other people.

'When I was lying in bed with two weeks to live,' he went on to say, 'people who came to see me thought they were saying goodbye. In actual fact, I have been to a few of their funerals since.' The room erupted with laughter, Ian apologised for his black sense of humour and the silent, stony sense of dread in the room disappeared.

Ian's joke had two messages. One, his own journey offers hope and, two, that death is a reality all of us have to face regardless of our apparent health. 'Just because you have cancer,' he added, 'it doesn't mean you aren't going to die of something else.'

By pointing out that death is something that happens to all of us, and at a time unknown, those in the room diagnosed with cancer—and given an apparent death sentence—suddenly felt no different from anybody else walking the earth. Better to be living with cancer, than dying with cancer.

Regardless, Ian's message was that death is a reality, and the sooner we get used to it then the sooner all of us—regardless of our relative health—can learn to really *live* for however long we have left.

Or as Ian writes in *You Can Conquer Cancer*:

Dying is a natural process. It is an integral part of life; we are all going to experience it during our lifetime. So you do not need a terminal illness to prepare for death. In fact, the terminally ill often see their condition as a blessing as it does give them just that opportunity. So often we become preoccupied with the mundane things of life and overlook what is happening inside. Who am I? Where am I going? What is life?

What if today was your last? Are you ready? Are you? Is your life's business complete? Have you used your life as you wanted? If this was your last day, would you be doing anything different? If you were run over by a bus tomorrow, would you die with a vulgar expletive on you lips, or could you produce an ineffable smile? The grace of a terminal illness lies in it providing the opportunity to focus on your self, to explore what is important for you and where your real priorities lie.

Some of the people who have found their way to The Foundation over the years come out of desperation, some reluctantly, others as a last resort. Others, at least in the past, came looking to be miraculously healed by a man they thought might be some kind of mystical saviour. 'They wanted to touch the hem of his gown and be cured,' says catering manager at The Foundation, Gail Lazenbury, 'but you don't get that so much now. For whatever reason this place has been turned around into a place of education and knowledge and healing, as opposed to a place to be miraculously cured.'

If you can characterise people who come to The Gawler Foundation it is very common, says Ian, for cancer patients to be described as 'fairly low-stress types. They often appear fairly relaxed on the outside, and they quite commonly seem to be coping with day-to-day events quite well.' What they typically are not so good at coping with, however, is a major life change, perhaps a bereavement, or a divorce or a sudden change of job. 'Well over 90 per cent of the people who come to our groups have felt that a major life-changing stress has been a significant factor in the development of their illness.'

A large proportion of the patients are women (the percentage is roughly 60 per cent female to 40 per cent male). Some bring their partners; others do not. They come from all strata of society and from all around Australia, New Zealand and sometimes further afield, looking for a better, more holistic way to heal their bodies.

Some go into remission, others do not: some add a number of years to their lives, others do not. Some have become remarkable long-term survivors like Ian.

Frank McClintock, 67, was one of the group on that hot and dry autumn day. Frank is from Maryborough, Queensland and an entrepreneur who has developed holiday resorts and run a charter boat firm in the warm blue waters of the sunshine state for the last 22 years. He was accompanied on the residential program by his wife, Dell.

Frank was diagnosed with prostate cancer and in 2001 had been called into the offices of his oncologist to discuss his latest tests. The oncologist broke the bad news that his cancer had spread significantly, told him that it was terminal and that he could be kept alive a little bit longer with radiotherapy. Frank's oncologist added there were no alternatives.

The McClintocks did not believe him. At the local library they found about six feet of shelving taken up with complementary and alternative therapies, headed home with a boxful and read like crazy. They were soon totally confused. Frank decided the best approach would be to determine who had the best track record and pursue it. Ignore the rest, he said. 'Ian's book stood out and so did Gerson's book. So we concentrated in those two areas.'

Taking Ian's advice that the Gerson diet was possibly a little extreme for most people, Frank used Ian's book, with some of the Gerson suggestions combined. Meditation proved more of a challenge than the diet.

'My brainbox goes at a hundred miles an hour day and night and I didn't find meditation easy at all,' says Frank, 'but we did concentrate on the diet program and the coffee enemas.'

Five weeks after the oncologist had first given Frank the bad news, he went to his GP to have the Prostate-Specific Antigen (PSA) levels in his blood tested.

PSA is a protein produced by the body and is a reasonably good marker for both prostate cancer and benign prostate enlargment. For someone in Frank's position a high level seemed a foregone conclusion.

On the contrary, Frank's PSA levels, following his strict adherence to a special diet, including the coffee enemas, had dropped significantly.

The following week he took the results to his oncologist. He was amazed. 'He opened it up and said: what have you done?' remembers Frank. 'Not wanting to pick an argument, I said, well, I did go on a diet. He said that wouldn't do you any good.'

Frank then asked his oncologist, a specialist in the field, what else he thought might have produced the result in light of the fact that lifestyle changes were the only ones he'd made. 'He said it might have been a spontaneous remission. You might be one of the lucky ones.'

Frank went home, continued on the Gawler maintenance diet and never went back to the oncologist. Frank went into full remission from cancer.

And then in January 2008, his PSA test escalated rapidly again. He went in for tests and discovered he had developed some bone problems. The cancer had returned. They booked in to The Gawler Foundation's next ten-day program. 'We'd always said we'd come and do the program if I had any more problems. I've got to knock it a second time and this time get into meditation.' Frank believes that the fact that he had not been using meditation to manage all the 'built-up stress and tensions and so on' had contributed to the cancer's return.

During the course meditation is led for three sessions per day, 45 minutes each, in a purpose-built six-sided mud brick building, just off the residential block. This meditation sanctuary is a two-storey structure—below is Ruth Gawler's consulting room and three massage rooms—and it has windows on all sides looking onto the treetops.

Residents sit on bench seating built around the room's perimeter or they can choose to lie down or sit on meditation cushions or stools. Participants are led —sometimes by Ian, other times by Ruth or one of the other therapists—through a series of relaxation and meditation techniques; techniques that Ian first learnt from Ainslie Meares and later expertly honed and developed over the years with other teachers and through personal experience for precise therapeutic effect.

Residents learn to progressively relax their bodies and to calm their minds. They learn to be spacious; learn to watch their thoughts come and go like clouds travelling across a clear blue sky. Instead of identifying with the clouds—which symbolise our thoughts, our hopes and our fears—the idea is to move into the simple, yet profound stillness beyond thoughts; to embark on the journey to discovering one's own intrinsic nature (the sky being the most simple and effective analogy) in all its pure, infinite peace and spaciousness. The idea is to let go of 'the busyness of life, the distractions, the pain and even the pleasantness,' writes Ian in his book *Meditation—Pure & Simple*.

> Let go of all you are familiar with on the surface, and delve deep into you own depths. And find out what is there. In your essence. In you own true heart . . .
>
> For lasting resolution, chronic illness requires that we regain a sense of balance, a balance which includes a healthy and active immune system. In the quest for Good Health therefore, many people are seeking a way to rebuild their immune systems. They are looking for healing from within. This then is why meditation has gained such recognition. It is almost as if meditation's 'calling card' has been its remarkable value as a self-help, self-healing technique. Quite simply, meditation—unequivocally and reliably—can transform disease into good health! And as people practise it more, equally clearly, the benefits of meditation extend far beyond 'just' physical healing. For the 'Good Health' we speak of will include emotional, mental and spiritual good health.

For many of the people who have passed through The Gawler Foundation, meditation has proven to be a crucial element in their healing and the understanding of their illness.

However, Ian is at pains to point out that the place of the mind in healing is not a passive thing. Many people make assumptions about calmness, peace and acceptance when the word meditation is mentioned. Profound healing requires acceptance, says Ian, but it also involves commitment; the commitment of treading a 'warrior's path. Getting well is not a casual thing, it is acceptance with resolve'.

Ian characterises this as the difference between a Rambo approach and a martial arts approach. 'Rambo represents the archetypal, Western, will-driven determination to prevail . . . there is a lot of hope and fear in it, particularly fear, so this drive comes out as being quite aggressive as well,' he says, adding that it is an approach that is high energy and taut and if it does not work 'there is often a real sense of disappointment'.

With the martial arts approach, on the other hand, there is an acceptance that not only is death real, but it is a real possibility. 'There is an acceptance of death and a preparedness for it,' he says. 'And what happens is that out of this acknowledgement of death, there comes a deeper peace.

'We help people get to understand the truth of how precious life is, and yet how impermanent it is. They come to realise that death is real. This leads to a state of mind which isn't a passive one.' People accept death, find an inner peace, and commit to living their lives with a determined, healthy resolve.

It is not, as some people suppose, that a meditation–based approach leads to passively giving up in some way, or that life simply does not matter. Quite the opposite, Ian says, 'In fact what it does is bring people to life. I think it makes people more awake, more present, more conscious that every moment is so precious and to make the most of it.'

If people take this martial arts-like approach to recovery, he says, then if they recover 'it is wonderful. But if they do die there's this deep knowing that they did the best that they could.' This Ian characterises as 'dying well, because they don't have this overwhelming fear or apprehension and they don't have regret. They do not have the feeling that they have let themselves down or others down, they know that they have honoured themselves by doing as much as they possibly can.'

Tens of thousands of lives have been profoundly touched by Ian's work over the years but of all the innumerable stories of triumph and tragedy, acceptance and transformation, one of the individuals who most inspired Ian personally has been Quentin, a remarkable young man brought to him in the early 1980s.

Quentin, then eleven, had undergone major brain surgery for cancer about six weeks earlier. The procedure had left him paralysed down his right side. The boy was withdrawn, traumatised and depressed following his recent experiences in hospital. He was positively terrified of anyone in a white coat—and was referred to Ian by a medical colleague to see if he could help.

Ian had always been interested in art therapy, and drawing with children in particular, which he found to be a skilful way for people to 'express themselves and a great catalyst for conversation'. So in their first meeting, Ian asked Quentin to do a drawing. Something spontaneous.

As Quentin began to make his first marks on the blank piece of paper it was already clear that he was quite an artist, says Ian, 'a prodigy really'. He drew a red dragon, simply but beautifully rendered, beside a village, a lake and, behind it, a mountain. On top of the mountain was a pagoda, or temple. Quentin was right-handed, but the tumour had rendered that side immobile. The work, Oriental in style, was being drawn by the boy using his left hand. It was exquisite in the simplicity and assuredness of its line. Ian asked Quentin to explain its meaning.

The dragon, Quentin went on to explain, had been living peacefully in the lake for ages past. In recent times he had become increasingly angry that the villagers were polluting the water and fishing 'too deep down' tangling his scales in their nets. So the dragon had risen up out of his lake to call upon the Emperor who lived in the pagoda on top of the mountain. He told the Emperor of his troubles and warned him to speak to the villagers urgently. If the villagers did not look after him better, the dragon roared, then he would destroy the village, the lake, the pagoda—everything.

'It was just such an extraordinary metaphor for cancer,' says Ian.

He was deeply touched by the boy's powerful images, not to mention his artistic skills. The drawing carried its message that cancer, as represented by the dragon, has its own 'claim to reality and, while it can appear imposing—scary and threatening—it can carry a blessing. The blessing,' he explains, 'is that you can get your house in order, . . . and not only can you regain your health but you can actually transform your life. For many people who take that view, cancer can be a transformative illness.'

This blessing—the dragon's blessing—this deep understanding that suffering can be transformed and be transformative, this is at the very core of both the work of The Gawler Foundation and of Ian Gawler himself.

For many years The Gawler Foundation and its Yarra Valley Living Centre has not only catered to those living with cancer and looking towards taking the first steps back to health. As well as the well-recognised programs for people dealing with major illnesses, there are programs for disease prevention and for fostering wellness. To this end Ian and Ruth Gawler lead meditation retreats. As well as those at the Yarra Valley Living Centre, the Gawlers have held several week-long meditation retreats in the desert near Alice Springs and one at a community on the north coast of New South Wales, working with local indigenous people and therapists from The Gawler Foundation.

Weekend meditation retreats are also held at the Living Centre as well as a five-day program called Living in Balance, a program that focuses more on emotional health.

The Foundation also offers professional training in the mind–body field. It is an endorsed provider of post-graduate medical education through the Royal Australian College of General Practitioners.

More than 12,000 people have attended residential programs at the Yarra Valley Living Centre over the years and around 100,000 have attended the other programs, public lectures, seminars and conferences run by Ian in the last 30 years.

If you count the people who have bought and read his books and listened to his CDs and the families and friends of the people who have benefited from The Foundation, the number of people that Ian's work has directly and indirectly touched, often profoundly, is a very big figure indeed.

Ian says that he can look back with confidence that virtually everybody his organisation has been directly involved with 'has experienced a significant increase in their quality of life,' he says. 'I just don't have any doubt about that at all. And for some of those dealing directly with cancer, this has translated into really good improvements in the length of their life. Also there have regularly been people who experience long-term recoveries like me.'

As for Quentin, while that gifted young man did not attend a formal program Ian did meet with him regularly after that first meeting when the dragon had been drawn. Quentin continued his extraordinary drawings in their sessions, while Ian taught him to meditate and he became committed to eating well. Quentin improved, went into remission and for a number of years enjoyed good health.

And then sadly, six or seven years later, the cancer recurred and slowly progressed to the point where Quentin lost his sight. Unable to draw anymore, he took up clay modelling. Ian has two of these works in his study at home, a camel and a bull. While their visual appeal is limited, their impact is felt, literally, if you close your eyes and touch them. They 'feel' remarkably like the animals they represent.

'The next thing he did was to take up the harmonica,' says Ian. 'Basically his capacity and senses were diminishing and disappearing, but he was remarkably unfazed. He carried it so well. And then he died [in 1993]. He had inspired so many people during the course of his short life and long illness. He died at peace, with no regrets. He was an extraordinary young fellow.'

Ian makes no grand or extravagant claims about the curative nature of his work, but there is an endless stream of patients queuing up to experience what his organisation proffers. Ian is committed to helping people with their quality of life and with their survival. 'People who come to us are usually interested in survival first and quality of life second,' he says. The Gawler Foundation meanwhile, although best known for offering hope, offers three things.

The first is indeed the *hope* of survival, of quality of life, but most of all, 'hope of finding peace of mind in this very moment'. The second is *choice*. 'For many these days the choices that are offered in the information age are overwhelming,' explains Ian. 'In earlier days people came thinking they had no choice and our groups were a revelation. Now there is so much available. We help people to make informed choices and help them follow through on their choices.' The third thing The Gawler Foundation offers is *peace of mind*. 'Find an inner peace that is real and independent of outer circumstances; find an inner peace which is sustainable—that is the real blessing.'

15

The Pioneer

Forget solid tumours shrinking to nothing under the sustained attention of directed meditation or bare fingers plunging through the skin and leaving no scars. Forget curative Bibles, coffee enemas and the effect of underground streams. The most puzzling thing of all in Ian Gawler's extraordinary story of healing, at least to Ian himself, is not some of these more astonishing turns and twists of his miraculous survival but the way his remarkable tale was received by his doctors.

One of the first things he did, as soon as he was well, was to write to all of the medical professionals that he had seen throughout his illness to set out the facts of his getting well. After all, even leaving some of the more mind-boggling events in the story aside, the very fact he was alive posed one very important question. Was he just lucky, or was there something repeatable in what had happened to him?

An essential element of the scientific method is observation. The history of antibiotics, for instance, can be traced to one remarkable observation. Perhaps Ian's story offered some crucial lessons, as yet unexamined, that could be learnt and applied in a therapeutic setting?

In 1928 British bacteriologist Alexander Fleming noticed that a random mould had begun growing on a culture dish containing a disease-causing bacteria with which he had been experimenting. The mould appeared to have killed the bacteria. Fleming had discovered—had observed—penicillin.

Great advances in science come when something is observed that does not fit with expected norms. From this observation, a hypothesis is formed and then tested. If the hypothesis holds true, then a new theory comes to light.

Fleming's hypothesis was that penicillin could treat bacterial infections. Although Fleming did not go on to test and prove his own hypothesis and develop it into a medicine (instead it was Australian Howard Florey and German Ernst Chain who in the 1940s went on to develop a useable product) it was this first observation that led to the development of penicillin. It would ultimately go on to treat bacterial infections and save countless millions of lives.

When Ian Gawler recovered, Ainslie Meares remarked that something 'only has to be done once to prove that it is possible'.

Back in 1978, Ian imagined that his doctors, professionals in the business of healing, would all be interested in his extraordinary story. Or at least curious. After all, was not this, too, the observation of something extraordinary outside of the expected norms—not unlike Fleming's mould—for which a hypothesis could be drawn and tested and results applied?

Instead most of them got angry. Only his surgeon, Mr John Doyle, the doctor who had shown Ian real compassion and care early in his story, took a more 'neutral stance,' says Ian. 'He said to me at the time that he couldn't think of any medical explanation for the fact that I'd recovered, but he said he was really pleased that I had and left it at that.'

Apparently his radiotherapist barely read a paragraph or two of Ian's letter before he screwed it up and threw it straight in a bin, muttering, 'He must have been misdiagnosed' under his breath—this according to the radiotherapist's receptionist. Ian's chemotherapist, Dr Ivon Burns, also reacted 'in a very lukewarm way', says Ian.

'He was always very objective, caring and reasonable during my illness,' Ian hastens to add. 'When I first consulted him he set out the possible benefits and side effects of the chemotherapy and was quite happy for me to go off for two weeks before deciding what to do. Later when I elected to stop the treatment so much sooner than he recommended, he was genuinely concerned for my welfare, advised me to continue, but accepted it well enough when I stopped.

'However, once I recovered, he seemed to me to be adamant that it was the chemo that led to my recovery. He was then, and continued for many years, to be very dismissive of all else I had done to recover personally and then went on to do with groups.

'It was very clear in those early days after my recovery and when the cancer groups first began that there was real antagonism amongst many medical people to things like nutritional therapy and meditation,' says Ian, adding, 'I suppose I could understand more easily that something like the Filipino healing was seen as being a bit flaky, but there was a real lack of enquiry generally.

'The thing that really disappointed me, was this lack of interest in the fact that by any estimate I had recovered in an extraordinary way. It was quite frustrating. I thought I had learnt something about what had happened to me; why I had recovered and I thought that there was something really valuable on offer for other people. I felt what had helped me could benefit many other people.'

Instead of the new groups being welcomed or supported, in the main they were attacked by the medical hierarchy. 'It seems the same thing happened with Alcoholics Anonymous,' says Ian. 'When it was first suggested that a group of alcoholics could get together and fix something that medicine was almost powerless in front of, it too had been attacked relentlessly.'

Even more, Ian soon observed that the doctors who had helped him—pioneers in this field, such as Ainslie Meares, John Piesse and Warren Hastings—were badly treated by their colleagues. 'In those early years they were subjected to attack and ridicule,' he says. 'Not long before he died, Ainslie Meares spoke to me of his disappointment with not being recognised or acknowledged by his medical peers for his pioneering work with therapeutic meditation.'

Ian soon realised that if he were to offer to help teach others about what had helped him, he was likely to receive little support and few referrals from the mainstream medical profession.

In that respect, Ian and Grace (or Gail as she was then) were on their own.

When they started holding groups in 1981, they were considered radical. Indeed their groups were the first of their type in Australia and one of the very first of their kind in the world. To get the message out about their work to those who needed it, Ian quite deliberately took the view that he had to go to the media and attempt to reach the community directly.

'Ian's engagement with the media has always been motivated by the desire to get his understandings about healing across to the maximum number of people,' says Ruth. 'His avenues to changing medical practice were initially limited by the parochial and sceptical response of the medical profession. In those early days he had to risk looking like a folk hero, guru type in order to have some impact. As time has gone on his methods have become more mainstream and he has been able to be more 'professional' in his methodology.'

One of the great constants in Ian's story is the indefatigable way that he has approached applying the lessons of his own story for the benefit of others. Ian's hard-won personal experience was a powerful thing indeed and it is this that he absorbed, analysed and honed and sought to share with anyone who was interested.

'It is helpful to be aware that when I began running cancer groups in 1981, I had nothing more than my own personal experience of recovery, along with a great deal of reading and contemplation,' says Ian. 'I had never been in a group myself. I had no training in running groups. Perhaps it is not surprising that the doctors were sceptical.'

Nevertheless, Ian is quite proud of this lack of apparent preparedness for the groups. The groups were something completely new, aiming as they were to help people with cancer, both patients and partners, to improve their quality of life and, more contentiously for the medical system of that day, improve survival.

'I was really clear in those early days—early years, really—that I did not know what I was doing. And there was no model for what

I was doing either. But because of this, I asked people continuously what they found to be helpful. What it was about each group meeting that was helpful; what they tried to do at home that was helpful. By responding to this feedback, the style of presenting the group sessions and the contents themselves, improved rapidly. The whole thing developed in a very practical, pragmatic way,' he says. 'Later on, I went to many workshops, read as much as I could and did a Masters in Counselling. However, the ongoing habit of continuing to ask people what works, is, I believe, one of the main reasons that the groups became and continue to be so useful.'

More specifically they were useful because they had a couple of very clear and powerful aims. First and foremost in Ian and Gail's minds, the groups were intended to improve the participants' prospects of survival. Secondly, they were designed to improve the quality of life, or as Ian puts it 'the experience of life living with cancer' for those who came.

When he wrote his first book, *You Can Conquer Cancer*, in 1984 Ian identified the common fears experienced by many when first diagnosed with cancer.

There can be personal fears such as: Why am I hurting? Is it going to get worse? Will I recover? Am I going to die? There can be financial fears: Can I pay my medical bills? Will I be able to work again? Will I get my job back? There can be social fears: Will I be rejected? What will my family do? What will my friends think? Am I to be an outcast? It does not take long to run up a list of horrors that are all too real in any disease, and in cancer especially.

Perhaps the greatest need in dealing with such fears is being able to accept our situation as it is. If we can do that, and through acceptance, deal with things as best we can, while at the same time avoiding worrying about what tomorrow may or may not bring, then we will be free of psychological pain. The 'if' that begins that last sentence may seem like a rather large one to begin with, but accepting our situation is something that can be done. Just realising the need to do it gets us halfway there. Then, identifying what causes pain to hurt shows us how to deal with it. Regular meditation and positive thinking definitely lead to a peace of mind which engenders acceptance. Many people have found this and by using the techniques have come to experience a calmness that has been followed by an automatic lessening in their pain.

Ian realised that people facing all these fears needed hope. Hope for survival. Sure, there was a recognition that quality of life was important, but for most of those who were facing the immediate prospect of a potentially difficult death from cancer, they were preoccupied with survival.

'That is why I chose such a strong title for *You Can Conquer Cancer*,' he says. 'There were plenty of reasons why not to use the *conquer* word, but I wanted to break through people's fears, society's fears, and plant a strong seed, that it was possible to recover—even if it was against the odds.'

This, it seems, is where the sticking point came with the medical profession and particularly its conservative hierarchy. They seemed adamant that the domain of curing cancer was theirs and the notion that people affected by cancer could influence the outcome of their own disease was radical indeed. This was exacerbated by the suggestion that what would make the difference were apparently fringe elements like nutrition, positive thinking and meditation. Throw in the hint of exotic forms of healing like psychic surgery and the initial scepticism of mainstream medicine becomes more understandable.

'Pretty much from the start, most doctors quickly recognised that our groups were helping people, both patients and families with their quality of life,' says Ian. 'But there were only a rare few doctors in those early days who embraced the idea that the things we were teaching could affect outcome and improve survival.'

What seems to have really frustrated and disappointed Ian was the lack of scientific enquiry.

'By any stretch of a medical imagination, I had recovered against the odds. Very quickly after the groups began we started to hear from people who reported how surprised their doctors were with their good progress and quite a few went on to have dramatic, unexpected recoveries.'

Instead of these observations being welcomed by the doctors, what happened was they were frequently dismissed as coincidences, anecdotes or 'just lucky'. Worse, the notion that the groups were helping people to survive, that individuals were helping themselves to survive, was commonly attacked.

'In cancer medicine, enquiry into the self-help approach has gone through a very long and arduous process. In those early days, most of the medical profession seem uninterested in ever admitting that people were getting well against the odds in a way that warranted investigation.'

Doctors were also suspicious that Ian's methods were in opposition to their own treatment regimes.

'In those early days, it seems many oncologists formed the view that we were suggesting people use our methods, not theirs. They were worried that people might forgo effective medical treatments.'

In fact, Ian has always emphasised the integrative approach. 'If people have curative cancer treatment available to them, we have always recommended they embrace that treatment and then use our methods to support their efforts. What we recommend can improve quality of life and may well reduce side effects and enhance the treatment outcome.'

Nonetheless, it is true that when people do not have a medically-based cancer cure available to them, Ian's views may be more challenging for all. 'In this situation what to do is often very difficult. If a cure is not possible medically, then any treatments offered are by definition palliative; that is, they need to be concerned with minimising side effects, extending life where possible and improving both the quality of life and death itself. Palliative treatments that, for example, include chemotherapy often pose challenging questions. How to balance their potential benefits with the potential side effects? Often these equations are difficult to resolve.'

Given all this, Ian's message has always been to suggest looking at techniques and therapies that can be used in *addition* to ones that are already readily available in mainstream practice. Early critics did not necessarily understand this point and they sometimes made the assumption he was setting himself up in critical opposition to established ways. Instead Ian's message was a powerfully inclusive and positive one.

Ian was and is motivated to help others to become empowered to use their own inner resources—to look at the whole of the body and the mind in their treatment; to be in a position to weigh up all of the available treatments, mainstream, lifestyle and complementary, and make an informed decision as to which choices to follow.

It seemed like a logical and common sense approach. It is little wonder, then, that Ian was so confused by the response and resistance he met when he first started talking to doctors about what he had discovered—particularly from oncologists.

It is also clear that some critics early on could not see beyond some of the more mystical elements of Ian's story—such as the Filipino faith healers. Perhaps they assumed he was looking to set himself up as a healer himself. How wrong they were.

Ian's interest was in distilling the universally applicable lessons he had learned about getting well. 'After my recovery first became public in '78,' Ian says, 'many other people contacted us who were going to the Philippines for healing. What we observed was that most had a good experience. Most felt benefit. However, of greater significance, if they did not change their lifestyle, they soon relapsed, commonly within three to six months. It became clear to us that while the Filipino healers, prayer, laying on of hands etcetera could be of significant benefit it was very, very rarely good enough on its own. It is the same with complementary therapies like herbs, Laetrile [a controversial anti-cancer drug], shark cartilage and the like. I do not know of any magic bullet out there. The real magic bullet is inside—in the power of the mind, in how it leads to good choices like eating well, exercising, meditating. Surgery may be necessary, drugs and radiotherapy useful. Use them for the benefits they offer and hope that they cure the immediate problem. But long-term good health is most benefited by a healthy lifestyle. And drugs will not bring peace of mind and lasting happiness. Peace of mind is an inner state. And that state can be learnt, developed and sustained.'

Dr Craig Hassed, one of Ian's key supporters in the medical community and one of the doctors who has worked in The Gawler Foundation's programs for many years, agrees that there often was, and in some quarters still is, a misunderstanding of what Ian was about.

'The message has always been to use the best of everything that's available,' says Dr Hassed, a senior lecturer at Monash University's medical school. 'I think there was also a misunderstanding that he might be making unsustainable promises.'

In fact Ian makes very clear promises.

'In those early days I told people very clearly that I felt that the things I did helped me to recover against the odds. I hoped they might help others and told them that I did not know if they would, but offered to share what I knew. As time went on, the quality of life benefits were very obvious and now we know from our own research and a solid body of evidence gathered around the world that those benefits are real. What is desperately needed is a major outcome study to answer the question everyone is interested in: does what we do extend life significantly? My strong impression is that it does, but that is a hypothesis that needs testing.'

Having trained in veterinary science, Ian's approach is very much rooted in the Western paradigm. He is critical and analytical and what he says and what he believes is based on logic and reason. His position is not influenced by drug companies, nor confined by oncology training. He is interested in, and committed to, what works for the patient. In the early days, it was perhaps the mere fact that he did not fall compliantly behind conventional medical ideas, as was the order of the day, that he was painted by the broad-brush term of 'alternative'.

'In the early days what I and others like me were offering was described as "Alternative Medicine",' Ian agrees, adding that 'In Australia this soon became a pejorative associated with quackery and charlatanism.'

In response, a new umbrella term was coined—complementary medicine. Complementary medicine and therapies usually involve more natural methods than their sister mainstream ones. And it is a massive field. Indeed both Americans and Australians now spend more out of their own pockets each year on complementary therapies than they do on the orthodox ones. Complementary therapies —including homoeopathy, herbalism, naturopathy, traditional Chinese medicine and acupuncture—are now so hugely popular that doctors are increasingly studying or practising them.

In Australia the word 'alternative' became such a derogatory expression in mainstream quarters that it fell into disuse. By contrast in the United States, there seems to be a more open, enquiring attitude. The Americans have a major body called the National Center for Complementary and Alternative Medicine (NCCAM). The word patently does not have the same loaded connotations in America as it does in the antipodes.

'As I understand it, a few years ago the US government began giving US$400 million annually to NCCAM for research in that field,' says Ian. By contrast it was not until 2007 that Australia established a similar body, calling it the National Institute of Integrative Medicine—leaving out any mention of 'alternative' and providing it with a $4 million budget.

In recent times, the term *integrative medicine* has become widely used and broadly accepted. Integrative is a term that fosters an atmosphere of mutual respect, understanding and cooperation—not to mention rigour.

Integrative medicine takes the whole of the body, the emotions, the mind and the spirit into consideration. The integrative approach is one that integrates a diverse team of health professionals, working cooperatively, and takes the best of mainstream, allied and natural therapeutic approaches on board. In Ian's view it is, in fact, what good medicine probably always was.

Ian was a key pioneer, and remains one of the most influential figures, in this field.

In 1995 Ian convened what was to become the annual Mind, Immunity & Health Conference. It was the very first integrative medicine conference in Australia. This innovation would later morph into the Holistic Health Conference and is now run under the auspices of the Australasian Integrative Medicine Association.

In 1988 Ian had started training people to lead cancer self-help groups and began to train meditation teachers as well that year. In the twenty years since, he has continued to be a principal leader and mentor in the integrative field, adding the Endorsed cancer teachers program in 2006 and the Endorsed meditation teachers program the following year, to his busy schedule. Currently a network of groups presenting The Gawler Foundation twelve-week lifestyle program, 'Cancer, Healing and Wellbeing', is developing across Australia and New Zealand.

One of the central tenets of the integrative approach to medicine is the importance of lifestyle factors for health and wellbeing. 'It would seem that there is great merit in differentiating between lifestyle factors and complementary medicine,' says Ian.

Complementary therapies involve visiting a health practitioner such as an acupuncturist, naturopath or traditional Chinese medicine practitioner. Complementary therapies often involve taking herbs or supplements. 'They rely on outside agencies for their benefits,' says Ian. 'On the other hand, lifestyle factors involve all the things that a person can do for themselves during daily life. These include exercise, what we eat, how we manage our relationships and our emotional and spiritual life; not to mention whether or not we use the power of our minds and practise things like relaxation and meditation techniques.'

The critical importance of lifestyle factors in good health and healing has always been the main focus of Ian Gawler and The Gawler Foundation. Important to note, too, is that the positive evidence for lifestyle factors in improving outcomes in healing and for wellbeing is very strong. For example, the effect of exercise on the prevention and treatment of breast cancer is particularly notable.

A study by Holmes et al. [*JAMA*, 2005 May 25; 293(20):2479–86] found that between three and nine hours of exercise per week halved the risk of dying in women with breast cancer whilst nine hours or more per week reduced the absolute mortality risk by 6 per cent at ten years. Exercising more is a simple and easily achievable lifestyle change and it is relatively cheap.

Ian goes on to point out that in contrast to lifestyle programs, the benefits of many complementary therapies are contentious. 'Some research has been done in this field that is both excellent and supportive, but the evidence base is patchy, claims are often exaggerated, and currently it is very difficult to be objective.'

Ian Gawler and The Gawler Foundation are 'committed to the integrated approach and we advocate, teach and support people to learn and sustain a healthy lifestyle. We use lifestyle factors to empower people to take more control of their own health.

'Clearly there is the potential within the human body to recover from cancer,' adds Ian, speaking with both the imposing authority gained from both his own experience and the countless cases he has observed in over three decades at The Gawler Foundation. That potential, he says, 'lies within our immune system specifically and the body's defence mechanism generally; and the best way to stimulate that potential for healing is through meditation, diet, exercise—all the lifestyle factors.'

When it comes to cancer medicine, Ian is of the view that lifestyle factors are being ignored to the detriment of all those diagnosed with the disease.

'If anyone is diagnosed with heart disease these days, their doctor would be virtually negligent if they did not ask that person about their lifestyle—at the first consultation. What are you eating? Do you exercise? How do you manage stress? Even how do you relax and do you meditate are becoming common questions.

'If someone is diagnosed with type 2 diabetes, the lifestyle questions are even more important. Yet with cancer there seems to be this huge error of omission. Very few doctors ask people diagnosed with cancer about their lifestyle, let alone give advice about it. Why is that? Why aren't lifestyle factors considered at the start of cancer management? In my opinion they need to be.'

Dr Hassed agrees that going into treatments with an informed and questioning mind, backed by a healthy lifestyle, is a critical factor on the road to good health. It's about getting the fundamentals—the lifestyle factors—of good health and wellbeing established and then being in a far better position and frame of mind to make informed choices about the best treatments.

'Sometimes the ones who are the critics can be the loudest and sometimes I am not sure that they have actually stopped to fully inform themselves of what it is being said,' says Dr Hassed. 'It has been hard to open up that dialogue for Ian, I think.'

Dr Hassed is one of a new breed of mainstream medical practitioners that now champion the efficacy of Ian's approach. But it has been a long road for Ian Gawler, the ex-vet, patiently and persistently convincing people to take the time to listen and absorb what he has to say—rather than make hasty, and often plainly wrong, assumptions.

His endurance has paid off handsomely. Today a significant number of GPs understand and support Ian's work and his inclusive approach. He is invited to speak at medical conferences worldwide.

The acceptance of his message amongst the decision makers in the larger institutions, however, has typically been a little more slow.

For instance in 1998 an invitation for Ian Gawler to present a talk to doctors on the subject of meditation at a major Australian children's hospital was cancelled suddenly at the last minute due to 'unforeseen circumstances' by a professor at the institution.

In a leaked email to a colleague at the hospital, who had protested at the visit's cancellation, the professor wrote that 'Ian Gawler advocates unproven methods of cancer therapy and I do not believe it is acceptable that such methods are marketed, within this institution, for use in children where conventional evidence-based practice offers a good chance of a cure. If you have evidence that his methods improve survival rates in children with leukaemia or cancer I would be delighted to see it.'

Many staff were appalled by the decision to 'censor' Ian's visit just on principle and wondered if the professor seriously thought that meditation was a threat to child health, not to mention that the professor had completely misunderstood the thrust of Ian's message. That conventional evidence-based practice 'offers a good chance of cure' was never in contention. The use of meditation was being advocated in *addition* to such treatment.

In Ian's letter of protest at the cancellation of his visit to the professor, he pointed out that he had presented the same topic as that proposed to be presented at the Children's Hospital, 'Meditation as a Therapy', earlier that year at the Australian Medical Association's Annual Convention in Perth and at the International Psychology Congress Convention in Melbourne. In September that year he also presented the topic at the International Psycho-oncology Society's Conference in Hamburg, Germany.

'You may also be aware that there are over 1000 references in the scientific literature attesting to the valid therapeutic use of meditation in a wide variety of situations,' Ian went on to say. 'Certainly there is a widespread interest in the subject amongst the professional and general community.'

Ten years later, in 2008, meditation is widely recognised for its therapeutic benefits in relation to many physical and psychological ailments. Now, there are over 2000 research studies published. 'Remarkably, however,' says Ian, 'despite Ainslie Meares reporting cases like mine of cancer recoveries following intensive meditation, and despite the huge public interest and uptake of meditation generally, we are still waiting for the first research study to thoroughly investigate whether meditation does improve survival from cancer. We know from many studies it can alleviate pain and improve quality of life in many ways. But what about survival?'

So while meditation remains a major focus of Ian's life and work, he has another major concern regarding current cancer management—and this one seems to be confronting a major modern-day taboo: the real concern he has that chemotherapy is being over-prescribed.

As Ian explains, chemotherapy can be given with two aims. One is curative—when there is the prospect of a full recovery—the other is palliative, when the treatment is not curative but where the aim is to improve quality of life and perhaps extend survival.

'In the early days of our groups, back in the '80s, most chemo-therapy seemed to have been given when a cure seemed feasible,' says Ian. 'These days it seems to be given much more often in a palliative situation.'

Ian has always maintained that if chemotherapy is potentially curative, then it makes sense to embrace it and do all the lifestyle and complementary options that will support it. However, what seems to really challenge some oncologists and even the public in general, is that if the aim of chemo is palliative 'there may be a difficult equation that needs examining,' he reiterates. 'Chemotherapy can involve serious side effects and the benefits need to be substantial to outweigh the risks.

'Unfortunately it seems from the evidence we hear of in our groups, and perhaps more importantly, the evidence that comes from research in mainstream and medical journals is that currently chemotherapy is being oversold and overused.'

In The Gawler Foundation's *Cancer, Lifestyle and Chemotherapy* report on its website Ian points out that, 'Chemotherapy is associated with significant cure rates for 50 per cent or more of childhood cancers, 50 per cent or more of Hodgkin Lymphoma and certain aggressive lymphomas, 75 per cent or more of carcinoma of the testes, 90 per cent of choriocarcinoma in women, 15 to 20 per cent of adult acute leukemia, and 15 to 20 per cent of ovarian carcinoma.'

There have been some real advances in chemotherapy protocols to treat particular cancers since Ian was ill, and for these cases chemotherapy treatment is highly effective.

What is not commonly understood, however, is that the overall benefit of chemotherapy for all cancers is not as high as we might be led to believe.

In 2004, a meticulous analysis of the published data by Morgan [Morgan, G. et al., *Clinical Oncologist* 2004; 16:549–60] of 22 types of cancer in adults, including breast, prostate, bowel and lung found that the overall benefit of chemotherapy to five-year survival was a mere 2.3 per cent in Australia.

The Morgan analysis found that 'the minimal impact on survival in the more common cancers conflicts with the perceptions of many people who feel they are receiving a treatment that will significantly enhance their chances of cure.'

Morgan's research showed that based on the evidence available in 2004, five-year survival from early breast cancer was increased by only 3.5 per cent by treating it with chemotherapy. No five-year survival benefits from secondary breast cancer have been shown from the use of chemotherapy. Yet is it still very commonly prescribed.

Perhaps the overuse of chemotherapy is indicative of modern mainstream medicine's over-dependence on drug-based strategies and the power of the pharmaceutical companies.

'It's very clear from the reviews of the medical literature that there's a huge publication bias in favour of drugs,' says Dr Hassed. 'What that means is that when research is funded by a pharmaceutical company, they are very unlikely to publish negative findings on the drugs,' he says. 'They readily publish positive trials, which means even the evidence that's out there, on a whole variety of drugs including chemotherapy, is probably significantly affected by publication bias in their favour. Who knows, the figures may be even worse than we think.'

However, Dr Hassed also points out the obvious: the 'vast majority of oncologists are very passionately interested in what is best for their patients'. But any independent research that throws up challenging findings puts them in a very difficult position.

'I think the medical profession is not questioning enough about what we do,' says Dr Hassed, 'nor do we appreciate the influence of marketing and pharmaceutical companies affecting not just what we do but our whole mentality about health care.'

When the Morgan study was released, one might have expected it to make front-page news. But no, it was hardly reported upon. Very few people noticed it.

For Ian, the issue is still a wider one. 'This is where the taboo lies,' he says. 'It is very difficult to even discuss the efficacy of chemotherapy, let alone challenge it. Believe me, I have tried!'

Ian presented the research both in public meetings and at two medical conferences—the Royal Australian College of General Practitioners and the Australasian Integrative Medical Association in 2006.

'Interestingly the doctors were very responsive,' he says. 'I had many coming up to me or writing, saying they had no idea of this literature and they thanked me for putting it together.' Professor John Murtagh, Australia's doyen of General Practice, encouraged Ian to write it up for a medical journal.

'Many GPs actually said how they felt badly as they saw people they had known for years being diagnosed with cancer then going off for chemotherapy. They seem to feel that often it makes people really sick for little benefit,' says Ian. 'What they told me was that previously if they were to question the treatments with oncologists, they were told to mind their own business.'

Now with the research Ian had brought to their attention, he says the GPs 'felt that they had the evidence to support those questions', adding that it is very important to underline that 'chemotherapy may well be useful—but there are many situations where its use needs to be questioned and considered more thoroughly, perhaps more objectively.'

During 2006, Ian collated the research findings on chemotherapy. 'The 2.3 per cent figure amazed me,' says Ian. 'I have been working in this field for a long time and the impression I had was that it would have been 15 or 20 per cent. Ten per cent would have been a low figure for me; 2.3 per cent is remarkably low.'

'It was not until 2006 that I came across Morgan's 2.3 per cent.' says Ian.

'For the five years prior to 2006 Ruth and I were concerned by what seemed to us to be a rapid rise in the number of people attending the residential cancer programs who were receiving palliative chemotherapy that was knocking them around. I searched the literature to find out what was happening.'

At this point Ian raises a challenging question—the very question his own case raises. If someone has been told their cancer is medically incurable, can they still recover?

'Clearly to recover against the odds is not easy,' says Ian. 'But we know it is possible. Remember Ainslie Meares—it only has to be done once to show that it is possible. I cannot heal someone else as such, but I do believe people can heal themselves. I can show them techniques, teach them skills and maybe, just maybe, remarkable things can happen.'

What concerns Ian is that if people are beyond a medical cure, palliative chemotherapy may impair their body's capacity to heal. 'We know chemo can have many side effects. This is a real taboo area. In fact it is a hugely difficult question. I myself had chemo in this situation and felt it was useful. But on a case-by-case basis, when and how much palliative chemotherapy to give someone is a vexed question. And if five-year survival is only increased on average for the common cancers by 2.3 per cent—and this figure may be over-inflated anyway—then by definition most chemotherapy is in fact palliative.'

There is even more to this. An additional study Ian has found—another that received very little press—investigated women who had primary breast cancer. The women studied all had surgery followed by chemotherapy. Three months later they were asked if they were to be offered another round of chemotherapy and it only added one extra day of survival to an imaginary five years, would they take it?

'Think of this,' says Ian, 'chemo for women with primary breast cancer is usually quite rugged. Another round for just one day—how many would take that on?

The research found that over 50 per cent would and when asked why they said things like: 'that extra day might be the day they discover a cure. That day might be the best of my life,' says Ian. 'But more importantly, perhaps, many said they would not like to think that they had not done enough, they would not like to let down their family or even their friends.

'This is the sort of pressure that worries me,' says Ian. 'The popular view currently is that if you get cancer you have chemotherapy. It is almost like "Why wouldn't you have it?" I am of the view that the right question for palliative chemotherapy is "Why should I have it?" If you can be convinced of its merits, then of course have it, but do your due diligence first.'

Perhaps part of the answer is for each patient to be empowered with all the information to make the right decision for *them*—without undue pressure and coercion of doctors, family and friends. However, this is made difficult by popular opinion and the fact that our medical institutions are better set up to support drug-based strategies rather than lifestyle ones.

During one ten-day residential program Ian remembers the case of two women, both with two children under ten, who sat next to each other. Both women had been diagnosed with primary breast cancer. Following surgery both had been offered chemotherapy and both had weighed up their options.

'Both had been advised by their doctors that the chemotherapy could improve their survival by 3 or 4 per cent, and had been told about the potential side effects,' says Ian. The doctors had told both women that they thought it a good idea that they opt for the chemotherapy.

'One woman said that she had gone away and thought about it, talked with her friends and her family, she'd taken her kids into account and she decided she was going to have the chemo,' says Ian. 'And the woman beside her said exactly the same thing—except for the last sentence. She decided not to have the chemo.

'And I think they were both right,' says Ian. 'They both made choices that were informed, they both weighed up the evidence. They were both exercising, meditating and they both made a choice about chemo that they thought they could live with.'

What happened next, however, was that the woman who decided to take the chemotherapy treatment continued to enjoy the raft of resources available to her through the hospital—breast care nurse, access to physios and social workers. The woman who declined chemotherapy meanwhile 'was shamed by her doctor, told she was making a really bad choice and told, "Don't bother to come back if things go badly",' says Ian. 'All the support that the other lady [who had chosen the chemotherapy treatment] enjoyed was unavailable to her. Even worse in her eyes, her friends all pressured her hard, insisting she had made a bad choice and should take up the chemotherapy. It was very hard for her to resist and stick to what she really believed in.'

The simple fact is that chemotherapy and any number of allied services, are paid for by the public health system, but if you choose to take a multidisciplinary approach to your illness—without chemo—then you are on your own.

Drug-based strategies are ascendant because pharmaceutical companies can wield stupendous amounts of money and resources to pump into research and marketing. With the research in place, and the argument that the pharmaceutical approach is evidence-based and credible—and other approaches are not—the drug companies' position is assured.

'Sooner or later a woman is going to get further down the track and realise that she has not been well advised and sue her doctor,' say Ian. 'And I reckon she will have good grounds on which to do it. Perhaps lawyers like Slater and Gordon will wake up to the fact that there is a class action possibility here. I really do not like the idea of suing doctors, and it must be a horrible experience to be sued, but perhaps that is what it will take to swing this around. Clearly, if research demonstrated that a new drug halved the risk of dying and it was not prescribed, doctors would be negligent. If you think about it, if there's an option like exercise with evidence that it has almost double the benefit of something like chemotherapy for women with early breast cancer—which has really tough side effects—and women aren't even being told about it or more importantly encouraged to exercise and being supported to exercise, then that is scandalous.'

Of equal concern is the scant regard good nutrition has been given in regard to health and healing. 'Doctors aren't taught nutrition,' says Ian, adding that when Ruth completed her medical training 25 years ago at Sydney University, one of the top institutions in the country, 'she did not receive one specific lecture on nutrition.' It is a state of affairs that is typical of doctors of Ruth's vintage, many of whom are now in positions of authority, so it is of little surprise that many do not emphasise the importance of diet.

'When you take your animals into the vet, one of the first things they ask is "What is it eating?",' says Ian. 'It seems that the average doctor rarely asks that question.'

For those in the mainstream, the basis for deciding what is acceptable hinges on the question of evidence and the issue of research. Without evidence from published research, there are those who say a medical intervention or procedure is invalid and should not be used. Yet evidence-based medicine has two components, not just one. The *British Medical Journal* published the definitive definition.

'Put simply, it stated that evidence-based medicine was medicine that made decisions on the best available evidence. That seems obvious enough!' says Ian. '[The journal] then said that the best evidence is made up of what is available via published research and clinical experience. In fact, many medical procedures, some say 75 per cent of them, are based on clinical experience. For example, there has never been a randomised trial to investigate if surgery to remove a lump is the best way to treat primary bowel cancer. Everyone assumes it is, it has been done for years, but it has never been "scientifically" tested.'

By the same token, when it comes to a therapeutic approach to nutrition and cancer there is very little published research, but plenty of clinical experience. In Australia, more to the point, The Gawler Foundation may well have more clinical experience applying an intensive nutritional approach than most. They may well have the best available evidence for what to do.

Nevertheless, as well as having nearly 30 years of clinical experience, Ian Gawler is passionately interested in research and regrets the lack of good research into what he does.

'It amazes me that huge amounts of money are raised each year for [cancer] research and no-one's said why don't we broaden the research,' says Ian. 'It is fine to look for a medical "magic bullet" for cancer. I am not sure one will be found, but let's continue to look. But at the same time, we need to investigate lifestyle factors and complementary therapies. These are in the public eye all the time, most patients who get cancer are quickly exposed to the thought that changing their diet might be useful, using the power of their mind might be useful, meditation might be useful, all sorts of other things that we are involved in might be useful. Why not have a definitive study which sorts out whether it is useful or not?'

It is a question Ian Gawler has wanted answered for decades, yet it is often the oncologists and cancer community leaders—the very people who most commonly use the lack of research as a criticism of Ian's work—that seem to be the ones positively reluctant to find out.

In 1989 on an hour-long debate on the ABC television show

Couchman, oncologist Dr Ray Lowenthal challenged Ian Gawler to present 50 of his best cancer recovery cases for review. Gawler was delighted to have the opportunity and agreed there and then on camera. Lowenthal had been one of Gawler's most ardent critics and to finally have the opportunity for some serious research was something Ian relished.

Nearly twenty years later the review still has not happened—and not from any unwillingness from Ian or The Gawler Foundation.

'We gathered together the 50 cases, they were ready to go', says Ian, 'but Ray said that he could not get funding for the study.'

In 1995 Ian edited and The Foundation published *Inspiring People*, a book that brought together 50 case stories of surviving against the odds, making the hope and the inspiration they offered available to the public.

'More recently, in 2008, this book has been replaced by *Surviving Cancer*, describing in detail the stories of 28 people's remarkable journeys through dealing with difficult cancer and again, surviving against the odds.'

Surviving Cancer was launched by the late top surgeon Professor Chris O'Brien, former director of the Sydney Cancer Centre, based at Royal Prince Alfred Hospital and the University of Sydney.

Professor O'Brien became well known in the wider community for his many appearances on the popular Australian reality television program *RPA*. In 2006 he was diagnosed with a malignant brain tumour and had three operations and underwent a number of radiotherapy and chemotherapy treatments. Later he took up meditation and embraced some complementary therapeutic approaches.

'In the last six months all I have taken is herbal medicine and homoeopathic medicine and I have meditated,' he said in 2008. 'My sense of wellbeing is excellent, my quality of life is great and I feel really well. Now what is contributing to that is a big unknown, but I'm comfortable doing what I am doing. The issue in my mind is returning the mind and body to harmony and balance.

'I was a cancer surgeon and the director of the Sydney Cancer Centre so my training and my thoughts have been very traditional,' he said, 'although I've always been open-minded to alternative and complementary therapies and the role of meditation. Now I'm using them myself. Ten years ago I would never have foreseen myself doing this but now that I am doing it, I am very comfortable with it and I think if anything is working, I believe those things are working.'

Professor O'Brien believed that the 'additive effects of meditation and nutrition and alternative medicine are really beneficial once the main tumour has been removed, because I think what they have the ability to then do is boost or empower the immune system and fight any microscopic disease that might be around and prevent it from coming back or spreading,' he said. 'That's the way I see it working.

'Meditation just creates a sense of peace and calm. I think that's the most important thing. I'm a type AA personality [driven, competitive, high achieving] and I've just been working incredibly hard and I now have a greater sense of peace and calm.'

That someone in such a position of authority and standing in conventional cancer medicine, such as Professor O'Brien, personally believed in the efficacy of meditation and an integrative approach that incorporates complementary therapies—and was willing to go on the public record—was an important breakthrough. Professor O'Brien's virulent brain tumour ultimately took his life in June 2009, but his legacy will be Lifehouse, The Chris O'Brien Cancer Centre, to be built at the Royal Prince Alfred Hospital in Sydney. Lifehouse will offer compassionate holistic care for cancer patients.

Gradually, the evidence is inexorably mounting as to the value of Ian's approach. In 2004 the preliminary findings of a study into the efficacy of The Gawler Foundation's programs were released by Melbourne's Swinburne University of Technology. The results showed a significant reduction in anxiety, depression, anger, fatigue and confusion amongst people who had attended The Gawler Foundation ten-day residential program. One hundred and thirty participants were tested on enrolment at The Foundation program, immediately afterwards and at intervals of three, six and twelve months.

The ten-day residential program run by The Foundation had, said the report's summary, 'beneficial effects on mood, mental adjustment to cancer, quality of life and salivary cortisol levels in cancer patients.'

'We've had a lot of success over the years, and I guess there has been the criticism that we haven't had any solid research done into the outcomes of our program,' said Ian, quoted at the time in the *Sydney Morning Herald*. 'And I've always felt bad about that, because for 20 years we've chased the mainstream bodies trying to get funding and it hasn't been forthcoming. This [research] has been a real breakthrough, and it's nice to see the results stand up.'

Meanwhile the clinical evidence of The Gawler Foundation's efficacy is mighty impressive too.

Surviving Cancer details 28 stories of remarkable recovery. Most of these fall into the category of what is commonly called 'spontaneous remission' or 'spontaneous regression'.

At the launch of the book in May 2008 Ian characterised spontaneous remission or regression as 'when a malignancy partially or completely disappears without medical treatment, or as a result of a therapy that is considered inadequate to exert a significant influence on neoplastic disease [tumors].'

Ian went on to put the achievements of the 28—all Gawler Foundation attendees—into the bigger picture by explaining that the going rate for spontaneous remission is generally accepted to be between one in 60 000 and one in 100 000.

In contrast, even taking only these 28 into account—'there are many others with similar stories that could have been told,' said Ian—this represents a rate of spontaneous remission from attendees at The Gawler Foundation at one in 500.

The figure was arrived at by dividing the total number of attendees at The Foundation's twelve-week program and it's ten-day residential program over the years combined—15 000 people.

Ian agreed this was 'playing with figures' rather than rigorous statistics, but added that from them you could comfortably draw the conclusion that: 'One in 500 people coming to us could be said to have a spontaneous regression, compared to the average of

1 in 60 000. That means that we have over 100 times the going average! Now, even if we are a factor of 10 out—and it is only 10 times greater—to my mind that is still remarkable and warrants deeper investigation. But in fact, we could have told many more similar stories than "just" the 28 presented in *Surviving Cancer*. Let's push for research into this area. Why do people survive against the odds? Were they just lucky? Is what they did repeatable?'

To help find out The Gawler Foundation recently added a research officer to its staff.

Another significant step forward has been a program for people dealing with multiple sclerosis, started in 2002, that was set up at The Gawler Foundation by Professor George Jelinek and Ian Gawler.

Professor Jelinek is the author of the groundbreaking self-help book *Taking Control of MS* and is Professor of Emergency Medicine at the Sir Charles Gairdner Hospital in Perth, Western Australia. Professor Jelinek has a background in medical research and has ensured that quantifiable findings from the program are being gathered in parallel.

Six years after the program's start 'it is clear that it is possible to stabilise MS with the lifestyle approach and good medical management,' says Ian. 'We are seeing people who are reversing symptoms, even more remarkably people are having MRI lesions disappear.'

Professor Jelinek was himself diagnosed with MS in 2000, but has been able to remain symptom-free using a lifestyle approach. Much as Ian had been inspired to do so over 30 years before, George Jelinek has sought to share his discoveries with others. The two combined forces and together they are doing some exciting, groundbreaking work by adding MS to the advances Ian had already made in cancer. Plans are now under way for Professor Jelinek and Ian Gawler to tackle diabetes using a similar lifestyle-based program. It's an exciting development as the integrative approach that takes lifestyle, the mind and the body into account goes ever more mainstream.

'What has happened is that a groundswell of public opinion has driven changes in attitudes,' Ian says. Just as he had hoped they would be when he first suggested they were needed all those years ago. It's an extension of the same groundswell that led to the 2005 Senate Enquiry into cancer medicine.

The enquiry looked into the 'services and treatment option for persons with cancer' and was instigated by a motion put to the Australian Senate by Labor Senator Peter Cook.

Cook had been diagnosed with melanoma, which had spread to other parts of his body, and was given the impression by his doctors that there was little or nothing that could be done for him.

'Peter went away, conducted his own research and discovered there were other lifestyle factors and complementary approaches he could try,' says Ian. 'He was ridiculed by his doctors.' Fortunately the senator was intelligent enough, says Ian, to realise the doctors were uninformed and were basing the dismissal on ignorance rather than evidence. 'That made him angry and fortunately he was in a position to do something about it.'

Cook had been a resident at one of The Gawler Foundation's programs and had discovered first-hand the enormous benefits it had offered. He subsequently pushed hard for a Senate enquiry to examine the efficacy of a multidisciplinary approach to cancer treatment, as well as the efficacy of complementary and 'less conventional' treatments. The enquiry also sought to discover to what extent less conventional and complementary cancer treatments are researched, or are supported by research.

When the enquiry handed down its findings in June 2005—receiving very little press at the time—among its recommendations were that funding be examined for 'programs and activities like those operated by The Gawler Foundation, which specialise in providing learning and self-help techniques based on an integrated approach for cancer patients and their carers.'

It recommended that the public health system under Medicare should consider covering the costs for cancer patients accessing these services from a 'health and equity point of view.'

Disappointingly the government of the day chose not to act on the report's recommendations. There is still time for the present Australian government to choose to breathe life into what was a landmark document in the provision of health care in the country.

If it does, it will finally give all Australians access to the latest and the most effective cancer care available—not just to those who have been fortunate enough to have stumbled upon the extraordinary work of Ian Gawler and that of the many others he has inspired.

Recently, a Canadian researcher told Ian that 'in America currently, a bone marrow transplant costs up to $150 000 per person. A course of chemotherapy for someone with secondary bowel cancer can also cost $150 000. Our twelve-week cancer lifestyle program costs us about $1000 per person to present,' says Ian. 'So for the cost of one bone marrow transplant, we could help 150 people to attend our program for free. Currently The Foundation subsidises this program heavily via fundraising. We charge $450 and have a program running for those who are financially limited. No-one disputes the value of bone marrow transplants being freely available, that is wonderful, but where is the equity? One hundred and fifty people could come to a program that offers so much for the same price.'

So what of the future?

Ian welcomes the progress that has been made, while remaining disappointed by how slow it has been and how much there still is to do.

'The inequity of how funds are used really disturbs me,' he says. 'If you consider how much money is raised from well-meaning people across the community and how many of those people use lifestyle factors and complementary therapies in their daily lives, why is there not more money going into researching these things? Most money still goes into searching for new drugs and how to improve radiotherapy. It is fine to continue to look for a magic bullet with a new wonder drug. I hope one is found but I think many researchers doubt that it will be. In the meantime we need equity and research into these other immediately promising areas.'

'Also there is inequity in how people are supported. A woman with early breast cancer can smoke, drink excessively, eat poorly, not exercise, take no interest in her own health at all, and still get $70 000 worth of Herceptin per year, freely on the PBS [Pharmaceutical Benefits Scheme],' he says. 'If another woman chooses to come to one of our groups and diligently applies herself by contributing her best efforts to her own healing then she has to pay for that privilege. The Foundation fundraises 25 per cent of our annual budget so we keep costs down as much as possible, but the programs still cost quite a deal to run and affordability is a real issue for many. The Senate Enquiry recognised the need for support for people who choose to support themselves and organisations like ours who teach them what to do and support them in doing it.'

There is still a lot of work to be done in reforming the cancer care and management field, in other words, but things are undeniably beginning to shift—and it is Ian Gawler's incredible survival, and the lessons he learnt and has selflessly shared along the way since, that have been a large and crucial factor in the change of the tide.

More than 30 years ago Ian conquered his 'incurable' cancer and has spent just about every waking hour since trying to communicate what he discovered. In the years since, against incredible odds, he has succeeded in spreading his message and has inspired and helped countless others. Ian is a true pioneer. Once considered a radical, ignored or criticised by the establishment, his methods are gradually, increasingly, being adopted by the mainstream.

One day in the not too distant future they will *be* the mainstream.

16

The Answer is Always Yes

If you ask Ruth Gawler today why she married Ian, she has at least one particular reason, beyond love, that she can easily articulate.

'I actually had my own uncompromising wish that I could develop into a better and more happy person,' she says. 'In a sense for me he was very much an opportunity and I am, in a sense, an opportunist.'

Ruth characterises Ian as 'no ordinary being' and a man who is clearly devoted to helping others with the sort of quiet, resolute intensity no self-centred society such as ours can really understand.

The moment Ruth *knew* she wanted to marry Ian, however, was the moment, for the very first time, she saw the depth of his humanity flash in his eyes. And this phenomenon is very much a sudden flash expressed in his pupils. It is like they suddenly appear to get bigger and then, like the wind on the surface of a lake, it passes. Something at once very strong, yet delicately human. She remembers it first when they drove back from Ooramina after the clinic conference in 1999.

I saw it for myself when he recounted the story of his son Peter's accident and his eyes glistened with the memory.

'He can be very open and one of the things I was attracted to in him was the actual capacity to show his vulnerability,' says Ruth. 'He sometimes has that sweeping expression in his eyes and . . . you see it and then you think: gosh, it's not hidden.'

It is the expression of a man in touch with his own suffering, his compassion. For Ruth this expression promised a relationship offering real depth, profundity and a chance for personal growth.

Ian has a singularly calm and unflustered manner, born, it would seem, of three decades of meditative practice and the cultivation of courage. On a broader scale, perhaps it is because of qualities like this, or perhaps it is his robe-like choice of clothing that gives the casual observer reason to suppose that Ian would lead an ascetic life of thrift, constant meditation and holy self-denial.

Not so. Ian is a very sensuous man, says Ruth. 'He loves sex, he loves good food, he loves gardens and he loves sport. He watches sport anytime, anywhere and becomes completely riveted.' When he is not working for The Foundation his greatest hobby is working in his extensive garden.

'We laugh a lot together, we share jokes,' says Ruth. 'The Melbourne Comedy Festival is an annual event with the family.'

At the reception following the recent wedding of some close friends, Ian and Ruth performed one of Peter Cook and Dudley Moore's classic *Beyond the Fringe* sketches from the 1960s, in which Mr Spiggott, a one-legged man, auditions for the role of Tarzan. Mr Spiggott, played by Moore, spends the entire sketch hopping around the room, as did Ian, much to the delight of Ian and Ruth's newly-wedded friends.

Inside the calm and kaftan-wearing exterior, a mischievous and fun-loving Ian Gawler is more than happy to explode any expectations or projections about how a respected cancer care pioneer and spiritual practitioner should behave.

'I remember learning something really important from Ainslie Meares,' says Ian. 'The importance of paradox. Ainslie was so paradoxical—very worldly, very mystical. Very much a pioneer and an innovator, yet in many ways deeply conservative, deeply affected by what his peers thought of him.

'What he helped me to realise was that if you only have one way of being, then it is very limited. So to get well I needed at times to be quite resolute. At others to surrender and yield. There were times when I was incredibly active, others quite lazy. So these apparent paradoxes are, in my view, vital.

'Some people do quite well sticking to one approach, one style, one way of doing things; but in my experience, really successful people have a range of responses. They can have the flexibility to respond appropriately to different circumstances and this gives the outward appearance of contradictory behaviour.'

Ian's illness and subsequent inner journey might have given him a tangible presence—one of serenity and equanimity—but it has also taught him to challenge the orthodoxy. Now if Ian gets a sniff of anything supposedly politically correct his immediate instinct is to quietly question it. It means he considers what other people think of him, but he places little stock in what might be considered 'acceptable behaviour'. Ian's overwhelming motivation might be the welfare of others—and he is the kindest, most considerate person you are ever likely to meet—but there is more than a touch of the rebel in him. How this typically manifests itself on any ordinary day is behind the wheel of his Subaru WRX.

Indeed, if there's something that really bothers Ruth about Ian, it is the velocity with which he chooses to drive. As she says, it has given a lot of people quite close to him a lot of fear and annoyance.

Ruth has tried every tactic she can to dissuade him from doing so. She has told him that it is not compassionate, or that it is egotistical and childish. Grace used to think that the fast driving was yet more evidence of Ian's love of risk-taking behaviour.

'He's a bad boy. There's a side to Ian that is this beautiful, boyish larrikin—and it's very appealing,' says Jamie Duff. 'Have you ever driven with him? Bloody hell, he likes to give it some stick.'

In his own defence Ian says he is not very good at doing things slowly, except meditating. He has always liked driving fast. He has never been good at doing cautious things. 'Actually I drive a helluva lot slower than I used to,' he adds.

On one hand Ian is an ordinary bloke with an ordinary love of watching sport on the television, sharing a joke and driving a powerful car too fast, yet the rigours of his life, his work and his spiritual engagement also lend him a tangible air of inner knowing. He is, in many ways, someone who has managed to stay in touch with his youthful enthusiasm, as well as to plug into something bigger and entirely more profound.

Friend Sally Browne says she has noticed that he is 'able to bring out the feminine in me. He's really able to bring out the softer side . . . It's just a talent he has. We all become more human'.

'Ian is absolutely passionate about his work and The Foundation,' says Siegfried Gutbrod. 'His stubbornness, his determination to realise a vision is extraordinarily strong. His ability to tune in to people, to run groups and to be compassionate is very good. He's a remarkable human being.'

'One of the things I used to notice when I was first married to him and we were living together,' adds Ruth, 'was that I used to look at him sitting on the lounge and see this old sage . . . and then I'd look at him a few moments later and he seemed about eight or nine years old and he would be laughing about something quite simple or silly.'

Ian Gawler lives life in the present moment. He has learnt to appreciate and savour every precious second of a life that very nearly did not stretch past 25 years of age.

Ian and Ruth Gawler share an L-shaped 1920s white weatherboard farmhouse, ringed by verandas, near a sleepy little settlement a couple of kilometres down the road from Yarra Junction. The house sits at the end of a narrow dirt road. The track wanders up the hill, over a grated steel bridge and through a mini-rainforest, flanked with tree ferns and agapanthus.

The first thing you notice about the house is its lilac-coloured corrugated steel roof, chosen to match the old wisteria that grows by the front gate and white picket fence. Just inside the front door, in the foyer on a brick chimney that backs a fireplace in the room beyond, is a personally signed photograph of His Holiness the Dalai Lama and a couple of Aboriginal works of art.

To the left of the hallway is the sitting room, hung with an

Australian landscape painting by Ian himself and more Aboriginal art.

The kitchen is country style, with a large timber rangehood and a large island bench. It overlooks the magnificent gardens where Ian spends most of his spare time. At one end of the space is a small round table, where Ian and Ruth eat on a daily basis. The table is overlooked by a myriad of framed photographs, including shots of their wedding, the family, one of Ian high in the Himalayas and shots of spiritual masters Sai Baba and Sogyal Rinpoche.

The blue-walled bedroom nearest the kitchen is where the kids stay on their visits. Dominating it are two large signed posters. The first is of Debbie Flintoff-King winning Olympic Gold at the Seoul Olympics 'To Ian, my mentor. Thanks Heaps. Love Debbie' and one of actor Will Smith in *Ali*, the film about the life of boxing superstar Muhammad Ali.

A friend, Robert Kirby, chairman of Village Roadshow, an ex board member and key supporter of The Foundation, had it signed by Will Smith.

'Ian loves stories of triumph against the odds,' says Ruth.

The garden meanwhile is perhaps Ian and Ruth's home's most impressive feature—and most of it is Ian's own work. There are no other gardeners. There is a comprehensive orchard which includes fig, avocado and olive trees and a magnificent vegetable patch featuring asparagus and artichokes, native spinach, cauliflower and eggplant. Whatever fresh vegetables happen to have ripened on that particular day often end up in a fresh and delicious sauce over pasta, or Asian noodles, for a simple dinner.

'It's more joyous for Ian to eat five asparagus that he's grown from the garden than if someone was to make some cordon bleu meal,' says Ruth. 'It's because he planted it, he's harvested it and it is part of the cycle of nature. It is a complete relationship with the earth for him.'

Ian and Ruth Gawler are self-evidently a couple who are in love and enormously good for each other. 'After my divorce, having reached a point where I broke the vow "for better or for worse", I thought a great deal about the possibility of another relationship,' says Ian. 'A part of me was seriously attracted to a celibate, monastic style of life. But then I concluded that one of the major things human life offered was that of an intimate relationship with a person of the opposite sex. The offer in such a union was to bring together, to unite, male and female. I decided to be open to the possibility again. And I knew there was only one type of relationship I was interested in.'

Before marrying Ruth, Ian realised that 'I only wanted the sort of relationship where the answer was always yes. So if Ruth asks me for anything, the answer is always yes. I'm not interested in anything else. Of course we discuss things where we might have a difference of opinion . . . and I don't always agree with her point of view, or follow her point of view, but I will always take account of it. But if she asks me for anything directly, then the answer is always yes. My idea of getting married was to share my life with another person and to be in an intimate relationship. The only sort of marriage that I am interested in, is when the answer is always yes.'

Interestingly, Ian says he has not asked Ruth for the same deal. 'From my point of view, that is a whole separate thing, and that is for her to work out.' Ian reveals that he has never had this sort of clarity in any of his other relationships.

It is also clear that his relationship with Ruth has allowed Ian to continue on the path to complete healing. It is easy to forget that this path is an ongoing one and not one that was over when he was declared cancer-free all those years ago.

Indeed the break-up of his family was a crisis, at least in Ruth's opinion, every bit as massive as the crisis he had to face with the amputation and then secondary cancer. But clearly by the age of 50 he was more prepared and wiser.

This is consistent with Ian's own sense that now his life can actually be divided into three. After the amputation of his leg he was reborn into his second life. After the equally traumatic end of his first marriage, Ian met Ruth, they married and he underwent, as he sees it, a 'reincarnation' of sorts into the third stage of what has been another most remarkable life.

In this phase of his second marriage, Ruth has been a catalyst to encourage Ian to try to heal some of the wounds that she saw as unhealed. One, in particular that she encouraged her husband to reconcile was the interference he had suffered at the hands of the teacher not long after his mother's death.

For Ian, the motivation to do this was fuelled by a sense that he needed to disclose what had happened to him for the sake of others who might have been affected similarly. Ian wondered if perhaps the teacher had done things to other children over the years and perhaps no-one had come forward.

'So when I was in Adelaide one day I made an appointment with the current headmaster and told him my story,' says Ian. 'He was terrific, he responded to it really well and he took it seriously.'

Ian could not remember the teacher's name but could clearly remember his face. He asked to look through old photographs and records and once he had identified the man, Ian also got in touch with the police.

'The police were very clear that what I had experienced was sexual assault,' he says. 'I had never put that name to it but they said that what I was describing was sexual assault. Also they said that if he was still alive, that they could and would charge him.'

The police tracked him down only to discover that he had died five years previously. Apparently there had been another question about him but nobody had made a formal complaint. The headmaster asked Ian what he would like to do about it.

'I thought about it a lot,' says Ian, adding that he came to the conclusion that it would be helpful if the school were to publish in their newsletter the fact that a complaint had been made about a teacher (without naming him) and that the school would undertake a review of its policy in this area. Which it duly did.

Ian says of the initial incident that it 'never really consciously bothered me, because at the time I was so naïve and didn't know what was going on,' he says. 'He didn't rape me or anything like that.' Although, with the death of his mother so recent and raw, Ian was particularly vulnerable. 'The bastard must have known,' he adds. 'It was wicked.' Clearly it must also have had some sort of detrimental effect on the young Ian, for him to want to investigate it so many years later—although you also get the sense that he would never have done so without Ruth's gentle insistence. Now, perhaps, the issue had been put to rest.

And then there are legacies of the past that simply come back unbidden.

Thirty years previously, Ian's osteogenic sarcoma had spread to his left lung and he had then contracted TB. Although the cancer had long since retreated, and the TB was cured, it was the TB that left Ian with a severely damaged left lung, filled with cavities and barely functioning. This meant that the lung would often became filled with mucus and was very susceptible to infection. 'Over the years he would take antibiotics from time to time to help manage it,' says Ruth. Despite such a healthy lifestyle, but perhaps exacerbated by the heavy workload, Ian's chest was a constant issue. He had a regular cough, infections would begin to occur more easily and Ian had pneumonia twice in 2004.

Something had to be done. Following a series of medical consultations and much reflection, it became clear that the only solution was a very difficult operation. It would fundamentally mean carefully dissecting Ian's entire left lung and removing it along with all traces of disease.

Ian and Ruth consulted with two top lung surgeons in Melbourne. One barely disguised his dread of the operation, says Ruth. 'The other, who was older and had performed this type of operation in his early days when TB was more prevalent, was quite confident. We chose him.'

It was not an immediate imperative, but Ian knew that if he did not undergo the operation the sickly lung could well have dire consequences for his continuing good health, if not his very survival.

The complex surgery, taking over five hours, was performed in December 2004. The left lung was dissected out of the pleural cavity, little by little. The surgeon had to open the pericardium—the heart sac—and tie off the major blood vessels to the lung.

Ian came very close to death once again, and afterwards he

needed several blood transfusions. 'It was a very difficult time. He lost a lot of weight,' says Ruth.

One of the key reasons Ian had opted to go through the operation was because he felt that he was still young enough and fit enough to recover, says Ruth. 'If we left it another five or ten years, we have no doubts he would have died. He left it as long as he could really.'

Ruth says she only became aware of the extent of the problem shortly before the operation. However, it had been bothering Ian for years and years. 'I think it got very much worse after the separation,' says Ruth. 'In terms of grief I think the divorce really affected that part of his body. Ian is not somebody who indulges in grief, but I'm sure there is a connection there.'

After the operation Ruth visited the hospital pathologist to have a look at the lung which had been removed. She was told that it was atrophied and completely non-functional. When the pathologist had cut the lung to examine it he had also discovered a 4 cm piece of bone that was wrapped around the left main bronchus. 'You don't normally have bone in the lung,' she says. 'The pathologist said it must have been the osteogenic sarcoma that had transformed back into ordinary bone and just lay dormant there.' It was also something the pathologist had never heard or read about before. 'He had to saw the lung in half to examine it.'

Meanwhile the recovery from the operation was 'long and it was horrible,' says Ruth, adding that the medications he took really affected him. 'He was quite detached and demanding and irritable and unlike himself. He was weak for months and was really flat.' Ruth remembers he would often just sit gazing out the window, clearly frustrated that his body was so weak and would not do what he wanted it to. 'That went on for a whole year and I got quite impatient with it,' she says.

From Ian's point of view he was slowly but steadily improving over this time, although he was still 'well below par'.

So in April 2005, more than eighteen months after the operation, Ruth took her husband off to New Zealand to see a Brazilian faith healer who was visiting the country.

Having spent so much time with the healers in the Philippines, Ian had a curiosity to investigate this healer as quite a few participants in their groups had made the effort to travel to Brazil seeking help. He was not expecting much personally, but now being the reconstructed spouse who always said yes, he agreed.

João Teixeira de Faria (aka John of God), is a famous psychic healer who works along similar lines to those Ian had visited nearly 30 years previously. John of God sometimes uses surgical instruments without anaesthetic.

Needless to say in New Zealand local laws prevented him performing the sort of surgery that reportedly includes scraping the eye with a kitchen knife and sticking artery forceps deep into the nose.

Held in the local town hall in Lower Hutt near Wellington, it was an 'unusual scene,' says Ruth, with people all wearing white gradually passing in front of John of God, all being blessed and some being chosen by the healer for further healing.

'It was quite novel and a little bit bizarre and I think Ian only did it because I was insisting. I was just hoping for anything to get this miserable spell broken.'

Ian was singled out for a psychic operation. This consisted of everyone, including John of God, meditating around him and a group of others for about twenty minutes. He was then instructed to go back to his hotel room and do nothing for 24 hours. 'I can't say I was in any way warmed by this fellow,' says Ruth. 'Nor did Ian or I have any particular conviction that any of this was meaningful or was going to work. It was definitely a dubious act of desperation to my way of thinking.'

That said, once back in Australia, Ian did improve radically and quickly. 'I don't know whether he was scared that I was going to take him to more unusual rituals,' says Ruth, 'but within a week he was back to his old self and within a month he was full bore again.'

And there was plenty to do, because it soon became obvious that The Foundation was teetering on the edge of collapse—or as the current chief executive officer of The Gawler Foundation, Karin Knoester, puts it, 'when I started in early 2005 I discovered we didn't have any money. We were nearly insolvent.'

The previous CEO (not Siegfried Gutbrod, who had moved on by this stage) had resigned shortly after Ian had gone into hospital for his operation. Before the operation Ian and The Foundation Board had been led to believe that The Foundation's financial situation was fine. In fact they were in dire straits. By the time Karin Knoester came on board, The Foundation was very nearly broke—and Ian was still out of the picture, recovering.

Karin prescribed a dose of fiscal medicine—some serious economising—and did not make herself very popular with the staff because of it. It had to be done. Ian made personal requests to influential friends and friends of The Foundation, for emergency donations. He then vowed to never do that again and to ensure that The Foundation worked towards financial sustainability.

Karin carried the day-to-day responsibilities of keeping things going and rebuilding. 'I said to myself if I can do this without sacking people, I'll be really happy, and that's what we did,' she says. 'Nobody left the organisation because of the financial position we were in.' More than that, though, she saw to it that the belt-tightening ensured that The Foundation would have an operating reserve of funds big enough to pay out all staff's entitlements should ever they be forced to close down in the future. 'We never had that before,' she says. 'But now it creates a more secure working environment which I think is really important.'

Karin is a firm, capable, strong-willed and compassionate pragmatist in a position that, in the past, has been held by individuals more in tune with Ian Gawler's original ideals for an organisation that runs on faith and a belief in the power of manifestation.

Since Karin started there has, she says, been a 'reasonable turnover of staff because people see that they do not fit in the organisation anymore. It's been a good thing in some ways.'

The organisation now has new computer equipment, new telephony, a new accounting system and a new business model. The Foundation is now on a very stable financial footing. In the past 'when money was short they all sat around and OM-ed until the money wasn't short. Whereas I come from a more pragmatic point of view. I think you have to do the right things right and do them at the right time. From that point of view I probably made a few enemies because everyone liked the old way . . .'

Karin reports direct to The Gawler Foundation's board (and not to Ian himself directly). They are both employees—contracted and salaried. 'I do what the board wants me to do, but it's difficult,' says Karin. 'I often feel like the meat in the sandwich.' She is head of the organisation. Ian goes under the title of Founder and Therapeutic Director. It's like having a 'two-headed dog', says Karin. 'It's a hard situation. Ian takes care of the entire therapeutic side of the organisation and I take care of the business—except where Ian has an opinion—more often than not Ian will get his way, because it's Ian's baby, even though Ian doesn't own it. It's a challenge for him to let it go. Yet he wants to let it go because he wants to see it bloom.'

It's clear Karin has an enormous amount of respect for Ian, but the management structure presents many challenges for them both. Sometimes when he comes into her office she says she could 'wring his neck'.

On the other hand, 'Ian's done a great job and he's done it because he has a very strong will. He knows exactly what he wants,' she says. 'Sometimes that makes him unbendable and sometimes he is perhaps so committed to his will that he doesn't actually take on board that there are other opinions. And sometimes he doesn't actually modernise his thinking. I don't mean that as a criticism, I mean that more as an observation because you don't get to where he got by being wishy-washy and not being committed to what you want. You get to it by being strong in your will and centred in your person. And that's everything that he is.'

Karin has also seen his 'inspiringly gentle' side in her tenure. 'When it comes to clients you cannot fault him,' she says.

Catering manager Gail Lazenbury says The Foundation has now hit a period in its history where it is 'working very well as a team. It's really great.' Although she says the two years of belt-tightening and budget constraints were a bit fractious. Lazenbury has lived in the valley for 28 years and first met the Gawlers when Ian was the local vet. She has worked for The Foundation, in the kitchen since

1992, first as an assistant cook and then as head cook when Dorothy Edgelow stepped down from the job around four years ago. She has seen a lot of changes in that time, not the least in the menu.

The food has changed dramatically over the years, she says. 'We have introduced lots of different things. We've introduced a lot more fancy sauces and a lot more Asian foods are coming into it.' There was a time, she adds, when the food was a bit stodgy and uninteresting. 'How many times can you serve steamed rice and vegies? Which is what Ian would like to live on, but the residents don't want steamed rice and vegies seven days per week.'

The arrival of Ruth has changed things considerably too, she says. 'When they were married we were told that Ruth was not going to have anything to do with The Foundation. She had her own practice and that was going to be it.'

Ian and Ruth were living in East Melbourne at the time—with Ruth working in a holistic medical practice in the city. Ian was commuting to Yarra Junction every day. They realised that long term they would need to move near The Foundation but Ruth was not keen to be a country doctor again. She wanted to work in a more integrative medical way and The Foundation was ideal. While Ian could anticipate all the benefits of having a highly qualified and experienced doctor working at The Foundation and was keen on working closely with Ruth, he did not openly encourage her; rather he left her to come to her own decision and apply for a job.

This she did in 2002 and now Ruth is The Foundation's medical practitioner, as well as a group leader and meditation and yoga teacher.

'Ruth has had quite a lot to do with the programs,' says Gail Lazenbury, 'and has inspired quite a dramatic change.' It was like a 'new wind blew in,' she adds. 'Young, intelligent, new ideas. A lot of the old stuff brushed out. It made you realise that a lot of the stuff that you did was just because that's what you did.'

At work people speak well of Ruth and her vitality, including those who were very close to Grace. Many friends who knew Grace were deeply saddened by her departure, but most have embraced

Ruth and can see the profoundly positive impact she has had on Ian since they got together.

But, Ruth did have her early doubts about her own capacity to manage living with such a strong and self-assured man. A man with a public profile and a way of working which was already both fully absorbing and unlimited.

It took a little while, she admits, to come to terms with the fact that Ian is, above all else, uncompromisingly committed to helping people. It means more to him than his own welfare and that of his marriage. 'I think now that the Bodhisattva Vow is the strongest intention he has,' says Ruth.

A Bodhisattva is someone who undertakes to work selflessly for the welfare and enlightenment of all beings. The Bodhisattva Vow, usually taken at the beginning of the Buddhist spiritual path and reconfirmed along it, is a vow to have the aspiration of a Bodhisattva. Ian first formally took this vow with the Dalai Lama in 1982.

Ruth is a highly independent woman used to having her own way. It came as a bit of a shock to discover that in marrying Ian things would be different. 'I think a lot of negativity came up for me when I realised I wasn't in control; perhaps I had some kind of illusion that I was going to be in control of the relationship. A bit amusing now when I see how it really is.'

Both Ruth and Ian would be described as strong characters with a firm but gentle way of seeing their suggestions are followed through. It is obvious that Ian has a deep respect for his wife's views—as well as his philosophical commitment to say yes to anything she asks for—and Ruth seems the driving force in the more practical and the day-to-day, but underlying this is Ian's quiet, unwavering wisdom, vision and will.

It is a part of Ian that even people at work do not necessarily understand. 'They keep trying to contain him in terms of his aspirations,' says Ruth. 'It's just not possible. Some people misinterpret his gentleness as weakness, but he's actually like titanium—light and very strong.'

On that score, however, things are now beginning to shift. As he approaches 60, which he will reach in 2010, Ian is gradually learning to let go (or at least toy with the idea of letting go) of some of his responsibilities at The Foundation and look towards entering a more actively spiritual phase of his life. 'It doesn't mean he won't work there after 2010,' says Ruth, 'but it may well be on an entirely different basis. This work at The Foundation has limited the possibility of his own spiritual development to some degree, it involves a lot of administration and personnel management. He seems ready for another change.'

Change is hard to visualise and it is hard to imagine Ian Gawler ever letting go of some sort of directorial contribution at The Gawler Foundation. But it is also clear that there is a profound yearning to devote more time to a contemplative, meditative life as he nears his seventh decade and his physical energy diminishes.

17

An Awakening

Every year, for a couple of weeks during the Australian summer, a large white marquee of the kind used for weddings is pitched on a stretch of lawn beside an idyllic tidal lake on the coast of New South Wales. The tent is flanked by a remnant forest of native palms; while a line of prayer flags—long bands of red, blue, yellow, green and white—ripple and flap on tall timber poles just outside.

Inside is Sogyal Rinpoche, eminent Tibetan master and author of the spiritual classic *The Tibetan Book of Living and Dying*. He teaches more than 300 people sitting in rapt and silent attention. The only sounds, apart from the master's voice, are the cicadas, the birds and, sometimes, the sing-song chatter of two or three youngsters playing nearby in the knee-deep waters of the warm, sandy-bottomed lake.

It is a mixed group of varying ages; nurses, teachers, doctors, lawyers, students, journalists, business folk, housewives, retirees. Some are relatively new to Buddhism, others have been coming for years, while some choose to spend an additional three or more weeks a year in the European summer at Rinpoche's main retreat centre, Lerab Ling, in the south of France near Montpellier.

In the summer of 2006, over 400 of the master's most devoted students began a three-year retreat at Lerab Ling.

A three-year retreat is something that many fully committed

students of Tibetan Buddhism traditionally undertake at least once in their lives. Some of the great masters of the past would spend up to twenty years in retreat. When it reached its conclusion at the end of 2009, the French retreat was the largest—by number of retreatants—ever completed in the West.

Inside the lakeside tent is a large timber shrine, coated a deep saffron colour and detailed in gold. On top are pictures of masters, living and dead, key to Sogyal Rinpoche's lineage of Tibetan Buddhism; together with intricate and vivid images of deities both wrathful and benevolent; as well as offering bowls and lamps, devotional objects, statuettes and fresh flowers.

In the centre of the shrine is a photograph of His Holiness the Dalai Lama and above, dominating the space, are rich tapestries of Buddha Shakyamuni, the buddha of our era who attained enlightenment around 2500 years ago and Guru Rinpoche, also known as Padmasambhava, Tibet's second buddha who brought the highest teachings of Buddhism to the roof of the world in the eighth century AD.

By mid-morning, as the humidity rises, Sogyal Rinpoche gently chides his students as one or two of them begin to nod their heads and close their eyes in the sticky, somnambulant air.

Sometimes relief from the heat of the sun beating down on the temporary temple comes by way of an afternoon storm and torrential rain. Other times a gentle cooling breeze, said to be the compassion of Padmasambhava himself, blows in off the surface of the lake and ripples the flaps of the tent and the thangkas— profoundly detailed and vivid Tibetan devotional paintings—inside.

One year, light rain drifted gently down as a vivid double rainbow, even more fleeting and impermanent than the tent itself, arched directly and perfectly above; just as the week's teachings concluded.

Sogyal Rinpoche is one of the most important and revered Tibetan masters alive and has played a central role in the spreading of the Tibetan Buddhist teachings to the modern world. Rinpoche fled to the West as a child in the Tibetan diaspora that followed the invasion and occupation of his country by China's communist forces in the 1950s.

He is founder and head of Rigpa, an international network of meditation centres and groups—over 100 centres in 23 countries—devoted to presenting the Buddhist tradition of Tibet in a way that is both completely authentic, but also relevant to modern lives. Rigpa has the patronage of His Holiness the Dalai Lama and is open to all schools of Buddhist Wisdom.

'Rigpa is a Tibetan word, which in general means "intelligence" or "awareness",'explains Rinpoche. Sogyal Rinpoche is a master of the Dzogchen lineage that carries the most profound teachings in the Buddhist tradition of Tibet. 'In Dzogchen rigpa has a deeper connotation, the innermost nature of the mind. The whole of the teaching of Buddha is directed towards realising this, our ultimate nature, the state of omniscience or enlightenment—a truth so universal, so primordial that it goes beyond all limits, and beyond even religion itself.'

Sogyal Rinpoche is an engaging and profoundly learned—not to mention witty and playful; occasionally witheringly serious—master of the Nyingma school. Tibetan Buddhism has four schools—Nyingma, Kagyu, Sakya and Gelugpa. Rinpoche reveals the Buddhist teachings to a modern Western audience with a remarkable and singular clarity.

At his annual Australian retreat, Rinpoche's students sit on chairs in the marquee, arranged four or five deep, with others, often his older students, sitting cross-legged on meditation cushions at his feet.

Every year, in the middle of the group, on cushions on the floor, are Ian and Ruth Gawler.

Ian first met Sogyal Rinpoche in 1984. Rinpoche, who travels the world teaching for most of the year, was speaking on death and dying at the University of Melbourne. Ian had been eager to attend because he was fascinated to hear what a practising Buddhist would say on the subject (the release of Rinpoche's bestselling book was then still eight years away).

'In the first few minutes of Rinpoche speaking,' says Ian, 'I had a recognition that here was a really authentic teacher with an authentic lineage, sharing authentic teachings.'

While Ian's other teachers, notably Ainslie Meares, had taught from a very deep personal experience about meditation, with Rinpoche Ian recognised that here was a man speaking with the profound authority of a long tradition of spiritual masters; a sacred lineage that had transmitted wisdom precisely and expertly down through the years, in an unbroken line, from master to student.

More than that, though, Ian says he felt an ease and familiarity with what Rinpoche was saying; he experienced a quality of remembering what was presented, rather than learning something new. 'There was a sense of coming to a spiritual home.'

In 1981 Ian had attended several days of teaching given by His Holiness the Dalai Lama—on one of his early visits to Australia. He had been deeply struck by His Holiness' personal presence and palpable wisdom and then, three years later, he had met a man from the same tradition, who again profoundly impressed Ian with his precise description of the ultimate nature of all things; with his intimate understanding of the relative and absolute.

Rinpoche and his words had a very deep, if initially a mostly intellectual, resonance for Ian.

Clearly, Ian was well aware that he was in the presence of an extraordinary spiritual teacher, but from his own side, there was a lot of reserve.

'When I first met Rinpoche, despite the recognition of what he had to offer, I was still cautious. In fact, to begin with I regarded him more as a university professor than a spiritual teacher,' adds Ian. 'While I felt a lot of warmth and enthusiasm for him as a teacher and a lot of respect, I was unsure about the relationship.'

Ian had, and still does have, a strong affinity with the Christianity of his youth and early adulthood. Then there is his connection with Sai Baba, a man whom he recognises, much as millions of others do, as an Avatar, a living manifestation of the Divine.

His unfolding relationship with, and devotion to, Sogyal Rinpoche meanwhile was a very slow process; a spiritual courtship that would unfold over the subsequent ten, or so, years.

When Rinpoche returned to Australia yearly, Ian would attend his teachings. He helped to organise retreats for Rinpoche in Victoria during the late 1980s and gradually his interest and knowledge deepened. 'Rinpoche has this incredibly generous nature,' he says. 'He would give me time each year to discuss my personal practice and what was relevant to my work. He was young and keen to share what he had. He was very patient with me.'

Ask Ian today if he is a Christian or Buddhist and he struggles for an answer. Brought up a Christian, having held a strong Christian faith and having prayed fervently through the early days of his illness, Ian characterises his relationship with Christianity and with Buddhism as 'a bit like having two wives,' he says. 'It's a bit like having had a close relationship, a marriage, that didn't end in divorce, and then developing another close relationship. If you do change religious traditions it's very important that you don't ditch the old one. So you are faced with issues of loyalty and allegiance. Perhaps the real issue is one of commitment . . . I can really relate to it when the Dalai Lama strongly recommends that people do not change traditions unless they are really very serious. I expect that there are many people like me who found Christianity limited or unsatisfactory in some way. But there is much that is good about it. These days if people have left the Church, spent time in some sort of spiritual limbo, then have a spiritual reawakening through illness like I did; I suggest to them that they start by revisiting their tradition of origin. To change traditions is quite a big deal!'

'Personally, however, I don't feel any contradiction,' he adds. 'I can go to church quite happily, although I don't do it very often because these days I am definitely more engaged in Buddhist spiritual practice, but I still find it very easy to relate to Christian iconography and Christian prayer.'

Being able to function with such ecumenical ease has, however, not been a straightforward road; rather it has been a road of inner questioning that began with his mother's death.

Manifesting initially as an abandonment of the simplistic world-view he held before his mum's passing, Ian's first tangible taste of transcendence had come at Melbourne Grammar's little old bluestone chapel in Year 7, the first time he went inside.

'I can remember the light shining through these stained-glass windows and it really hit me. I was blessed with one of those mystical experiences,' he says. 'It was a really transcendent moment where time stood still.'

He had another similar taste at seventeen years of age on a darkening winter's evening in August. Ian had gone into Melbourne city at around five in the afternoon, just as most other people were leaving work and were coming the other way. The streets were wet and the light was glistening and bouncing off the road as a sea of humanity advanced towards him.

'I had this dramatic shift in conscious awareness: what I was seeing and what I was experiencing shifted,' he says. 'Rather than seeing this mass of individuals coming towards me, it felt like all these people were the one entity, as it were; one sort of interconnected mass of humanity. I had a sort of mystical glimpse of the interconnectedness of beings and some sort of brief insight into this essential nature we have.'

He kept the experience very much to himself at the time, but it confirmed, just as he suspected deep inside, the realisation that there was a 'whole other dimension to life and a whole other layer of experience.' It also inspired a new direction in his reading and Ian subsequently became much more intent on pursuing spiritual themes—particularly anything that touched on a sense of unification, unity and oneness.

Later, as a curious, if essentially conservative, veterinary science student, he thought Muktananda might have some further answers and attended a teaching by the Hindu guru on a visit to Australia from his home in India. Ian went on his own to the lecture theatre, at Melbourne University and made a 'very conscious decision to sit up the back,' he remembers. 'I was very suspicious'. Muktananda was the founder of Siddha Yoga, who during his life (he died in 1982) established hundreds of meditation centres around the world.

Ian positioned himself as close to the rear exit as possible and had told himself, 'If there's any funny stuff, if anyone tries to mess with my mind, I'm out of here.'

He need not have worried. Ian was deeply impressed by Muktananda's presence.

Even from the back of the room he felt the sense of 'serenity and the ease which he displayed,' he says. 'I was really drawn to that ... at the same time here was Muktananda, dressed up like an Indian yogi and representing something quite foreign to me, I had too many obstacles in my way because of my cultural background to approach something like that at that particular point in my life.'

The following year Raynor Johnson's series of lectures, covering karma and reincarnation, eloquently explaining them within a Western scientific paradigm, had transfixed Ian.

After graduation the drive for answers on the meaning of life were close at hand, but Ian consciously parked his quest in a quiet corner of his psyche, and got down to what seemed like more pressing business at the time: making a comfortable living. Every week, however, the nagging sense that he was ignoring his true calling would come looming into his consciousness, particularly while he was standing at the counter depositing his earnings at the Bacchus Marsh bank.

'Every week I would go off to the bank with all this money and see the bank account going up in a straight line and think how wonderful it was,' he says. 'But then in the same moment I would have this real existential dilemma. I would think, well, what have I done that is of any real meaning or purpose in terms of my personal and spiritual development? But I would dismiss these thoughts, stifle them and engage with working full-on for the next week.'

And then came the cancer, the amputation of his right leg, and a real sense of urgency to tap into the inner nature that he already knew was burning insistently deep inside and waiting to be awakened.

Initially he was led, and identified deeply, with his new understanding of Eastern philosophy—taking in reincarnation and karma as self-evident truths—but he nonetheless retained his Christian faith.

When Ian had first begun meditation he did it 'looking for some sort of spiritual experience,' he says. All that first year none came—until one month before the terrible arrival of secondaries.

Sitting quietly in the dark of the evening, with his eyes closed in meditation, Ian had thought Gail must have come into the room and turned the light on. 'And then I realised what I was seeing, what I was experiencing, was an internal light, not an external one,' he says. 'A fairly intense light had formed in front of my eyes. It was a real luminosity. I got excited, but as soon as I got excited and tried to analyse it, it disappeared.' At all his subsequent meditation sessions, Ian tried to recreate the experience, but to no avail. 'The harder I tried, the less it happened.'

A couple of months later, learning meditation with Ainslie Meares, he discovered that the eminent psychiatrist's approach was shorn of any overt spirituality. While profoundly spiritual in his own right, Meares was not openly aligned to any religious tradition. Nevertheless, using the technique Meares had taught for five hours per day, Ian framed his meditation in a Christian context. He invoked the presence of Christ and used The Lord's Prayer as a mantra.

In the Philippines, the venerable faith healer Mr Terte further deepened Ian's connection with Christ by way of the two Bibles he instructed the young man to buy. Mr Terte blessed both the Bibles. One was to be given to someone in need and the other Ian took home with the intention of reading every year. Mr Terte gave Ian a passage from Ephesians to read as a contemplation for daily practice, which he did for about a year.

'He basically introduced me to analytical contemplation, where you take a passage and you repeat it over and over,' he says. 'You actively contemplate the obvious meaning, but it's almost like a deeper meaning reveals itself through insight. For me this was really helpful. It was remarkable how much I learnt from just this one passage.'

Mr Terte had also instructed Ian to put the open Bible that he had blessed for him, on any area of his body that was giving him trouble and Terte told him that if he did so, then he, Terte, could send him some absent healing.

Around six weeks after Ian had returned from the first trip to the Philippines, he was experiencing a great deal of pain across the top of his chest. He struggled with it for a few days and then remembering what Terte had suggested, he opened up the Bible and put it on his chest.

'It was the most extraordinary experience,' he says. 'It was like someone had put a vacuum cleaner on my chest and just sucked all this pain out . . . In a couple of minutes it was like all this pain had been drained out of me and gone into the Bible. To this day I have no idea if it was psychosomatic or something extraordinary. But it certainly happened and I was totally relieved.'

Also around the same time—upon Ian and Gail's return from the first trip to Philippines—Norma Pelic had put Ian in touch with the Christian mystic, Reverend Mario Schoenmaker, founder of the Independent Church of Australia and the Order of the Mystic Christ.

Reverend Schoenmaker had emigrated from Holland and had begun his ecclesiastical career as a Protestant minister in Western Australia. He later claimed to have developed clairvoyant gifts. Schoenmaker's progressive brand of Christian worship also included meditation and embraced reincarnation.

'He was a very colourful character and really quite extraordinary,' says Ian, adding that he was reputed to have the capacity to see people's past lives and relate them to their present situation. Ian sent him a lock of hair and a photograph, as he required, for a life reading. 'I still had a very over-healthy scepticism,' he says, so he sent him a photo that was taken before the amputation and that also showed only his head and shoulders. Schoenmaker sent him back a quite remarkable cassette.

'Mario spent the first half an hour of the cassette describing my character and my life in amazing detail. I think he picked up on my scepticism. He said that if you were ever to take notice of something a psychic says to you, they should first establish their bona fides by telling you things that you know, but that they could not know in the ordinary course of events. What he said about me was very convincing. Then he proceeded to tell me something about how he perceived my past lives to have been, and how these related to my current situation.'

Ian found all this somewhat interesting and helpful but not revelatory. However, he also sent for some cassettes of Schoenmaker's sermons. 'He really had a wonderful way of interpreting Christian scripture in a mystical context,' he says.

In Torquay Ian attended the local Anglican Church on a regular basis, enjoying the company and fellowship of the small and predominantly elderly congregation.

'Relating to Christ and seeing Christ as a Divine incarnation and a representation of Divine love was very powerful for me through that time,' explains Ian. 'And I didn't find any conflict with holding a strong Christian view and with being interested in the notion of reincarnation and karma. They all seemed to me like they were real possibilities.'

'Schoenmaker had an incredible gift for bringing the mystical side of Christianity alive,' says Ian. 'He interpreted all the New Testament in a mystical way and gave it a whole new dimension. When I went to church I was hearing the same actual words as the old ladies,' he says, 'but I suspect I was interpreting a little differently.'

At the same time Ian and Gail were involved with a Yogananda group who used to meet locally once a week. Yogananda was a Hindu saint who lived in the early part of last century. The Gawlers would regularly meet with a group of like-minded people at a house where they would talk, meditate and chant. It felt like a 'spiritually orientated social gathering,' says Ian, adding that he had no direct relationship with Yogananda as a person, but found his teachings useful and the chanting wonderful. Nor did he feel any inherent conflict between his core Christian beliefs and the philosophical framework of Hinduism. 'Yoga has a lot to do with living well within a spiritual framework.' The study of yoga began to inform Ian and Gail's own way of life.

On the other hand, Ian had no fixed or solid devotion to any single dogma, set of teachings or teacher. His commitment was to seeking the spiritual essence of life, our ultimate nature, wherever it might be found—and he felt no self- or institutionally-imposed parameters or restrictions.

It was only when he met Sai Baba that the conflict posed by both faith and devotion powerfully made their presence felt.

On the second trip to the Philippines to visit the psychic surgeons, just before he headed for India and Sai Baba, he was told time and again that he had a mental block to getting well. 'I knew in myself that this was true and that it related to the fact that, while I believed it was possible to get well, I didn't have a real conviction, I didn't have a real faith.'

Ian was all too aware that his way of viewing the world was grounded in the Western paradigm of science and medicine.

'While I believed that you could get well from cancer, I still had doubt about whether things like diet and meditation and healing— both the ordinary things that we were doing and extraordinary ones—could actually bring about a complete cure. I feel that at this point in my healing saga, the doubt was the thing that was holding me back from actually getting well.

'Belief involves a balance of evidence. You can have a weak belief with a lot of doubts; or a strong belief with little doubt. While Faith is a word most often used in a spiritual context, in this healing context it is where you have no doubts. Instead you have conviction. At this point I had strong belief, not faith. And I felt sure that the doubts I had were what was holding me back.'

Visiting Sai Baba caused something to shift. 'The meeting was pivotal in two ways,' he says. 'The first thing I got was a strong sense of his presence . . . a very strong and spiritual presence.'

Then, when Sai Baba said words to the effect of 'You are already healed, don't worry', Ian says, 'it basically essentialised where I was at that point. I had done all the things I needed to be healed and it was actually my worry, my lack of conviction, that was holding me back.'

Ian had gone to Sai Baba hoping for some sort of 'profound mystical experience, altered consciousness and, you know, a few flashing lights', but instead what he received had the air of the ordinary about it. 'It was ordinary in the sense that it was so matter of fact. Yet there was such a clarity.' Ian saw clearly that he had two potential paths stretching out in front of him. One was the path of belief where he could continue believing it was *possible* to get well, but continue also to doubt it would actually happen. The other was the road of absolute faith, one of 100 per cent conviction that he *would* be well.

'There was this choice that I had to make—and I realised that an internal shift was actually possible. Being in the atmosphere that Sai Baba created catalysed that shift,' he says. 'For me it was a fairly deliberate process. While I had expected something mystical, something magical; it was far more deliberate—like a choice of my mind. But I think this is often what real healing is all about, where you actually shift some fundamental attitude inside and go from a belief in something to a point of faith.'

Regardless of what it actually was that healed him—and it was likely a complex matrix of many things—once Ian made the conscious decision to go forward with faith he *knew* his ultimate good health was assured; even if there were still many challenges ahead. Everything now had this added dimension of certainty. It was as if rather than believing he could recover, now he knew that he would.

During the 1980s, in the years following his return to health, Ian's spiritual search then took on elements of a number of different spiritual traditions.

One particularly influential meeting, in the early 1980s, was with renowned mystic and spiritual teacher Father Bede Griffiths on one of his visits to Melbourne. Ian had the good fortune to be invited to dinner with Father Bede, and on another one of his trips to Australia, Father Bede was invited to speak to one of the cancer support groups at The Foundation.

Bede Griffiths was a Benedictine monk, born in Britain, who spent much of his life living and working in India. Although a Christian, he had adopted Hindu teachings into his devotional practice and was also known as Swami Dayananda. He wrote many books expertly interpreting Eastern religion for a Western audience. Ian felt an enormous sense of kinship with Father Bede and his ecumenical approach.

Like Father Bede, Ian's spiritual interests were wide and he voraciously studied as much as he could about everything from progressive Christianity, to Hinduism and Tibetan Buddhism. 'It seemed to me that when you looked into all these traditions, when you went past the dogma or the fundamentalism, and when you got into their more esoteric side,' says Ian, 'they were all speaking the same language and had all the same essential elements.'

He was, however, particularly attracted to Buddhism and its pursuit of the truth. Buddhism also offered very clear and precise meditation practices as an integral part of its teaching.

'As a Buddhist it makes a lot of sense not to describe yourself as a Buddhist but as someone who is seeking the truth,' he explains. 'What the Buddhist teachings do is to give you a reliable pathway to follow that leads to a direct experience of that truth. There aren't any articles of faith in Buddhism. You don't get to the point where you can only move forward with a leap of blind faith. You are encouraged to be intellectually critical and only adopt what resonates for you and makes sense.'

What he found so impressive about both Sai Baba and Sogyal Rinpoche was that there was an experiential element to their presence and their teachings that came across quite clearly. Tibetan Buddhist masters typically practise meditation for a number of hours a day—and have done so for most of their lives. Their meditative practice, and the realisation and awakening it has brought them, imbues their every moment, their every action.

'It's not that there aren't people in Christianity like that. Of course there are,' adds Ian. 'But I think there's a real problem that many of the spiritual leaders in Christianity don't speak from that place, or they don't have that presence that comes with a lot of practice.' There can be a concern, he says, that they have learnt a lot from books, but maybe missed out on sitting quietly in prayer, contemplation and meditation.

What particularly attracted Ian to Sogyal Rinpoche, he adds, was not only that he had an extraordinary presence, based on a profound experiential understanding of the Buddhist teachings, but he also had the intellectual capacity and the fluency in English to speak clearly about the path.

'He spoke very thoroughly about meditation, about training the mind, about dealing with difficult emotions,' he said. More specifically, he had very great, very profound insights into a subject dear to Ian's heart; dear to his life's work: how to help the dying and to help people caring for the dying.

And so it was at the annual retreat in 1988, after a few years of exploring and sampling the spiritual path, Ian formally asked Rinpoche if he would accept him as his student.

Rinpoche did not answer him directly. In fact, as Ian puts it, 'he fobbed me off. In a way I was quite comfortable with this and a bit relieved. But not put off.'

In Tibetan Buddhism the relationship between teacher and student is a vital one. Devotion to the teacher, along with an ego-less profound compassion for all beings, is the fastest and the most skilful way to fully understand and to realise the teachings and, ultimately, the true nature of all things. Devotion is the very foundation upon which the living lineage between master and student is built. The compassion Ian had; the devotion he found a more fraught idea to commit to.

Devotion to a teacher is not something that comes very easily to Westerners—and Ian was no different. Ego-bound, proud and deeply suspicious of the guru principle, Westerners do not easily grasp the meaning of devotion.

Then in the mid-1990s, at another of the annual retreats, Rinpoche taught in great depth about devotion and 'spoke in a way that helped me to clarify it a lot,' Ian says. 'In effect it was a simple clarification, but it really made a huge difference. Rinpoche made it clear that the devotion was actually to the teachings and that the teacher embodies the teachings, and in doing so, warrants devotion. He is devoted not to the personality of the teacher but to the teachings that they impart and embody. Perhaps in a way this is obvious, but after that retreat I really got it. I really knew it and that allowed a whole deeper level of commitment to Rinpoche as my main teacher.'

Based on this understanding, and with Ian's determination for a deeper spiritual commitment, from that moment on Sogyal Rinpoche became his main teacher. This was clearly relevant on two levels: not only was Rinpoche now the guiding light for Ian's own personal spiritual path, but also the understanding of the mind and meditation techniques Rinpoche was teaching proved to have a very practical application in Ian's work.

For Ian, Tibetan Buddhism is particular attractive because of its teachings. It is an enormously precise and practical 'mind science'; a great spiritual tradition, exacting and detailed in its understanding of the profound subtleties of the nature of existence; and one that appeals to the modern intellect trained in the sciences and psychology. More specifically, right from his early exposure to these teachings, it was clear it offered some validation and clarification of Ian's work.

'It reinforced a lot of that work and deepened it,' he says. 'Buddhism has been studying the mind for thousands of years. When it comes to mind–body medicine, they have such a lot to offer about how the mind works and how we can heal using the power of the mind. There is so much to offer regarding transforming destructive emotions into joy and happiness and then the real depth of knowledge about how to teach and practise meditation.'

When Ian now attends any of Rinpoche's retreats, sitting on a deep blue cushion in the humidity under the white marquee with Ruth alongside him, he says that one of the things at the front of his mind is how he can learn, how he can express the things that Rinpoche teaches in a way that is going to help other people.

Ian seeks to distil what he learns and communicate it in such a way that is 'going to be accessible to people who don't necessarily share my enthusiasm for Tibetan Buddhism as a spiritual path,' he says, adding that he tries to take the principles that stand independently 'that can be applied as a mind science and can be taken up if you are a Christian, Jew, Muslim or even sceptical atheist.'

As Ian writes in *You Can Conquer Cancer*,

I hesitate because I do not want to be labelled, nor do I want to run the risk of having good straightforward techniques like meditation labelled. All these techniques stand independently in their own right and are quite free of spiritual bias. They can be judged on their own merits.

The Gawler Foundation's Yarra Valley Living Centre is a non-denominational place of healing and refuge, a place open to absolutely everyone. Ian Gawler is a deeply spiritual man, but he is also a pragmatist. He understands that many people seek therapy in this day and age foremost, before they seek spiritual understanding. Many people come knowing that the meditation techniques Ian teaches can have a therapeutic effect.

For some the act of sitting quietly and stilling the mind, is merely a key vehicle on the road to good health and wellbeing. For others, like Ian, it is also the path to awakening.

Ian's life thus far has been a truly remarkable, inspiring and classic tale of triumph against incredible odds. That he lives and thrives more than 30 years after he was given less than a couple of weeks to live, riddled with the end-stages of 'terminal' cancer, is indeed one of the most incredible survival stories of modern times.

In the same situation, even if we had the same superhuman application, intelligence, intuition, willpower, courage and faith that Ian embodies, most of us would no doubt have justifiably chosen to tread an easier path after winning such a miraculous second chance.

Instead, Ian chose with extraordinary resilience and grit, to push relentlessly, with positivism and good humour against a medical establishment that refused to accept the incredible lessons he had learnt and was so selflessly offering to others. Meanwhile mainstream health care is in crisis, as expenditure on it grows exponentially.

Generally Ian holds a respected place in the wider medical community and it is a testament to the power of his message and to his extraordinary tenacity. But there is work to be done—many others are yet to be convinced.

Ian Gawler is one of the great pioneers of our age. Future generations of health care professionals will, one suspects, shake their heads in disbelief that some of their colleagues of the day could not see that much of Ian's message was straightforward, if hard-won, common sense.

Ian Gawler's story is primarily one of hope. It is a benchmark of possibility against which any of us, however hopeless our situation might appear, can look to and be inspired.

Something only has to be done once to show that it is possible.

Ian has had the courage and openness to embrace the lessons of his life's experiences—extraordinary and fantastic and miraculous as they have been—and has made it his life's work to offer what he has discovered, humbly and utterly selflessly to others.

Ian's life story is a teaching. A teaching offering some powerful and universal truths about who we are and who we can be.

Resources

Gawler, Grace, *Women of Silence*, Highclere Limited, 2003

Gawler, Ian, *You Can Conquer Cancer*, Michelle Anderson Publishing, 2001

Gawler, Ian, *Meditation—Pure & Simple*, Michelle Anderson Publishing, 2004

Gerson, Max, *A Cancer Therapy: Results of Fifty Cases*, Totality Books, 1977

Haraldsson, Erlunder, *Modern Miracles*, Hastings House, 1997

Johnson, Raynor C, *The Imprisoned Splendour*, Hodder & Stoughton, 1969

Kraus (ed.), Paul, *Surviving Cancer*, Michelle Anderson Publishing, Pty Ltd, 2008,

Meares, Ainslie, *Relief Without Drugs*, HarperCollins Publishers Ltd, 1970

Meares, Ainslie, *Strange Places and Simple Truths*, Souvenir Press Ltd, 1971

Moody, Ray, *Life after Life: The Investigation of a Phenomenon—Survival of Bodily Death*, HarperOne, 2001

Ormond, Ron, *Into the Strange Unknown*, Esoteric Foundation, 1959

Rinpoche, Sogyal, *The Tibetan Book of Living and Dying*, Harper Collins, 1992

Trungpa, Chogyam, *The Collected Works of Chogyam Trungpa*, vol.1, Shambala, 2003 [containing *Meditation in Action*]

Yutang, Lin, (ed.), *The Wisdom of China and India, an anthology* Modern Library 1955

CA, 'Psychic Surgery' in *A Cancer Journal for Clinicians*, CA Cancer J Clin 1990;40; 184–188

Interview with Ian Gawler, Director of Australian Cancer Patients' Foundation [sound recording] / interviewer: Barbara Blackman, 1986 May 28–Aug. 12. 6 sound cassettes (ca. 540 min.): 1 7/8 ips, mono. ORAL TRC 2023 (2252331), Oral History Section, The National Library of Australia

Permissions

Acknowledgements

I would like to offer my heartfelt thanks and appreciation to everyone who has made this book possible. Thanks to Lolita, my wife, and Tam and Jasper, my sons, for putting up with me while I wrote it (and talked about little else for 18 months). Thanks to Siobhan Hannan at Camerons Management for her advice, enthusiasm and support, and to Jane Palfreyman and everyone at Allen & Unwin for their diligence and foresight. Thanks to the National Library of Australia for making available the transcripts to Ian Gawler's oral history recordings. Thanks to Kris Kepars for her tireless efforts transcribing the countless hours of interviews. Thanks to Grace Gawler and many others for sharing their thoughts and memories. And thanks especially to Ian and Ruth Gawler for so frankly and generously letting us all into their lives.

Guy Allenby
Sydney, NSW

Index